## UCLA Symposia on Molecular and Cellular Biology, New Series

*Series Editor*
C. Fred Fox

RECENT TITLES

*Volume 13*
**Molecular Biology of Host–Parasite Interactions,** Nina Agabian and Harvey Eisen, *Editors*

*Volume 14*
**Biosynthesis of the Photosynthetic Apparatus: Molecular Biology, Development and Regulation,** J. Philip Thornber, L. Andrew Staehelin, and Richard B. Hallick, *Editors*

*Volume 15*
**Protein Transport and Secretion,** Dale L. Oxender, *Editor*

*Volume 16*
**Acquired Immune Deficiency Syndrome,** Michael S. Gottlieb and Jerome E. Groopman, *Editors*

*Volume 17*
**Genes and Cancer,** J. Michael Bishop, Janet D. Rowley, and Mel Greaves, *Editors*

*Volume 18*
**Regulation of the Immune System,** Harvey Cantor, Leonard Chess, and Eli Sercarz, *Editors*

*Volume 19*
**Molecular Biology of Development,** Eric H. Davidson and Richard A. Firtel, *Editors*

*Volume 20*
**Genome Rearrangement,** Melvin Simon and Ira Herskowitz, *Editors*

*Volume 21*
**Herpesvirus,** Fred Rapp, *Editor*

*Volume 22*
**Cellular and Molecular Biology of Plant Stress**, Joe L. Key and Tsune Kosuge, *Editors*

*Volume 23*
**Membrane Receptors and Cellular Regulation**, Michael P. Czech and C. Ronald Kahn, *Editors*

*Volume 24*
**Neurobiology: Molecular Biological Approaches to Understanding Neuronal Function and Development**, Paul O'Lague, *Editor*

*Volume 25*
**Extracellular Matrix: Structure and Function**, A. Hari Reddi, *Editor*

*Volume 26*
**Nuclear Envelope Structure and RNA Maturation,** Edward A. Smuckler and Gary A. Clawson, *Editors*

*Volume 27*
**Monoclonal Antibodies and Cancer Therapy**, Ralph A. Reisfeld and Stewart Sell, *Editors*

*Volume 28*
**Leukemia: Recent Advances in Biology and Treatment,** David W. Golde and Robert Peter Gale, *Editors*

*Volume 29*
**Molecular Biology of Muscle Development,** Charles Emerson, Donald Fischman, Bernardo Nadal-Ginard, and M.A.Q. Siddiqui, *Editors*

*Volume 30*
**Sequence Specificity in Transcription and Translation,** Richard Calendar and Larry Gold, *Editors*

*Volume 31*
**Molecular Determinants of Animal Form,** Gerald M. Edelman, *Editor*

*Volume 32*
**Papillomaviruses: Molecular and Clinical Aspects,** Peter M. Howley and Thomas R. Broker, *Editors*

*Volume 33*
**Yeast Cell Biology,** James Hicks, *Editor*

*Volume 34*
**Molecular Genetics of Filamentous Fungi,** William Timberlake, *Editor*

Volume 35
**Plant Genetics,** Michael Freeling, *Editor*

# UCLA Symposia Published Prior to 1983

(Numbers refer to the publishers listed below.)

**1972**
Membrane Research **(2)**

**1973**
Membranes **(1)**
Virus Research **(2)**

**1974**
Molecular Mechanisms for the Repair of DNA **(4)**
Membranes **(1)**
Assembly Mechanisms **(1)**
The Immune System: Genes, Receptors, Signals **(2)**
Mechanisms of Virus Disease **(3)**

**1975**
Energy Transducing Mechanisms **(1)**
Cell Surface Receptors **(1)**
Developmental Biology **(3)**
DNA Synthesis and Its Regulation **(3)**

**1976**
Cellular Neurobiology **(1)**
Cell Shape and Surface Architecture **(1)**
Animal Virology **(2)**
Molecular Mechanisms in the Control of Gene Expression **(2)**

**1977**
Cell Surface Carbohydrates and Biological Recognition **(1)**
Molecular Approaches to Eucaryotic Genetic Systems **(2)**
Molecular Human Cytogenetics **(2)**
Molecular Aspects of Membrane Transport **(1)**
Immune System: Genetics and Regulation **(2)**

**1978**
DNA Repair Mechanisms **(2)**
Transmembrane Signaling **(1)**
Hematopoietic Cell Differentiation **(2)**
Normal and Abnormal Red Cell Membranes **(1)**
Persistent Viruses **(2)**
Cell Reproduction: Daniel Mazia Dedicatory Volume **(2)**

**1979**
Covalent and Non-Covalent Modulation of Protein Function ***(2)***
Eucaryotic Gene Regulation **(2)**
Biological Recognition and Assembly **(1)**
Extrachromosomal DNA **(2)**
Tumor Cell Surfaces and Malignancy **(1)**
T and B Lymphocytes: Recognition and Function **(2)**

**1980**
Biology of Bone Marrow Transplantation **(2)**
Membrane Transport and Neuroreceptors **(1)**
Control of Cellular Division and Development **(1)**
Animal Virus Genetics **(2)**
Mechanistic Studies of DNA Replication and Genetic Recombination **(2)**

**1981**
Immunoglobulin Idiotypes **(2)**
Initiation of DNA Replication **(2)**
Genetic Variation Among Influenza Viruses **(2)**
Developmental Biology Using Purified Genes **(2)**
Differentiation and Function of Hematopoietic Cell Surfaces **(1)**
Mechanisms of Chemical Carcinogenesis **(1)**
Cellular Recognition **(1)**

**1982**
B and T Cell Tumors **(2)**
Interferon **(2)**
Rational Basis for Chemotherapy **(1)**
Gene Regulation **(2)**
Tumor Viruses and Differentiation **(1)**
Evolution of Hormone-Receptor Systems **(1)**

## Publishers

**(1)** Alan R. Liss, Inc.
41 E. 11th Street
New York, NY 10003

**(2)** Academic Press, Inc.
111 Fifth Avenue
New York, NY 10003

**(3)** W.A. Benjamin, Inc.
2725 Sand Hill Road
Menlo Park, CA 94025

**(4)** Plenum Publishing Corp.
227 W. 17th Street
New York, NY 10011

# PAPILLOMAVIRUSES
## MOLECULAR AND CLINICAL ASPECTS

# PAPILLOMAVIRUSES
## MOLECULAR AND CLINICAL ASPECTS

**Proceedings of the Burroughs-Wellcome–UCLA Symposium**
**Held in Steamboat Springs, Colorado**
**April 8–14, 1985**

**Editors**

**Peter M. Howley**
National Institutes of Health
Bethesda, Maryland

**Thomas R. Broker**
Department of Biochemistry
University of Rochester
Rochester, New York

**Alan R. Liss, Inc. • New York**

**Address all Inquiries to the Publisher**
**Alan R. Liss, Inc., 41 East 11th Street, New York, NY 10003**



**Printed in the United States of America.**



**Library of Congress Cataloging-in-Publication Data**
Main entry under title:

Papillomaviruses : molecular and clinical aspects.

"Represents a series of papers presented at the Burroughs-Wellcome-UCLA Symposium on "Papillomaviruses: Molecular and Clinical Aspects"—Pref.
Meeting held concurrently with the UCLA Symposium on "Biochemical and molecular Epidemology of Cancer."
Includes index.
1. Papillomavirus diseases—Congresses. 2. Papillomaviruses—Congresses. I. Howley, Peter M. II. Broker, Thomas R. III. Burroughs Wellcome Company. IV. University of California, Los Angeles. V. Burroughs-Wellcome-UCLA Symposium on "Papillomaviruses: Molecular and Clinical Aspects" (1985 : Steamboat Springs, Colo.) VI. UCLA Symposium on "Biochemical and Molecular Epidemiology of Cancer" (1985 : Steamboat Springs, Colo.) [DNLM: 1. Papillomaviruses—genetics—congresses. 2. Tumor Virus Infections —congresses. W3 U17N new ser. v.32 / QW 165.5.P2 P216 1985]
RC186.P15P37 1985 616.9'25 85-24029
ISBN 0-8451-2631-8

# Contents

## VIII. PAPILLOMAVIRUS TRANSFORMATION



## IX. VIRAL VECTORS

# Contributors

**Allan L. Abramson,** Department of Otolaryngology, Long Island Jewish Medical Center, 270-05 76th Avenue, New Hyde Park, NY 11042 **[413]**

**Kathryn M. Albers,** Department of Oral Biology and Pathology, School of Dental Medicine, State University of New York at Stony Brook, Stony Brook, NY 11794 **[427]**

**Dave S. Alberts,** Department of Internal Medicine, University of Arizona and Arizona Cancer Center, Tucson, AZ 85724 **[249]**

**Elliot J. Androphy,** Laboratory of Cellular Oncology, National Cancer Institute, Bethesda, MD 20205 **[457]**

**Helen Badiak,** Interferon Sciences, Inc., 783 Jersey Avenue, New Brunswick, NJ 08901 **[217]**

**M. Barrois,** Laboratoire de Pharmacologie Clinique et Moléculaire, Institut Gustave Roussy, 94800 Villejuif, France **[47]**

**Bernard Binétruy,** INSERM U273 and CNRS LP7300, Centre de Biochimie, Université de Nice, 06034, Nice, France **[473]**

**Thomas R. Broker,** Cold Spring Harbor Laboratory, Cold Spring Harbor, NY 11724; present address: Department of Biochemistry, University of Rochester, Rochester, NY 14642 **[501]**

**M.S. Campo,** The Beatson Institute for Cancer Research, Garscube Estate, Bearsden, Glasgow, G61 1BD, UK **[305]**

**O. Castren,** Department of Pathology, Gynecology and Obstetrics, and Clinical Microbiology, University of Kuopio, POB 6, SF-70211 Kuopio, Finland **[31]**

**Brenda Castro,** Department of Dermatology and Microbiology, New York University Medical Center, 550 First Avenue, New York, NY 10016 **[217]**

**Christa Cerni,** Institute for Tumor Biology, Cancer Research Center, University of Vienna, A-1090 Vienna, Austria **[473]**

**Louise T. Chow,** Cold Spring Harbor Laboratory, Cold Spring Harbor, NY 11724; present address: Department of Biochemistry, University of Rochester, Rochester, NY 14642 **[501]**

**Barbara A. Clark,** Departments of Obstetrics and Gynecology and Laboratory Medicine and Pathology, University of Minnesota, Minneapolis, MN 55455 **[101]**

**Gisèle Connan,** INSERM U273 and CNRS LP7300, Centre de Biochimie, Université de Nice, 06034, Nice, France **[473]**

**Patricia Cremin,** Department of Dermatology and Microbiology, New York University Medical Center, 500 First Avenue, New York, NY 10016 **[217]**

**Odile Croissant,** Institut Pasteur, 75-724, Paris, France **[69]**

**C.P. Crum,** Department of Ob/Gyn, Columbia University, 630 W. 168th Street, New York, NY 10032 **[19]**

**François Cuzin,** INSERM U273 and CNRS LP7300, Centre de Biochimie, Université de Nice, 06034, Nice, France **[473]**

The number in brackets is the opening page number of the contributor's article.

**Olivier Danos,** Unité des Virus Oncogènes, Département de Biologie Moléculaire, Institut Pasteur, 25 rue de Docteur Roux, 75724 Paris Cedex 15, France **[379]**

**Frank Dean,** Graduate Program in Molecular Biology and Virology, Sloan-Kettering Institute for Cancer Research, New York, NY 10021 **[397]**

**Herbert Dedo,** Department of Otolaryngology, School of Medicine, University of California, San Francisco, CA 94143 **[137, 273]**

**Odile de Lapeyrière,** INSERM U199, 27 bd Lei Roure, 13009 Marseille, France **[473]**

**Daniel DiMaio,** Department of Human Genetics, Yale University School of Medicine, New Haven, CT 06510 **[437]**

**William N. Drohan,** Department of Molecular Biology, Revlon Health Care Research and Development, Springfield, VA **[515]**

**V. Dutronquay,** Unite de Papillomavirus (INSERM U 190), Institut Pasteur, 75015 Paris, France **[47]**

**Ronald M. Evans,** Molecular Biology and Virology Laboratory, The Salk Institute, San Diego, CA 92138 **[545]**

**Anthony J. Faras,** Department of Microbiology, University of Minnesota, Minneapolis, MN 55455 **[101,501]**

**David Fedorczyk,** Interferon Sciences, Inc., 783 Jersey Avenue, New Brunswick, NJ 08901 **[217]**

**Mark A. Feitelson,** Department of Microbiology and Immunology, UCLA School of Medicine, Los Angeles, CA 90024; present address: Fox Chase Cancer Center, Philadelphia, PA 19111 **[327]**

**Simon Ford,** Department of Microbiology, University of Southern California School of Medicine, 2011 Zonal Avenue, Los Angeles, CA 90033 **[529]**

**Alvin E. Friedman-Kien,** Department of Dermatology and Microbiology, New York University Medical Center, 550 First Avenue, New York, NY 10016 **[217]**

**Pawel G. Fuchs,** Institut für Klinische Virologie der Universität Erlangen-Nürnberg, D-8520 Erlangen, F.R. Germany **[85]**

**Michio Fukushima,** Departments of Obstetrics and Gynecology and Laboratory Medicine and Pathology, University of Minnesota, Minneapolis, MN 55455 **[101]**

**Stanley A. Gall,** Department of Obstetrics and Gynecology, Duke University Medical Center, Durham, NC 27710; present address: Department of Obstetrics and Gynecology, University of Illinois—Chicago, 840 S. Wood Street, Chicago, IL 60612 **[137, 201]**

**Jeremy R. Geffen,** Interferon Sciences, Inc., 783 Jersey Avenue, New Brunswick, NJ 08901 **[217]**

**Elisabeth Georges,** Unité des Papillomavirus, Département de Virologie, Institut Pasteur, 25 rue du Docteur Roux, 75724 Paris Cedex 15, France **[379]**

**Isabelle Giri,** Unité des Virus Oncogènes, Département de Biologie Moléculaire, Institut Pasteur, 25 rue Docteur Roux, 75724 Paris Cedex 15, France **[379]**

**Donald L. Glassman,** Molecular Genetics, Inc., Minnetonka, MN 55343; present address: College of Veterinary Medicine, University of Minnesota, St. Paul, MN 55108 **[257]**

**Kimberly F. Glassman,** Molecular Genetics, Inc., Minnetonka, MN 55343 **[257]**

**Milaine Grisoni,** INSERM U273 and CNRS LP7300, Centre de Biochimie, Université de Nice, 06034, Nice, France **[473]**

**Donna Guralski,** Department of Human Genetics, Yale University School of Medicine, New Haven, CT 06510 **[437]**

**Stig Haglund,** Radiumhemmet and Department of Oto-Rhino-Laryngology, Karolinska Hospital, 104 01 Stockholm, Sweden **[165]**

**Alois Haslinger,** Department of Microbiology, University of Southern California School of Medicine, 2011 Zonal Avenue, Los Angeles, CA 90033 **[529]**

**G.B. Healy,** Department of Otolaryngology, The Children's Hospital, 300 Longwood Avenue, Boston, MA 02115 **[181]**

**Adriana Heguy,** Department of Microbiology, University of Southern California School of Medicine, 2011 Zonal Avenue, Los Angeles, CA 90033 **[529]**

**Heidi Holtgreve,** Department of Microbiology, University of Southern California School of Medicine, 2011 Zonal Avenue, Los Angeles, CA 90033 **[529]**

**Margaret Hood,** Department of Molecular Biology, Revlon Health Care Research and Development, Springfield, VA 22151 **[515]**

**Bernard Horowitz,** Blood Derivatives Program, New York Blood Center, 310 East 67th Street, New York, NY 11042 **[413]**

**Peter M. Howley,** Laboratory of Tumor Virus Biology, National Cancer Institute, Bethesda, MD 20205 **[343, 363]**

**Connie E. Hughes,** Department of Obstetrics and Gynecology, Duke University Medical Center, Durham, NC 27710 **[201]**

**Jerard Hurwitz,** Graduate Program in Molecular Biology and Virology, Sloan-Kettering Institute for Cancer Research, New York, NY 10021 **[397]**

**Thomas Iftner,** Institut für Klinische Virologie der Universität Erlangen-Nürnberg, D-8520 Erlangen, F.R. Germany **[85]**

**Stefania Jablonska,** Department of Dermatology, Warsaw School of Medicine, 02-008 Warsaw, Poland **[69]**

**W.F.H. Jarrett,** University of Glasgow Veterinary School, Department of Veterinary Pathology, Garscube Estate, Bearsden, Glasgow G61 1BD, UK **[299, 305]**

**A. Bennett Jenson,** Departments of Pathology and Obstetrics and Gynecology, Georgetown University, School of Medicine, Washington, DC 20007 **[3]**

**M. Jacqueline Johnson,** Molecular Biology and Virology Laboratory, The Salk Institute, San Diego, CA 92138 **[545]**

**Michael Karin,** Department of Microbiology, University of Southern California School of Medicine, 2011 Zonal Avenue, Los Angeles, CA 90033 **[529]**

**Haskins Kashima,** Department of Otolaryngology—Head and Neck Surgery, Johns Hopkins Medical Institutions, Baltimore, MD 21205 **[125, 137, 235]**

**Gunter Krämmer,** German Cancer Research Center, Institute of Cell and Tumor Biology, Im Neuenheimer Feld 280, D-6900 Heidelberg, F.R.G. **[391]**

**Robert J. Kurman,** Departments of Pathology and Obstetrics and Gynecology, Georgetown University, School of Medicine, Washington, DC 20007 **[3]**

**Mark J. Kutcher,** School of Dentistry, University of Maryland, Baltimore, MD 21205 **[155]**

**Wayne D. Lancaster,** Departments of Pathology and Obstetrics and Gynecology, Georgetown University, School of Medicine, Washington, DC 20007 **[3]**

**Ming Fan Law,** Molecular Biology and Virology Laboratory, The Salk Institute, San Diego, CA 92138; present addres: Sibia, La Jolla, CA 92037 **[545]**

**Hermann Lehn,** Institute for Virus Research, German Cancer Research Center, 6900 Heidelberg, FRG **[57]**

**Brigid Leventhal,** Department of Pediatric Oncology, Johns Hopkins Medical Institutions, Baltimore, MD 21205 **[125,137,235]**

**Norman S. Levine,** Department of Internal Medicine, Univeristy of Arizona and Arizona Cancer Center, Tucson, AZ 85724 **[249]**

**R.U. Levine,** Department of Ob/Gyn, Columbia University, 630 W. 168th Street, New York NY, 10032 **[19]**

**John Link,** Department of Molecular Biology, Revlon Health Care Research and Development, Springfield, VA 22151 **[515]**

**Douglas R. Lowy,** Laboratory of Cellular Oncology, National Cancer Institute, Bethesda, MD 20205 **[457]**

**Melissa A. Lum,** Molecular Genetics, Inc., Minnetonka, MN 55343 **[257]**

**P.-G. Lundquist,** Radiumhemmet and Department of Oto-Rhino-Laryngology, Karolinska Hospital, 104 01 Stockholm, Sweden **[165]**

**R. Mäntyjärvi,** Departments of Pathology, Gynecology and Obstetrics, and Clinical Microbiology, University of Kuopio, POB 6, SF-70211 Kuopio, Finland **[31]**

**Richard F. Marshall,** Molecular Genetics, Inc., Minnetonka, MN 55343 **[257]**

**Guerrino Meneguzzi,** INSERM U273 and CNRS LP7300, Centre de Biochimie, Université de Nice, 06034, Nice, France **[473]**

**James Metherall,** Department of Human Genetics, Yale University School of Medicine, New Haven, CT 06510 **[437]**

**Frank L. Meyskens, Jr.,** Department of Internal Medicine, University of Arizona and Arizona Cancer Center, Tucson, AZ 85724 **[249]**

**A. Dusty Miller,** Molecular Biology and Virology Laboratory, The Salk Institute, San Diego, CA 92138; present address: Fred Hutchinson Cancer Center, Seattle, WA 98104 **[545]**

**M. Mitao,** Department of Ob/Gyn, Hiroshima University School of Medicine, Hiroshima, Japan **[19]**

**M.H. Moar,** Department of Zoology, University of Edinburgh, West Mains Road, Edinburgh EH9 3JN, UK **[305]**

**Phoebe Mounts,** Department of Immunology and Infectious Diseases, Johns Hopkins Medical Institutions, Baltimore, MD 21205 **[125, 137]**

**Yasufumi Murakami,** Graduate Program in Molecular Biology and Virology, Sloan-Kettering Institute for Cancer Research, New York, NY 10021 **[397]**

**Charles C. Muscoplat,** Molecular Genetics, Inc., Minnetonka, MN 55343 **[257]**

**N. Nagai,** Department of Ob/Gyn, Hiroshima University School of Medicine, Hiroshima, Japan **[19]**

**Zohreh Naghashfar,** Department of Immunology and Infectious Diseases, School of Hygiene and Public Health, The Johns Hopkins University, Baltimore, MD 21205 **[155]**

**Mohammed Nasseri,** Department of Microbiology and Immunology, UCLA School of Medicine, and Molecular Biology Institute, University of California, Los Angeles, CA 90024; present address: Department of Biological Chemistry, University of Rochester Medical Center, Rochester, NY 14642 **[487]**

**Kathryn Neary,** Department of Human Genetics, Yale University School of Medicine, New Haven, CT 06510 **[437]**

**Slavomir Obalek,** Department of Dermatology, Warsaw School of Medicine, 02-088 Warsaw, Poland **[69]**

**Takashi Okagaki,** Departments of Obstetrics and Gynecology and Laboratory Medicine and Pathology, University of Minnesota, Minneapolis, MN 55455 **[101]**

**Hiroto Okayama,** Laboratory of Molecular Genetics, National Institute of Child Health and Development, Bethesda, MD 20205 **[363]**

**Carl Olson,** Department of Veterinary Science, University of Wisconsin-Madison, WI 53706 **[279]**

**Robert O. Olson,** Department of Veterinary Science, University of Wisconsin-Madison, WI 53706 **[279]**

**Gerard Orth,** Unité des Papillomavirus, Département de Virologie, Institut Pasteur, 25 rue du Docteur Roux, 75724 Paris Cedex 15, France **[47, 69, 379]**

**Ronald S. Ostrow,** Department of Microbiology, University of Minnesota, Minneapolis, MN 55455 **[101, 501]**

**S. Parkkinen,** Departments of Pathology, Gynecology and Obstetrics, and Clinical Microbiology, University of Kuopio, POB 6, SF-70211 Kuopio, Finland **[31]**

**Herbert Pfister,** Institut für Klinische Virologie der Universität Erlangen-Nürnberg, D-8520 Erlangen, F.R. Germany **[85]**

**William P. Pilacinski,** Molecular Genetics, Inc., Minnetonka, MN 55343 **[257]**

**Terry F. Plasse,** Interferon Sciences, Inc., New Brunswick, NJ 08901 **[217]**

**David E. Reed,** Molecular Genetics, Inc., Minnetonka, MN 55343 **[257]**

**Sheila S. Reilly,** Department of Oral Biology and Pathology, School of Dental Medicine, State University of New York at Stony Brook, Stony Brook, NY 11794 **[427]**

**George A. Ricca,** Department of Molecular Biology, Revlon Health Care Research and Development, Springfield, VA 22151 **[515]**

**G.F. Riou,** Laboratoire de Pharmacologie Clinique et Moléculaire, Institut Gustave Roussy, 94800 Villejuif, France **[47]**

**Walter G. Röwekamp,** German Cancer Research Center, Institute of Cell and Tumor Biology, Im Neuenheimer Feld 280, D-6900 Heidelberg, F.R.G. **[391]**

**S. Saarikoski,** Departments of Pathology, Gynecology and Obstetrics, and Clinical Microbiology, University of Kuopio, POB 6, SF-70211 Kuopio, Finland **[31]**

**Nava Sarver,** Department of Molecular Biology, Revlon Health Care Research and Development, Springfield, VA 22151 **[515]**

**Gerhard Sauer,** Institute for Virus Research, German Cancer Research Center, 6900 Heidelberg, FRG **[57]**

**Edward Sawada,** Maryland State Cancer Control Unit, Baltimore, MD 21201 **[155]**

**John T. Schiller,** Laboratory of Cellular Oncology, National Cancer Institute, Bethesda, MD 20205 **[457]**

**Klaus Seedorf,** German Cancer Research Center, Institute of Cell and Tumor Biology, Im Neuenheimer Feld 280, D - 6900 Heidelberg, F.R.G. **[391]**

**Keerti V. Shah,** Department of Immunology and Infectious Deisease, School of Hygiene and Public Health, The Johns Hopkins University, Baltimore, MD 21205 **[155]**

**S. Silverstein,** Department of Microbiology and the Cancer Research Center, Columbia University, 630 W. 168th Street, New York, NY 10032 **[19]**

**George Singleton,** Divsion of Otolaryngology, College of Medicine, University of Florida, Gainesville, FL 32610 **[137]**

**K.T. Smith,** The Beatson Institute for Cancer Research, Garscube Estate, Bearsden, Glasgow G61 1BD, UK **[305]**

**C. Daniel Sooy,** Department of Otolaryngology, University of California, San Francisco, CA 94143 **[273]**

**Barbara A. Spalholz,** Laboratory of Tumor Virus Biology, National Cancer Institute, Bethesda, MD 20205 **[343]**

**Bettie M. Steinberg,** Department of Otolaryngology, Long Island Jewish Medical Center, 270-05 76th Avenue, New Hyde Park, NY 11042 **[413]**

**Jack G. Stevens,** Department of Microbiology and Immunology, UCLA School of Medicine, Los Angeles, CA 90024 **[327]**

**Hans Strander,** Radiumhemmet and Department of Oto-Rhino-Laryngology, Karolinska Hospital, 104 01 Stockholm, Sweden **[165]**

**Earl A. Surwit,** Departments of Obstetrics and Gynecology, University of Arizona and Arizona Cancer Center, Tucson, AZ 85724 **[249]**

**Kari Syrjänen,** Departments of Pathology, Gynecology and Obstetrics, and Clinical Microbiology, University of Kuopio, POB 6, SF-70211 Kuopio, Finland; present address: Laboratory of Pathology and Cancer Research, Finnish Cancer Society, POB 25, SF-70200 Kuopio, Finland **[31]**

**S. Syrjänen,** Department of Pathology, Gynecology and Obstetrics, and Clinical Microbiology, University of Kuopio, POB 6, SF-70211 Kuopio, Finland **[31]**

**Lorne B. Taichman,** Department of Oral Biology and Pathology, School of Dental Medicine, State University of New York at Stony Brook, Stony Brook, NY 11794 **[409,427]**

**G. Criss Tarr,** Department of Molecular Biology, Revlon Health Care Research and Development, Springfield, VA 22151 **[515]**

**Françoise Thierry,** Unité des Virus Oncogènes, Département de Biologie Moléculaire, Institut Pasteur, 25 rue du Docteur Roux, 75724 Paris Cedex 15, France **[379]**

**Kenneth Trofatter, Jr.,** Department of Obstetrics and Gynecology, Duke University Medical Center, Durham, NC 27710 **[201]**

**J. Richard Trout,** Department of Statistics, Cook College, Rutgers University, New Brunswick, NJ 08903 **[217]**

**A.L. Trowbridge,** Department of Otolaryngology, The Children's Hospital, 300 Longwood Avenue, Boston MA 02115 **[181]**

**Leo B. Twiggs,** Departments of Obstetrics and Gynecology and Laboratory Medicine and Pathology, University of Minnesota, Minneapolis, MN 55455 **[101]**

**William C. Vass,** Laboratory of Cellular Oncology, National Cancer Institute, Bethesda, MD 20205 **[457]**

**M. Väyrynen,** Departments of Pathology, Gynecology and Obstetrics, and Clinical Microbiology, University of Kuopio, POB 6, SF-70211 Kuopio, Finland **[31]**

**Inder M. Verma,** Molecular Biology and Virology Laboratory, The Salk Institute, San Diego, CA 92138 **[545]**

**Susan L. Watts,** Cold Spring Harbor Laboratory, Cold Spring Harbor, NY 11724; present address: Department of Surgery, University of North Carolina, Chapel Hill, NC 27514 **[501]**

**Dawn Weber,** Department of Microbiology, University of Minnesota, Minneapolis, MN 55455 **[101]**

**Phillip K. Weck,** Department of Obstetrics and Gynecology, Duke University Medical Center, Durham, NC 27710; present address: Burroughs Wellcome Co., Research Triangle Park, NC 27709 **[137,185,201]**

**Sheldon A. Weiner,** Department of Obstetrics and Gynecology, University of Arizona and Arizona Cancer Center, Tucson, AZ 85724 **[249]**

**Lawrence Weissbach,** Graduate Program in Molecular Biology and Virology, Sloan-Kettering Institute for Cancer Research, New York, NY 10021 **[397]**

**Felix O. Wettstein,** Department of Microbiology and Immunology, UCLA School of Medicine, and Molecular Biology Institute, University of California, Los Angeles, CA 90024 **[327,487]**

**John K. Whisnant,** Department of Immunology and Oncology, Burroughs Wellcome Co., Research Triangle Park, NC 27709 **[137,185,201]**

**C. Richard Wobbe,** Graduate Program in Molecular Biology and Virology, Sloan-Kettering Institute for Cancer Research, New York, NY 10021 **[397]**

**Tzyy-Choou Wu,** Department of Immunology and Infectious Diseases, School of Public Health, The Johns Hopkins University, Baltimore, MD 21205 **[135]**

**Yu-Chung Yang,** Laboratory of Tumor Virus Biology, National Cancer Institute, Bethesda, MD 20205 **[343, 363]**

**Moshe Yaniv,** Unité des Virus Oncogènes, Département de Biologie Moléculaire, Institut Pasteur, 25 rue du Docteur Roux, 75724 Paris Cedex 15, France **[379]**

**Karen Zachow,** Department of Microbiology, University of Minnesota, Minneapolis, MN 55455 **[101]**

# Preface

This volume represents a series of papers presented at the Burroughs-Wellcome-UCLA Symposium on "Papillomaviruses: Molecular and Clinical Aspects" held at Steamboat Springs, Colorado, April 8–14, 1985. The meeting was attended by nearly 180 participants, and was held concurrently with the UCLA Symposium on "Biochemical and Molecular Epidemiology of Cancer". Due to the rapidly growing awareness of the potential role of papillomaviruses in human as well as animal cell cancers, this meeting was most timely. Papers were presented on (1) the molecular biology of papillomaviruses; (2) the clinical spectrum of human papillomavirus associated diseases; (3) the animal papillomaviruses: (4) viral spectors; and (5) the transforming functions and carcinogenic potential of papillomaviruses. In addition to the plenary sessions, there were two poster sessions and two workshops: one dealt with epithelial cell culture and the second examined the immunology and therapeutic modalities being investigated in papillomavirus associated illnesses.

The chapters document many of the talks delivered in the plenary sessions and workshops, although not all of the presentations are included. Contributions to the volume were made voluntary in order to encourage presentation of unpublished data at the Symposium and to foster widespread participation. In addition, a number of poster session presentations were selected for inclusion in this volume. The papers are arranged in the volume roughly according to the session organization of the meeting.

The success of this meeting was in large part due to the diversity in the backgrounds and in the interests of the participants. The program included basic scientists as well as clinical investigators and the topics ranged from the biochemistry of DNA replication to the discussion of clinical trials involving treatment of papillomavirus associated illnesses. Many of those attending the Symposium were from Europe, and participants were from government research laboratories and industry, as well as from medical schools and universities. The spectrum of those at the Symposium ranged from graduate students to established investigators, and included many new to the field. A very successful feature of the program was the inclusion of one or two talks in each session reviewing related viral or cellular systems to broaden the discussion and to provoke thought about the directions that future research on the papillomaviruses might take. We are particularly grateful to

Howard Green who presented the Keynote Address and to Tom Banjamen, Bill Sugden, George Khoury, Jerry Hurwitz, Stu Yuspa, Henry Sun, and Yakov Gluzman for providing this perspective to the meeting. Because of the diversity of the clinical as well as the basic science problems associated with the papillomaviruses, multidisciplinary gatherings such as this symposium are critical in order to promote free exchange of scientific information and advancements in this field. The abstracts for the Symposium are published in the *Journal of Cellular Biochemistry* (Supplement 9C, 65-100, 1985).

This meeting was generously supported by Burroughs-Wellcome and the editors are especially grateful to Drs. John Whisnant and Phillip Weck of Burroughs-Wellcome for their input into the planning of the Symposium. The editors wish to acknowledge the skilled assistance of Dr. Robin Yeaton and the UCLA Symposia staff in organizing this meeting.

**Peter M. Howley**
National Institutes of Health
Bethesda, Maryland

**Thomas R. Broker**
Department of Biochemistry
University of Rochester
Rochester, New York

# I. PAPILLOMAVIRUSES AND HUMAN GENITAL TRACT DISEASES

**Papillomaviruses: Molecular and Clinical Aspects, pages 3–18**


# PAPILLOMAVIRUSES AND CERVICAL NEOPLASIA REFLECTIONS ON THE PAST, PERCEPTIONS OF THE PRESENT AND SPECULATIONS FOR THE FUTURE[1]

Robert J. Kurman, A. Bennett Jenson and Wayne D. Lancaster

Departments of Pathology and
Obstetrics and Gynecology
Georgetown University
School of Medicine
Washington, D.C. 20007

ABSTRACT The recognition that human (H) papillomaviruses (PV) are associated with benign genital warts (condyloma acuminata), precancerous lesions of the cervix (dysplasia, carcinoma-in-situ [CIS] or alternatively cervical intraepithelial neoplasia [CIN]), and invasive cervical carcinoma has raised a number of questions concerning the etiology, pathologic diagnosis, and management of this disease. Traditionally, cervical dysplasia was regarded as a precancerous lesion although it was recognized that a high proportion of these lesions spontaneously regress or persist and only a minority progress to invasive cancer. Moreover, the behavior of a particular dysplastic lesion based on its histologic appearance has been notoriously unpredictable and consequently clinical management has ranged from observation to hysterectomy.

The evidence relating PV to cervical neoplasia is based on morphologic, immunocytochemical and molecular virologic data. Thus, dysplasia is composed of a group of lesions that form a morphologic continuum ranging from mild to severe dysplasia merging imperceptibly with CIS. HPV-specific structural antigens have been identified within all phases of the intraepithelial process leading up to CIS and HPV-DNA sequences have been detected in a high proportion of cervical dysplasias and invasive cervical cancers. These data provide further evidence implicating PV with cervical neoplasia and also suggest that cervical abnormalities traditionally classified as "dysplasia" may be composed of a heterogeneous group of lesions that are induced by a limited number of PV types of varying oncogenic potential. Perhaps only a subset of PV types acting in concert with other factors such as herpes infection or cigarette smoking induce neoplastic transformation whereas the majority of PVs produce lesions with little or no oncogenic potential that persist as chronic infections or regress spontaneously.

[1]This work was supported by NCI Contract No. CN-17501 and grants CA32603 and CA32638.

## INTRODUCTION

In the last five years mounting evidence has associated human (H) papillomaviruses (PV) with cervical cancer and its precursor, dysplasia and carcinoma-in-situ (CIS). In order to more clearly elucidate the role of HPV in cervical neoplasia (dysplasia and carcinoma) it is necessary to correlate the clinical behavior, pathology, and epidemiology of the neoplastic process with the biology of HPV infection of the female genital tract.

## DEFINITION OF DYSPLASIA AND CIS

The term "dysplasia" was introduced independently by Ober (1) and Reagen (2) but it was not until the First International Congress of Exfoliative Cytology in 1961 that it was officially sanctioned (3). Dysplasia is defined as a proliferation of atypical cells that do not involve the full thickness of the squamous epithelium of the cervix. In the deeper levels the cells are undifferentiated but near the surface, maturation is evident. The cells vary considerably in size and shape and the nuclei are hyperchromatic and exhibit coarse chromatin clumping. Dysplasia is subclassified further as mild, moderate, or severe based on the extent to which the squamous epithelium is replaced by undifferentiated basal cells. In mild dysplasia these cells occupy the deepest level but do not exceed one-third the thickness of the epithelium. In moderate dysplasia undifferentiated basal cells occupy between one-half to three-quarters of the thickness of the epithelium and in severe dysplasia they replace almost the full thickness except for the most superficial layer which still shows evidence of maturation. In CIS replacement of the epithelium is complete. All of these lesions may involve endocervical glands.

## NATURAL HISTORY OF DYSPLASIA

Considerable variation has been reported in the proportion of patients with dysplasia whose lesions regress, persist, or progress to CIS or invasive carcinoma. The mean figures from five different series totaling 1035 patients indicates that 55% regress, 27% persist, 19% progress to a higher level of dysplasia, 10% progress to CIS, and 1% progress to invasive carcinoma. In contrast, in another study (4) over 90% of all grades of dysplasia progressed to CIS if the patients were followed by cytologic smears and were not biopsied. A recent long-term follow-up study (5) of 894 patients with moderate dysplasia showed that regression occurred in 54%, persistence in 16%, and progression in 30%. Based on these follow-up studies as well as the similar morphologic features of dysplasia, CIS, and invasive cancer, dysplasia has been regarded as a transitional stage of carcinogenesis.

## MORPHOLOGIC, IMMUNOCYTOCHEMICAL AND MOLECULAR VIROLOGIC EVIDENCE ASSOCIATING HPV WITH CERVICAL CANCER

Evidence for HPV in cervical dysplasia was first inferential, based on studies showing a close cytologic and histologic similarity to vulvar and perianal condylomas, lesions known to be caused by HPV (6,7). The identification of viral particles by electon microscopy in cervical dysplasia compatible with PV ultrastructure (8) added weight to this argument but the demonstration of PV structural proteins by immunocytochemistry (9-12) and DNA sequences by molecular hybridization (13-16) has provided the most convincing evidence supporting this view.

The immunocytochemical studies have shown that PV capsid antigen is present directly within mild, moderate, and severe dysplasia in 30%, 15% and 3% of cases respectively. Capsid antigen has not been found in normal metaplastic squamous epithelium or in CIS (12). Using Southern blot hybridization techniques PV-DNA has been identified in 80-90% of all grades of dysplasia including CIS and invasive carcinoma (17,19). Several types of HPV including HPV-6, 11, 16, 18 and others not yet completely characterized, have been identified in these lesions (19). HPV-6 or HPV-11 are found in over 90% of benign genital condylomas and only rarely in cancers. In contrast, HPV-16 and HPV-18 are found in over 80% of invasive cervical cancers (17,19) and rarely in condylomas. These findings suggest that the oncongenic potential of a particular dysplasia may, in part, depend on the HPV type (20).

A possible source of error in studies that utilize Southern blot hybridization is that the PV-DNA identified may represent a contaminant from the vagina and not truly reflect viral DNA within a particular cervical lesion. This concern has been disspelled by in situ hybridization studies demonstrating viral DNA directly within dysplastic lesions (21). Further evidence associating HPV directly with the neoplastic process has been the demonstration of the same type of HPV-DNA within metastatic carcinoma in pelvic lymph nodes and in the primary cervical tumor from the same patient (22). The recent report of transcription of specific HPV-18 sequences in cervical cancer cell lines and the identification of HPV-16 RNA species in extracts from invasive cervical cancers is cogent evidence supporting an active as opposed to a passenger role of PV in this disease (23).

## CORRELATION OF THE HISTOLOGY AND BIOLOGY OF HPV INFECTION AND CERVICAL NEOPLASIA

Correlation of the histologic, immunocytochemical and molecular hybrIdization findings reveals that the histologic appearance of cervical dysplasia reflects the biologic behavior of HPV. The various grades of dysplasia comprise a spectrum of subtle morphologic transitions ranging from very mild and mild dysplasia to severe dysplasia and CIS. These transitions are frequently observed within the same specimen (Figs. 1,2). Lesions at the

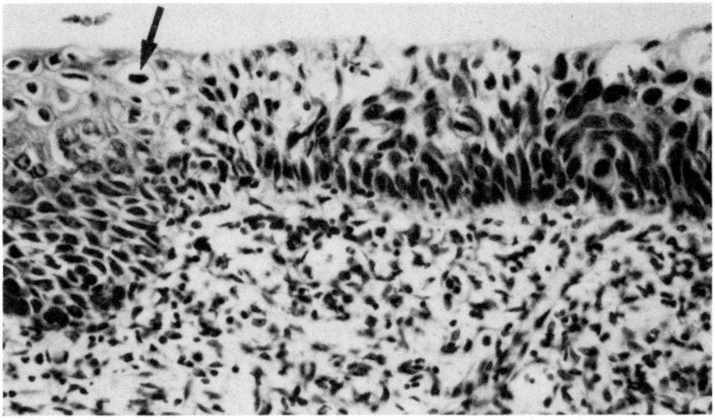

Fig.1 Very mild to mild dysplasia on left merging into moderate dysplasia. PV capsid antigens are frequently localized in koilocytotic cells (arrow) (Hematoxylin and eosin).

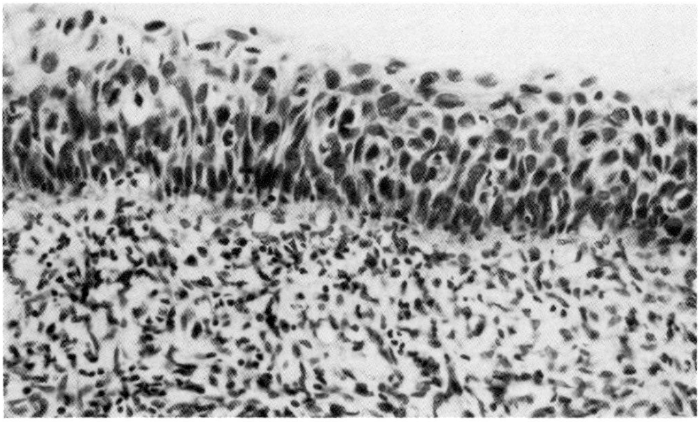

Fig.2 This field is immediately adjacent to Fig. 1 and illustrates moderate dysplasia on the left merging into severe dysplasia and CIS. Note that the basal and parabasal cells in this part of the lesion are similar to those in the areas of mild and moderate dysplasia in Fig. 1 (Hematoxylin and eosin).

mild end of the spectrum represent viral infections since PV capsid antigens can be demonstrated by immunocytochemistry and intact viral particles can be demonstrated by electron microscopy. At the other end of the spectrum, CIS is an intraepithelial neoplasm composed of cells which morphologically resemble the cells of invasive squamous carcinoma. Lesions in the intermediate range (moderate and severe dysplasia) are composed of a heterogenous population of cells. Among these are differentiated squamous cells in the superficial layers of the epithelium that display degenerative changes characteristic of PV infection and in which PV antigens can be identified. Underlying these cells are undifferentiated basal cells that occupy a half to three quarters of the epithelium and closely resemble the neoplastic cells of CIS. Based on autoradiographic studies of other PV-induced lesions (24-26) it seems likely that this proliferation of basal cells is due to a stable and heritable transformation induced by PV-DNA. Molecular hybridization and immunocytochemistry studies of cervical dysplasia (12,13) have confirmed that PV-specific DNA sequences and PV structural proteins are found in lesions in which a proliferation of basal and parabasal cells is present. Furthermore, in 85% of PV positive cases this proliferation occurs immediately beneath superficial squamous cells containing PV antigens (12). It therefore appears that the basal cell proliferation is due to an early gene expression of HPV occuring prior to vegetative viral DNA synthesis. In contrast, the synthesis of viral capsid proteins appears to be a function of late gene expression that occurs only in terminally differentiated squamous cells in the superficial layers. The nuclei of the squamous cells in this location show signs of degeneration manifested by wrinkling, angulation, smudging, and clumping of chromatin. Vacuolation of the cytoplasm, so-called koilocytosis, is typically present. These cellular changes constitute what has been generally recognized morphologically as papillomavirus infection but in fact represent only the final stage of the viral life cycle.

A recent immunocytochemical study (27), correlating the expression of the cellular structural protein involucrin and HPV, sheds further light on the role of squamous differentiation and HPV expression. Involucrin is a non-filamentous protein, unrelated to cytokeratins, that is a precursor for a cross-linked protein that envelops squamous epithelial cells. In the normal cervix involucrin is first observed in the parabasal cells with progressive increased intensity and distribution in the superficial layers. It is absent in the basal cells suggesting that there is a coordination between cellular DNA synthesis and involucrin expression. Immunocytochemical localization of involucrin therefore serves as a marker of squamous differentiation. Comparison of cervical dysplasias matched according to grade reveals that expression of HPV structural antigens occurs only in lesions displaying an abnormal distribution of involucrin that involves the full thickness of the epithelium including the basal layer (Fig. 3). These

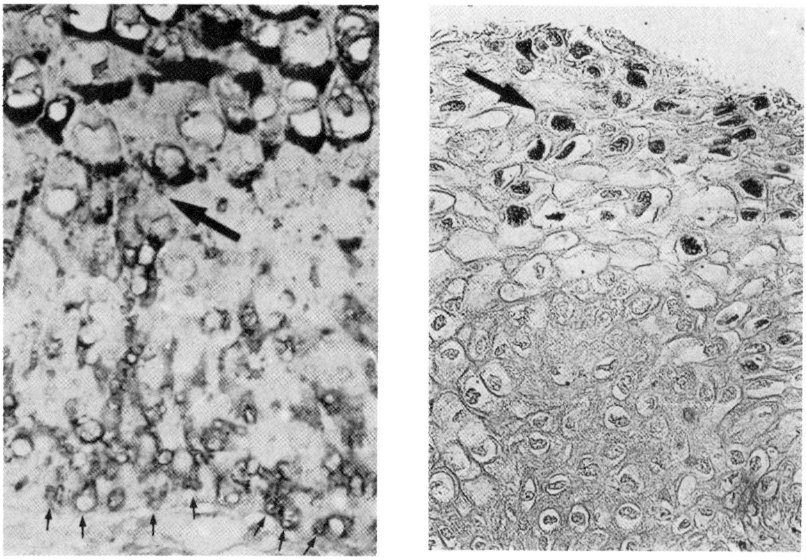

Fig.3 A. Mild dysplasia showing full thickness staining for involucrin (granular black deposit), in koilocytotic cells (large arrow) and basal cells (small arrows) (Immunoperoxidase-involucrin and methyl green counterstain). B. A step section showing localization of papillomavirus antigens (black deposit) in nuclei of superficial cells (arrow) (Immunoperoxidase-papillomavirus antigens, no counterstain).

findings suggest that HPV infection of squamous epithelium "uncouples" cellular DNA synthesis and differentiation inducing premature maturation of the squamous epithelium which appears to be a necessary prerequiste for capsid protein synthesis and virion assembly. This sequence of events underscores the close interaction between PV gene expression and the cellular proliferation and differentiation of the squamous epithelium that characterizes cervical dysplasia.

## EPIDEMIOLOGIC ASPECTS OF HPV INFECTION AND CERVICAL NEOPLASIA

Epidemiologic studies have shown that CIS and invasive carcinoma show strong correlations with the sexual history of the patient as well as with that of her partner (28). Rotkin (29) concludes on the basis of a review of 17 epidemiologic studies that sexual intercourse before the age of 17 years and multiple sexual partners are the most important risk factors in the development of cervical cancer. In contrast, in a case-control study (30) it was found that for several characteristics, including age at first coitus, women with cervical dysplasia showed no difference compared to controls whereas women with CIS and invasive carcinoma were younger than the control group. These data were interpretated as indicating that CIS and invasive cancer are different forms of the same disease but that dysplasia represents a diverse disease composed of some lesions that are precancerous and some that are not.

Over the last two decades cervical neoplasia has been related to sexually transmitted diseases with most of the attention directed to Herpes simplex virus 2 (HSV-2) based on retrospective seroepidemiologic studies. In a prospective study involving more than 10,000 women, however, Vonka et al. (31) found no difference in the serum level of HSV-2 antibodies in patients with preinvasive and invasive cervical neoplasms compared to matched controls. Since HPV has been only recently implicated with cervical neoplasia and since a reliable serologic assay for HPV antibodies is not available, similar epidemiologic studies for HPV have not been performed. A recent clinicopathologic study (32), however, provides evidence linking preinvasive cervical lesions with HPV-related penile lesions such as Bowenoid papulosis and dysplasia. In this study it was shown that more than half of the male sexual partners of women with all grades of cervical dysplasia had either a history of genital warts (12%) or presently had Bowenoid papulosis or dysplasia (41%). The latter lesions were typically occult and were detected only after careful examination using a magnifying lens.

## TERMINOLOGY OF HPV-INFECTION AND CERVICAL NEOPLASIA

Considerable confusion exists over the terminology of the various types of intraepithelial lesions. The crux of the problem revolves around the distinction of lesions that have been shown to contain PV antigens and therefore qualify as PV infection and those that are truly neoplastic i.e., capable of autonomous growth, in which PV antigens are not found. In the past, all of the intraepithelial lesions were included in the category of dysplasia and CIS or cervical intraepithelial neoplasia (CIN) and were regarded as precursors of squamous carcinoma. It is of interest to consider the classification of intraepithelial lesions in the light of what is presently known about the biology of HPV infection. Depending on the extent of the basal cell proliferation relative to the extent of squamous differentiation in which the morphologic manifestations of HPV infection (koilocytosis) are evident, these lesions have been traditionally classified as mild, moderate, or severe dysplasia and CIS or alternatively CIN I, II, or III.

The term "flat condyloma" has been applied to cervical lesions, previously classified as mild dysplasia, to draw attention to their cytologic similarity to the classic condyloma acuminatum (33). The term "atypical flat condyloma" was introduced to describe high grade dysplasias with morphologic evidence of HPV infection. Implicit in the use of this terminology is the ability to distinguish, on strictly morphologic grounds, a benign viral infection (flat condyloma) from a "true dysplasia" (atypical flat condyloma) which is precancerous. The use of different terms for these lesions also implies that they are discrete entities, however, considerable overlap in their morphology exists and their behavior is uncertain. A clear-cut distinction can not always be made between atypical proliferating cells underlying areas of viral-induced atypia in which PV antigens can be identified (infection) and proliferating cells in intraepithelial lesions displaying cytologic features similar to those of invasive cancer (neoplasia). Furthermore, PV-DNA sequences have been detected by molecular hybridization in more than 80% of all grades of intraepithelial lesions ranging from mild dysplasia to CIS (18). It appears, therefore, that the present terminology of cervical dysplasia or CIN subsumes both a morphologic continuum and a biologic dichotomy, i.e., an infectious and a neoplastic process linked through a proliferation of atypical basal and parabasal cells (Fig. 4) This proliferation characterizes

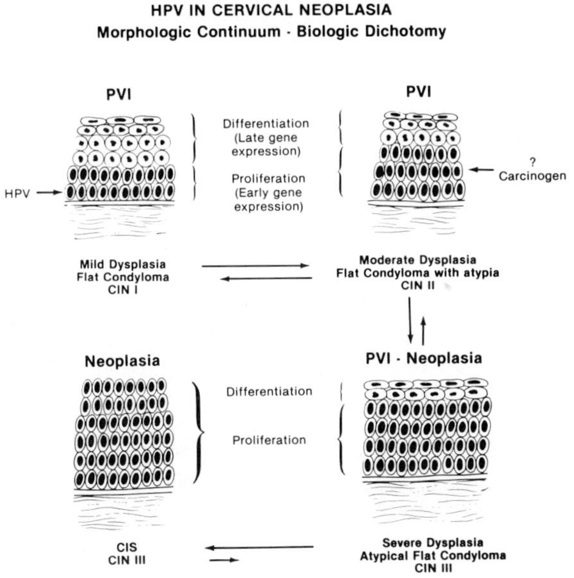


Fig. 4 (Legend on next page)

Fig.4 Schema depicting the relationship of papillomavirus infection (PVI) to cervical intraepithelial neoplasia (CIN) and various diagnostic terms. Lesions have been traditionally graded according to the degree of proliferation, probably induced by PV, relative to the degree of differentiation. The morphologic manifestations of productive PV infection (koilocytosis) and PV capsid antigens are found in the differentiated squamous cells. The progression and regression of these lesions (shown by arrows) may depend on the varying oncogenic potential of specific HPV types, other extrinsic factors i.e., envirnmental carcinogens. Although there is a morphologic continuum, the ends of the spectrum, papillomavirus infection and neoplasia, represent a biologic dichotomy.

cervical dysplasia and can also be observed in PV-induced lesions in other sites. Since at present it is not clear whether all lesions that predominantly display the morphologic features of PV infection are benign or whether a subset of these may progress to carcinoma it is prudent to retain the traditional classification of dysplasia or CIN. The presence of morphologic changes indicative of PV infection can be noted.

## SUMMARY

Review of the available data suggests that dysplasia is a sexually transmitted disease composed of a heterogeneous group of lesions of varying oncogenic potential. The presence of HPV-DNA in the vast majority of dysplasia and invasive cancer provides compelling evidence linking HPV with cervical neoplasia. The finding of multiple HPV types in dysplasia and their different distribution in benign and malignant lesions suggests that certain HPV types may be associated with dysplasias that have a low risk of progression to carcinoma whereas others may have a high risk of progression. Correlation of specific HPV types with the histopathologic features of cervical dysplasia and other host factors may permit distinction of true precancerous lesions from benign viral infections in the future.

## REFERENCES

1. Papanicolaou, GN (1949). A survey of the actualities and potentialities of exfoliative cytology in cancer diagnosis. Ann Int Med 31:6614.
2. Koss, LG (1978). Dysplasia: A real concept or a misnomer. Obstet Gynecol 51:374.
3. Weid, GL (1962) (Editorial). Proceedings of the First International Congress of Exfoliative Cytology, Vienna, Austria. Appleton-Century-Crofts, Philadelphia, Pa. p 297.
4. Richart, RM, Barron, BA (1969). A follow-up study of patients with cervical dysplasia. Am J Obstet Gynecol 105:386.
5. Nasiell, K, Nasiell, M, Vaclavinkova, V (1983). Behavior of moderate cervical dysplasia during long-term follow-up. Obstet Gynecol 61:609.
6. Ludwig, ME, Lowell, DM, LiVolsi, VA (1981). Cervical condylomatous atypia and its relationship to cervical neoplasia. Am J Clin Pathol 76:255.
7. Meisels, A, Fortin, R, Roy, M (1977). Condylomatous lesions of the cervix II. Cytologic, colposcopic and histologic study. Acta Cytol 21:379.
8. Reid, R, Laverty, CR, Coppleson, M, Isarangkul, W, Hills, E (1980). Noncondylomatous cervical wart virus infection. Obstet Gynecol 55:476.
9. Woodruff, JD, Braun, L, Cavalieri, R, Gupta, P, Pass, F, Shah, KV (1980). Immunologic identification of papillomavirus antigen in condyloma tissues from the female genital tract. Obstet Gynecol 56:727.
10. Kurman, RJ, Shah, KH, Lancaster, WD, Jenson, AB (1981). Immunoperoxidase localization of papillomavirus antigens in

cervical dysplasia and vulvar condylomas. Am J Obstet Gynecol 40:931.
11. Morin, C, Braun, L, Casas-Cordero, M, Shah, K.V, Roy, M, Fortier, M, Meisels, A (1981). Confirmation of papillomavirus etiology of condylomatous of the cervix by the peroxidase-antiperoxidase technique. J Natl Cancer Inst 66:831.
12. Kurman, RJ, Jenson, AB, Lancaster, WD (1983). Papillomavirus infection of the cervix II. Relationship to intraepithelial neoplasia based on the presence of specific viral structural proteins. Am J Surg Pathol 7:39.
13. Kurman, RJ, Sanz, LE, Jenson, AB, Perry, S, Lancaster, WD (1982). Papillomavirus infection of the cervix I. Correlation of histology with specific structural antigens and DNA sequences. Int. J Gynecol Pathol 1:17.
14. Gissmann, L, Wolnik, L, Ikenberg, H, Koldovsky, U, Schursh, HG, zur Hausen, H (1983). Human papillomavirus types 6 and 11 DNA sequences in genital and laryngeal papillomas and some cervical cancers. Proc Natl Acad Sci USA 80:560.
15. Okagaki, T, Twiggs, LB, Zachow, KR, Lark, BA, Ostrow, RS, Faras, AJ (1983). Identification of human papillomavirus DNA in cervical and vaginal intraepithelial neoplasia and molecularly cloned virus-specific DNA probes. Int J Gynecol Pathol 2:153.
16. Lancaster, WD, Kurman, RJ, Sanz, LE, Perry, S, Jenson, AB (1983). Human Papillomavirus: Detection of viral DNA sequences and evidence of molecular heterogeneity in metaplasias and dysplasias of the uterine cervix. Intervirology 20:202.
17. Durst, M, Gissman, L, Ikenberg, H, zur Hausen, H (1983). A papillomavirus DNA from a cervical carcinoma and its prevalence in cancer biopsy specimens from different geographic regions. Proc Natl Acad Sci USA 80:3812.

18. Lorincz, A, Temple, G, Santos, C, Castellano, C, Lemos, L, Delgado, G, Petrilli, Hummel, S, Kurman, RJ, Jenson, AB, Lancaster, WE (1985). Identification of human papillomavirus (HPV) DNA sequences in female genital tract neoplasms. Gynecol Oncol 20:252.
19. Gissmann, L, Wolnik, L, Ikenberg, H, Koldovsky, U, Schursh, HG, zur Hausen, H (1983). Human papillomaviruses types 6 and 11 DNA sequences in genital and laryngeal papillomas and some cervical cancers. Proc Natl Acad Sci USA 80:560.
20. Crum, CP, Ikenberg, F, Richart, RM, Gissman, L (1984). Human papillomavirus type 16 and early cervical neoplasia. N Engl J Med 310:880.
21. Crum, CP (Unpublished data).
22. Lancaster, WD, Castellano, C, Santos, C, Delgado, G, Kurman, RJ, Jenson, AB (Unpublished data).
23. Schwarz, E, Freese, UK, Grismann, L, Mayer, W, Roggenbuck, B, Stremlau A, zur Hausen, H (1985). Structure and transcription of human papillomavirus sequences in cervical carcinoma cells. Nature 314:111.
24. Rashad, AL (1969). Radioautographic evidence of DNA synthesis in well differentiated cells of human skin papillomas. J Invest Dermatol 53:356.
25. Orth, G, Breitburd, F, Favre, M, Croissant, O (1977). Papillomaviruses: Possible role in human cancer. Cold Spring Harbor Conference Cell Prolif 4:1043.
26. Delescluse, C (1975). Incorporation of thymidine and uridine in the epidermis of epidermodysplasia verruciformis. In Biomedical Aspects of Human Wart Virus Infection, M Pruneiras, (eds), Merieux Foundation, Lyon, p 171-179.
27. Warhol, MJ, Pinkus, GS, Rice, RH, El-Tawil, GH, Lancaster, WD, Jenson, AB, Kurman, RJ (1984). Papillomavirus infection of the cervix III. Relationship of the presence of viral structural proteins to

the expression of involucrin. Int J Gynecol Pathol 3:71.
28. Beral, V (1974). Cancer of the cervix: A sexually transmitted infection. Lancet 1: 1037.
29. Rotkin, IA (1973). A comparison review of key epidemiological studies in cervical cancer related to current searches for transmissable agents. Cancer Res 33:1353.
30. Terris, M, Wilson, F, Nelson, JH, Jr (1980). Comparative epidemiology of invasive carcinoma of the cervix, carcinoma in situ, and cervical dysplasia. Am J Epidemiol 112:253.
31. Vonka, V, Kanka, V, Hirsch, I, et al. (1984). Prospective study on the relationship between cervical neoplasia and herpes simplex virus type-2 virus. II. Herpes simplex type-2 antibody presence in sera taken at enrollment. Int J Cancer 33:61.
32. Levine, RU, Crum, CP, Herman, E, Silvers, D, Ferenczy, A, Richart, RM (1984). Cervical Papillomavirus infection and intraepithelial neoplasia. A study of male sexual partners. Obstet Gynecol 64:16.
33. Meisels, A, Morin, C, Casas-Cordero, M (1982). Human papillomavirus infection of the uterine cervix. Int J Gynecol Pathol 1:75.

**Papillomaviruses: Molecular and Clinical Aspects, pages 19–29**


# Histological and Molecular Analysis of Early Cervical Neoplasia(1)

C.P. Crum,(2) N. Nagai,(3), M. Mitao,(3), R.U. Levine,(2) and S. Silverstein (4)

Departments of Ob/Gyn, Pathology, Microbiology, and the Cancer Research Center, Columbia University, New York, N.Y., and the Department of Ob/Gyn, Hiroshima University School of Medicine, Hiroshima, Japan

ABSTRACT We combined systematic histological analysis with Southern blot hybridization and DNA in-situ hybridization to correlate the presence of certain human papillomavirus (HPV) strains with specific precancerous cervical lesions and to pinpoint the distribution of HPV's in these lesions. In a series of 69 biopsies, HPV sequences were detected in 81% of samples with abnormal histology; HPV 16 was detected in 71% of precancers which contained abnormal mitoses and/or diffuse nuclear atypia(Cervical intraepithelial neoplasia). Seventy five percent of condylomata contained HPV sequences; of these 56% contained HPV 6 or 11. Mixed infections were uncommon. DNA in-situ hybridization of tissue sections from CIN and condylomata localized HPV sequences within nuclei, primarily in the superficial cell layers. However, in some lesions posi-

(1) This work was supported by grants from the NIH (CA 23767, to SJS) and the American Cancer Society (to CPC and SJS).

(2) Department of Ob/Gyn, Columbia University, 630 W. 168th Street, New York, N.Y. 10032

(3) Department of Ob/Gyn, Hiroshima University School of Medicine, Hiroshima, Japan

(4) Department of Microbiology and the Cancer Research Center, Columbia University, 701 W. 168th Street, New York, N.Y. 10032

tive nuclei were found in both mature and immature appearing neoplastic cells. This study indicates that these viruses segregate within lesions which exhibit strikingly different histological changes. However, in neoplastic epithelium as in condylomata, replication of HPV appears to be maturation dependent.

## INTRODUCTION

Human papillomaviruses have been detected in more than 80% of precancerous lesions of the uterine cervix(1-4). Furthermore, specific HPV strains have been associated with certain histological changes. HPV 6 and 11 have been found primarily in condylomata, whereas HPV 16 associates primarily with invasive carcinomas and high grade precancers (carcinoma in-situ) and HPV 18 almost exclusively with invasive carcinoma(3-5). We have previously demonstrated that HPV 16 is present in poorly differentiated precancers and in lesions which contain characteristics common to both condylomata(koilocytotic atypia) and carcinoma in-situ(abnormal mitoses)(6). This suggests that HPV 16 may influence the development of a form of "condyloma" which may progress to carcinoma in-situ and/or invasive carcinoma.

We have found that certain histological criteria, specifically abnormal mitoses and diffuse nuclear atypia, will define precancers with an aneuploid DNA content(7,8). Aneuploidy correlates closely with persistence of the lesion or its progression to cancer, and such lesions are empirically termed cervical intraepithelial neoplasia (CIN)(9). In contrast, condylomata are generally diploid or polyploid, frequently regress, and infrequently progress to invasive carcinoma(10). The present study was designed to determine if these histological criteria would consistently identify lesions containing HPV 16 as determined by Southern blot hybridization, and segregate them from lesions containing other viruses, including HPV's 6 and 11. More recently, we employed DNA in-situ hybridization to compare the distribution of HPV 16 in neoplastic epithelium to that of HPV 6 or 11 in condylomata in selected lesions. We present evidence that HPV's segregate within distinctly different lesions, but that in neoplastic epithelium, replication of HPV 16 appears to be closely linked to epithelial maturation, similar to that observed in condylomata.

## MATERIALS AND METHODS

Sample collection and histological classification. Colposcopically-directed biopsies were obtained from patients with abnormal Papanicolau smears, divided and one half frozen on a cryostat chuck. The other half was fixed for histology. Frozen sections were obtained to confirm the lesion was present in the frozen specimen and the remainder was stored at -70 deg C. for DNA extraction and in-situ hybridization. The frozen and permanent sections were reviewed and the lesions were classified into one of 4 groups; 1) Normal squamous epithelium, 2) condyloma, 3) Well differentiated CIN with koilocytotic atypia(CINK),and 4) classical CIN, analagous to carcinoma in-situ(Fig 1). CIN lesions contained either abnormal mitoses or diffuse nuclear atypia; the group resembling condyloma (CINK) were identified in order to compare the HPV sequences and their distribution in these lesions to both condylomata and classical CIN(11).

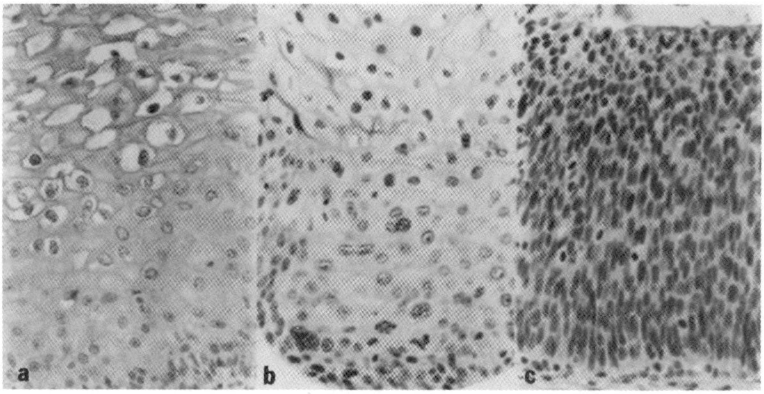


Figure 1. Classification of lesions: a) Conventional condyloma, b) CIN with koilocytotic atypia, c) Classical CIN (Carcinoma in-situ).

Southern blot hybridization. DNA was extracted from biopsies as previously described(11). Five to 10 ug of DNA was electrophoresed on agarose gels, and transferred to nitrocellulose filters(12). Hybridization probes specific for virus sequences prepared from gel-purified fragments from HPV's 6c,11a, and 16. The plasmids containing these clones were kindly provided by L. Gissman, H. zur Hausen, and their colleagues at Heidelberg, W. Germany(1-4). The strategy for hybridization was based upon the marked differences in sequence homology between the group of HPV's 6 and 11, and HPV 16 and has been described(11). Using this strategy, the HPV's present were classified into the following groups; 1) No HPV detected, 2) HPV 6 or 11, 3) HPV 16, 4) Other HPV (ie. positive with the probes under low stringent conditions only), and 5) mixtures of more than one HPV.

In-situ hybridization. In selected cases of CIN and condylomata, serial sections were removed from the frozen tissue prior to DNA extraction, fixed in Carnoys fixative, 100% ethanol, and stored at -70 deg.C. Serial sections were then incubated sequentially in 0.1M HCL, Proteinase K (5ug/ml in 2X SSC), and fixed in 5% paraformaldehyde for 2 hrs., using a modification of previously published methods(13, H. Gendelman, personal communication). Sections were then dehydrated in graded alcohols, dried briefly, then incubated with a hybridization cocktail containing 2X SSC, 10mm Tris, 5mm EDTA, 5% dextran sulfate, 50% formamide, and 400 ng/ml of a HPV DNA probe. The DNA was biotinylated by nick translation using the procedure suggested by the supplier(Bethesda Research Laboratories). Thirty ul of cocktail was placed on the slide, the coverslips were sealed with rubber cement and heated to 80 deg C. for 15 minutes. After rapid cooling, the slides were incubated for 18 hours at 42 deg C.(Tm-18). The coverslips were then removed, the slides were washed sequentially in 2X SSC(2 hrs) and 0.2X SSC(3 hrs) and then incubated serially with streptavidin, biotinylated alkaline phosphatase, and nitro-blue tetrazolium and bromo-chloro- indolyl phosphate(Bethesda Research Labs). The sections were then washed, counterstained with eosin, dehydrated in alcohols and mounted.

Each section was incubated with both HPV 16 and a mixed probe of HPV 6 and 11, one serving as a control for the other under the stringent hybridization conditions. In addition, the remainder of each biopsy was analyzed by Southern hybridization as described above. Sensitivity and specificity of the biotinylated system were further established by comparison with SV-40 infected monolayers of CV-1 cells, which were infected at different multiplicities of infection and analyzed by both Southern and in-situ hybridization with SV-40 DNA probes. Using this approach the threshold of sensitivity was estimated to be between 100 and 200 copies per cell.

## RESULTS

Correlation of viral strain with lesion type. Table I summarizes the relationship between HPV strain and morphology. Excluding 5 cases of negative epithelium, 64 lesions were analyzed and of these 52 or 81% contained HPV sequences. Seventy five, 96 and 55% of condylomata, CINK and CIN lesions resepectively contained HPV sequences. Fifty seven percent of HPV-positive condylomata contained HPV 6 or 11, 28% contained other HPV's and 14% contained more than one HPV. Two of these samples hybridized strongly with the HPV 6/11 probe as well as weakly with HPV 16 probes under stringent conditions. Seventy Three percent of CINK lesions contained HPV 16 alone and 19% contained other HPV's of undetermined type. Two biopsies from the same case hybridized to HPV 16 and weakly to HPV 6/11 probes. Fifty-five percent of CIN lesions contained HPV, 3 of which contained HPV 16. HPV 6/11 alone was not detected in any CIN lesion, and HPV 16 alone was not found in any classical condyloma.

Table I

Correlation of Virus Strain with Diagnosis

| Lesion | Number | HPV+ | HPV 6/11 | HPV 16 | Mixed | Other |
|---|---|---|---|---|---|---|
| Neg | 5 | 0 | - | - | - | - |
| Condy | 28 | 21 | 12 | 0 | 3 | 6 |
| CIN K | 27 | 26 | 0 | 19 | 2 | 5 |
| CIN | 9 | 5 | 0 | 3 | 2 | 0 |

In-Situ hybridization. A total of 21 cases of CIN were analyzed by both in-situ and Southern blot hybridization. Sixteen were positive for HPV 16 by blot hybridization and one contained a novel HPV strain. Ten were positive by in-situ hybridization. Nine of the ten were also positive by blot hybridization, in contrast to 6 of 11 which were negative by ISH.

The distribution of staining for HPV nucleic acids is illustrated in the figures. In condylomata which contained sequences hybridizing with HPV 6/11 probes, the staining usually concentrated in areas of maturation and koilocytotic atypia. Staining was intense in the superficial cells and less so in the deeper layers of the epithelium, usually being absent within two cell layers from the basal lamina(Fig 2).

In the well differentiated CIN lesions which hybridized with HPV 16 probe, positive staining was strongest in the mature cells, concentrating in the koilocytes. However, the hybridization signal varied considerably between cells, and the morphology of the nuclei which stained varied, ranging from small uniform nuclei in koilocytotic cells, to larger, irregular nuclei within cells in the middle and superficial areas of the epithelium. In some lesions, staining was present in nuclei near the basal lamina (Fig 3).

In high grade CIN lesions which contained sequences hy bridizing to the HPV 16 probe, staining was limited to very few nuclei and these nuclei were invariably located in the most superficial cells of the epithelium(Fig 4).

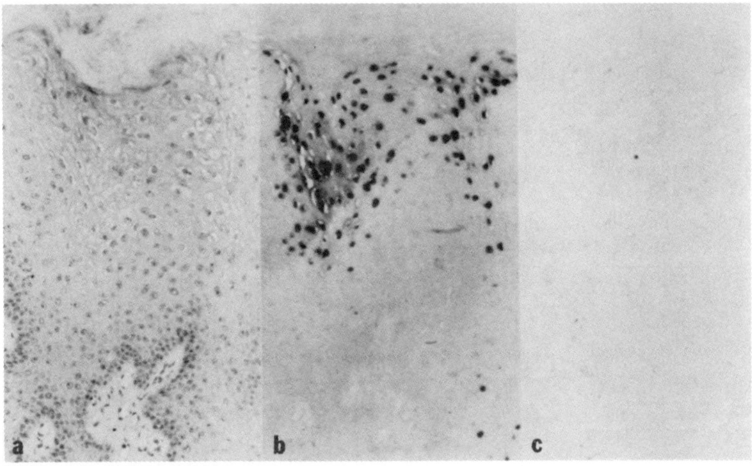


Figure 2. In-situ hybridization of classical condyloma. a) H&E stained section; b) following stringent hybridization with HPV 6/11 probe and c) HPV 16 probe.

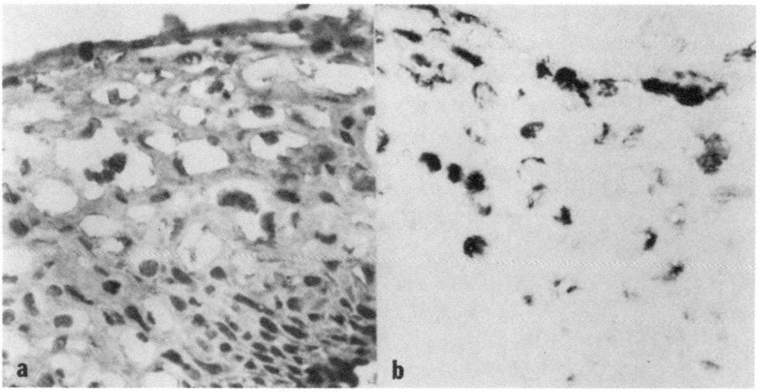


Figure 3. CINK lesion which contained HPV 16 by blot hybridization. a) H&E stained frozen section; b) following in-situ hybridization with HPV 16 probe. There is strong staining in the superficial cells and weak staining in a few cells near the basal layer.

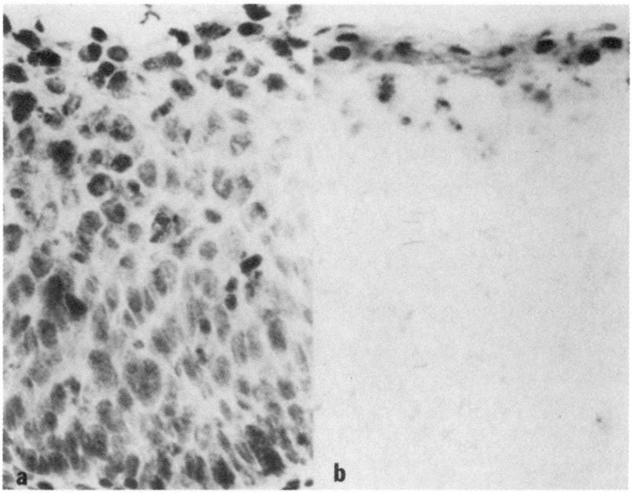


Figure 4. High grade CIN lesion which was positive for HPV 16 by blot hybridization. a) H&E stained frozen section; b) following in-situ hybridization with HPV 16 probe.

Serial sections of all CIN cases which hybridized to HPV 16 probes were analyzed with HPV 6/11 probes under stringent conditions. All were negative. Nine of the ten lesions positive for HPV 16 sequences by in-situ hybridization were positive for HPV 16 by blot hybridization.

## DISCUSSION

This study and others indicate that HPV 16 segregates within a distinct class of precancerous lesions and that the viral sequences are distributed in a pattern which reflects a dependency of viral replication upon maturation, similar to that observed with other HPV´s in warts. THe association of HPV 16 with the histological features of aneuploidy (abnormal mitoses and diffuse nuclear atypia) suggests that this HPV may influence the development of aneuploid lesions, which in turn are at high risk for progressing to invasive carcinoma(7,8,10). Histological criteria can be used to pinpoint these lesions, and may be of further value for identifying other HPV´s which may be associated with neoplasia.

The marked differences between lesions associated with HPV 16 and other HPV´s such as HPV 6 or 11 suggest that the interaction between HPV 16 and the host epithelium is unique, and may include genomic integration of its DNA sequences and/or expression of sequences important for neoplastic change(14). Whatever the mechanism for these changes, it is clear that lesions containing HPV 16 exhibit many features of conventional HPV infections. Lesions containing HPV 16 often contain koilocytosis and nearly half contain focal areas of epithelium indistinguishable from conventional condyloma(15). We have found that most of these lesions contain HPV 16 sequences only, and that the diversity of morphological patterns in one lesion cannot be attributed to multiple HPV strains in most cases(15). This concept is supported further by the data from in-situ hybridization. For example, HPV 16 related sequences were isolated in some lesions within nuclei in areas closely resembling condyloma as well as areas of definite CIN. The distribution of the HPV 16 sequences in CIN correlated closely with the extent of epithelial maturation. Positive nuclei were most prominent in the mid and superficial regions of the epithelium.

The close correlation between maturation and replication of HPV 16 may explain the higher frequency of detection of HPV´s in these lesions. Ninety six percent of CIN lesions containing maturation or koilocytosis were positive by Southern blot hybridization, in contrast to 55% of classical high grade CIN(carcioma in situ), the latter of which are by definition undifferentiated.

A major problem with in-situ hybridization is sensitivity. Several cases were blot positive and ISH-negative, suggesting that many cells may contain HPV sequences which are either not accessible to the probes, or are present in a copy number below the minimum detectible level(ie less than 150 copies per genome) for the biotinylated probes. This may be particularly true in lesions which contain mimimal maturation and a low copy number by Southern blot hybridization. Conversely, it is possible that in-situ hybridization will occasionally detect }ences which are limited to a few cells, and which would be missed by blot hybridization.

It is of interest that despite a close relationship between HPV 16 replication and epithelium maturation, and despite the fact that large amounts of viral DNA are present in some of the mature cells, there is little evidence for production of mature HPV 16 virus. We stained all 21 CIN lesions using antisera to human plantar warts and bovine warts and detected evidence of capsid antigens(late gene expression) in only one case. Whether the lack of detectible structural antigens is related to defective virus, the neoplastic environment, or the production of gene products by HPV 16 which do not cross react with these antisera is unclear.

The close link beteen HPV 16 DNA replication and maturation supports the observation that most of the DNA detected exists in an episomal replicating form(11). Genomic integration of HPV 16 and expression have been documented in cancers(14). The possibility that genomic integration and transcription occur in early precancerous lesions is currently under study.

ACKNOWLEDGMENTS

We gratefully acknowledge the help of Ms. Betsy Nutt and Dr. Daniel Friedman for their technical assistance; Dr. Maria Schevchuk for providing additional case material; and Dr. Harold Ginsberg and Dr. Ralph M. Richart for their support.

REFERENCES

1. Gissman L, de Villiers E-M, zur Hausen H (1982), Analysis of human genital warts (condyloma acuminatum) and other genital tumors for human papillomavirus type 6 DNA. Int J Cancer 29: 143
2. de Villiers E-M, Gissman L, zur Hausen H (1981). Molecular cloning of viral DNA from human genital warts. J Virol 40: 932
3. Gissman L, Wolnik H, Ikenberg H, Koldovsky U, Schnurch HG, zur Hausen H (1983). Human papillomavirus types 6 and 11 DNA sequences in genital and laryngeal papillomas and in some cervical cancers. Proc Natl Acad Sci USA 80: 560
4. Durst M, Gissman L, Ikenberg H, zur Hausen H (1983). A papillomavirus DNA from a cervical carcinoma and its prevalence in cancer biopsy samples from different geographic regions. Proc Natl Acad Sci USA 80: 3812
5. Boshart M, Gissman L, Ikenberg H, Kleinheinz A, Scheurlen W, zur Hausen H (1984). A new type of papillomavirus DNA, its presence in genital cancer biopsies and in cell lines derived from cervical cancer. EMBO J 3: 1151
6. Crum CP, Ikenberg H, Richart RM, Gissman L (1984). Human papillomavirus type 16 and early cervical neoplasia, New Engl J Med 310: 880
7. Crum CP, Fu YS, Levine RU, Richart RM, Townsend DE, Fenoglio CM (1982). Intraepithelial squamous lesions of the vulva: biologic and histologic criteria for the distinction of condylomas from vulvar intraepithelial neoplasia. Am J Obstet Gynecol 144: 77
8. Winkler B, Crum CP, Fujii T, Ferenczy A, Boon M, Braun L, Lancaster WD, Richart RM (1984). Koilocytotic lesions of the cervix: the relationship of mitotic abnormalities to nuclear DNA content. Cancer 53: 1081
9. Richart RM (1973). Cervical intraepithelial neoplasia. In Sommers, SC(ed); "Pathology Annual." New York, Appleton Century Crofts, p 301
10. Fu YS, Regan J, Richart RM (1981). Definition of precursors. Gynecol Oncol 12: s220
11. Crum CP, Mitao M, Levine RU, Silverstein S (1985). Cervical papillomaviruses segregate within morphologically distinct precancerous lesions. J Virol (in press)
12. Southern EM (1975). Detection of specific sequences among DNA fragments separated by gel electrophoresis. J Mol Biol 98: 503

13. Myerson D, Hackman RC, Nelson JA, Ward DC, McDougall JK (1984). Widespread presence of histologically occult cytomegalovirus. Human Pathol 15: 430
14. Schwarz E, Freese UK, Gissman L, Mayer W, Roggenbuck B, Stremlau A, zur Hausen H (1985). Structure and transcription of human papillomavirus sequences in cervical carcinoma cells. Nature 314: 111
15. Mitao M, Nagai N, Levine RU, Silverstein S, Crum CP (1985). Human papillomavirus type 16 infection of the cervix: a morphological spectrum with evidence of late gene expression. Obstet Gynecol (submitted).

**Papillomaviruses: Molecular and Clinical Aspects, pages 31–45**


# NATURAL HISTORY OF HPV INFECTIONS IN UTERINE CERVIX AS DETERMINED BY PROSPECTIVE FOLLOW-UP[1]

Kari Syrjänen,[2] M. Väyrynen, R. Mäntyjärvi, S. Parkkinen, S. Saarikoski, S. Syrjänen and O. Castrén

Department of Pathology, Gynecology & Obstetrics, and Clinical Microbiology, University of Kuopio, POB 6, SF-70211 Kuopio, Finland

ABSTRACT To assess the natural history of cervical HPV lesions, i.e. flat, inverted and papillomatous condylomas, a long-term prospective follow-up study was started in October 1981. At this writing, a total of 343 women have been followed-up for a mean of 18±15 (M ± SD) months, either by cervical punch biopsy or Papanicolaou (PAP) smears, repeated at 6-month intervals. On each attendance at the Clinic, the patient is subjected to colposcopy accompanied by cervical swabs ( for isolation of Chlamydia trachomatis ), and by blood samples for viral ( HPV, HSV, CMV ) serology. PAP smears and punch biopsies are analysed for the cytopathic changes of HPV, and for concomitant CIN, and the biopsies also for HPV particles on TEM, for HPV structural proteins with IP-PAP technique and for the local immune reactivity using monoclonal antibodies (McAb) to define T cell subsets, NK ( natural killer ) cells and Langerhans cells. HPV typing was accomplished by DNA probes for HPV 6, 11, 16 and 18. All patients are requested for their sexual habits by a detailed questionnaire. Serological (CF-test) evidence was found for the coexistent HSV infection in 10% of the females during the

[1]This work was supported by Research Grants from the Medical Research Council of the Academy of Finland and from the Finnish Cancer Society
[2]Present address: Laboratory of Pathology & Cancer Research, Finnish Cancer Society, POB 25, SF-70200 Kuopio, Finland

follow-up. Chlamydial cervicitis was detectable in 10.4% of the patients. In HPV patients, the questionnaires disclosed the same risk factors ( i.e. early onset of sexual activity, poor hygiene, and multiple partnerships ) as shown to be associated with the development of cervical cancer, thus emphasizing the STD nature of these two diseases. Only minor fluctuations in the relative levels of NK (HNK-1$^+$) cells and Langerhans (OKT-6$^+$) cells were observed between the different types of HPV lesions, between various grades of HPV-CIN, and related to their different natural history. The same was true with the T helper/ T suppressor cell ratio, being lowest (0.93) in progressed lesions and highest (1.07) in the regressed ones. HPV particles were discovered on TEM with equal frequency in all types of lesions, including the regressed ones. On DNA hybridization, HPV 6 was found in 8%, HPV 11 in 33%, HPV 16 in 10% and HPV 18 in 8% of the 49 lesions typed for HPV DNA so far. During the follow-up, 86/343 (25.1%) of the HPV lesions regressed (RE), 209 (60.9%) remained persistent (PE), and 48 (14.0%) progressed (PR), 14 (4.1%) having been coned due to progression into CIS. The clinical course was most powerfully influenced by the grade of HPV-associated CIN, to which RE was inversely and PR directly related. The results unequivocally confirm that cervical HPV infections being capable of progressing into CIS present with the natural history quite comparable to that of classical CIN. Therefore, cervical HPV infections should be regarded as truly precancerous lesions, and they should be examined, treated and followed-up with the same concern as the classical CIN.

## INTRODUCTION

Recent data on Human papillomaviruses (HPV) strongly suggest an intimate association of certain HPV types ( HPV 6, 10, 11, 16 and 18 ) with cervical intraepithelial neoplasia (CIN) and with frankly invasive cervical carcinomas as well ( 1-7 ). Evidence has been provided by the reports on frequent association of HPV lesions ( flat, inverted and papillomatous condylomas ) with CIN in punch biopsy ( 3-7 ), as well as by epidemiological studies showing the same risk factors for HPV infection and cervical cancer, both being currently regarded as sexually transmitted diseases (STD) ( 8 ). Furthermore, HPV structural proteins ( HPV antigens ) have been repeatedly demonstrated by IP-PAP technique in a substantial percentage of CIN biopsies ( 4,5,9 ). Finally, HPV 16 and 18 DNA sequences were recently discovered in the CIN lesions and in invasive cervical carcinomas, sometimes integrated in the host cell genome by DNA-hybridization technique ( 1,2 ).

Despite the circumstantial evidence, the final proof of HPV as an etiological agent of cervical cancer still remains to be established ( 5,7 ), especially because of the lack of data on the natural history of cervical HPV infections. Study on this line has been neglected so far, although the natural history of the classical CIN has been well characterized by a number of carefully conducted follow-up studies ( 10-15 ). Accordingly, CIN lesions may progress to CIS and eventually to an invasive carcinoma ( 11,15 ). Observations on a short-term follow-up of a limited number of cervical HPV lesions as well as retrospective analysis of an extensive series of such cases suggest similarities in their behaviour to that of classical CIN ( 9,16,17 ). To elucidate the natural history of cervical HPV infections, a prospective follow-up study of these women has been conducted in our Clinic since October 1981 ( 16,18 ).

One of the major aims of the current follow-up study is to analyse the factors possibly modifying the clinical course of the disease, including the immune reaction in situ in the HPV-lesions. Indeed, both humoral and cell-mediated immunity have been amply demonstrated against a variety of HPV infections ( 20,23 ). It is agreed that skin warts frequently disappear spontaneously, the regressing lesions showing an intense immunocompetent cell (ICC) infiltration ( 20,22 ). In cervical HPV lesions, some preliminary analyses of the in situ ICC infiltrates have been published quite lately ( 16,24,25,26 ). In such infiltrates, OKT-8$^+$ T cells seemed to outnumber the OKT-4$^+$ T cells ( 16,25 ). The large granular lymphocytes (LGL), shown to possess the NK (natural killer cell) function, were recently shown to bear surface determinants definable by the monoclonal antibody HNK-1 ( Leu-7 ) ( 29 ). So far, no data are available on NK cells in cervical HPV lesions, albeit these cells are thought to be involved in surveillance of malignant tumors and viral diseases ( 27 ), including those due to Herpes simplex virus (HSV) ( 28 ).

Similarly, practically no data concerning the cervix are available on Langerhans ( OKT-6+ ) cells, the important role of which was recently emphasized as antigen presenting cells, (APC) in the in situ immunological reactions of the skin ( 25, 30 ).

The natural cycle of HPV in the target cell (keratinocyte) is far from being clarified ( 5,32 ). It is well established by animal experiments that viral particles disappear in the squamous cells upon malignant transformation ( 5,7,32 ). Only a limited number of studies at ultrastructural level have been done to clarify this issue in cervical HPV lesions, however ( 33-35 ). So far, no attempts have been made to correlate the presence of HPV particles with the data relevant to the behaviour of these lesions, i.e. with the lesion type, severity of HPV-associated CIN, or with the presence of HPV structural proteins ( 5,16,18 ).

The present communication based on data from 343 women prospectively followed-up for cervical HPV-infections summarizes the current findings on the phenotypic characterization ( with monoclonal antibodies Leu-10, OKT3, OKT4, OKT6, OKT8 and HNK-1 ) of the in situ ICCs, on TEM, and on HPV typing by DNA hybridization, pertinent to the natural history of this disease.

## METHODS

The present series consists of 343 consecutive women currently included in a prospective follow-up study conducted for cervical HPV lesions since 1981. The women are invited to participate in the follow-up whenever HPV-induced cytopathic changes are found in their routine cervical Papanicolaou smears, ( 3-6,9 ). All the patients are examined at the Outpatient Department of Gynaecology and Obstetrics, Kuopio University Central Hospital, Kuopio, Finland, at 6-month intervals, as detailed recently ( 14,29 ). At each attendance, the patient is subjected to careful gynaecological examination including colposcopy and PAP smears with or without directed punch biopsy. This depends on whether or not the patient presents with cytological changes consistent with CIN ( 8,16 ). The lesions are eradicated by conization, whenever progression to carcinoma in situ ( CIS ) had been established. The details of the study outline and the techniques used have been given in previous papers ( 8,16,18,29 ), to which the reader is referred.

In HE-stained sections, each lesion is classified into one of three categories: flat, inverted or papillomatous condyloma ( 3-6,9 ). The grade of CIN is assessed using commonly accepted criteria for CIN I, II and III ( 12,15 ).

HPV structural proteins ( viral antigens ) are demonstrated in paraffin sections using a commercially available immunoperoxidase (IP-PAP) kit with the primary antiserum raised against the PV genus specific capsid antigens ( DAKOPATTS ) ( 4,5 ).

Antibody titres to HSV (HSV 1 and 2) and CMV are determined using the Complement-fixation (CF) tests in routine use for this purpose. At each visit, a cervical swab is taken for isolation of Chlamydia, using the standard culture system in McCoy cells grown in MEM.

Cryostat sections are stained for the ICC phenotypes using monoclonal antibodies and the avidin-biotin peroxidase complex (ABC) technique, as detailed previously ( 16 ). Following monoclonal antibodies are used; Leu-10 known to define B lymphocytes, OKT-3 known to react with all peripheral T lymphocytes, OKT-4 for T inducer/helper cells, and OKT-8 for T suppressor/cytotoxic cells ( 37 ), HNK-1 ( Leu-7 ) to define the NK cells ( 29 ), and OKT-6 for Langerhans cells ( 31 ).

The samples of biopsy-derived DNA ( each 2-3 ug ) are digested with Bam H1 enzyme and the Southern blots are each hybridized under stringent conditions with $^{32}$P-labelled HPV 6, 11, 16 and HPV 18 DNA, according to the standard DNA-hybridization technique. ( 1,2,38,40 ).

The clinical course of the HPV lesions is classified as either regressed (RE), persistent (PE), or progressed (PR) ( 8,16 ), depending on presence or absence of the cytopathic changes of HPV in PAP smear or in biopsy.

## RESULTS

Table 1 shows the percentages of the lymphocyte subsets related to the clinical course of the HPV lesions. The relative levels of OKT-8$^+$ T cells are elevated in progressed lesions, being responsible for the lowest OKT-4$^+$/OKT-8$^+$ ratio in these HPV lesions.

Table 2 gives the relation between the proportions of HNK-1$^+$ cells and the clinical course of the HPV lesions. The HPV lesion was shown regressed in 47 ( 28.8% ) of these females, persistent in 85 ( 52.1% ) cases, and progressed in 31 ( 19.1% ). The percentage of HNK-1$^+$ cells was highest in regressed lesions, and practically equal in persistent and progressed ones.

TABLE 1
LYMPHOCYTE SUBSETS AND CLINICAL COURSE

| Clinical course | No. of Cases | Lymphocyte subsets ( Mean % ) Leu-10 | OKT-3 | OKT-4 | OKT-8 | OKT-4/OKT-8 |
|---|---|---|---|---|---|---|
| Regressed | 47 | 55.6 | 21.1 | 8.5 | 9.2 | 1.07 |
| Persistent | 85 | 52.5 | 20.1 | 9.1 | 11.0 | 1.04 |
| Progressed | 31 | 52.5 | 21.2 | 8.9 | 11.2 | 0.93 |

TABLE 2
NK CELLS AND CLINICAL COURSE

| Order of biopsy | No. of biopsy | HNK-1$^+$ Cells ( Mean % ) Regressed | Persistent | Progressed |
|---|---|---|---|---|
| First | 163 | 2.5 | 1.7 | 1.8 |
| Second | 69 | 1.4 | 1.4 | 1.8 |
| Third | 27 | 1.6 | 2.5 | 2.5 |

Table 3 shows the levels of Langerhans cells in HPV lesions with different clinical course. The numbers of RE, PE and PR lesions are those given in Table 1. The levels of OKT-6$^+$ cells in the first biopsies of RE, PE and PR lesions are identical, and remained so also in the second biopsies. The relative levels of Langerhans cells do not seem to bear any direct correlation to the clinical course of the HPV lesions.

TABLE 3
LANGERHANS CELLS AND CLINICAL COURSE

| Order of biopsy | No.of biopsy | $OKT\text{-}6^{+}$ Langerhans cells ( Mean % ) Regressed | Persistent | Progressed |
|---|---|---|---|---|
| First | 163 | 1.6 | 1.7 | 1.7 |
| Second | 69 | 1.9 | 2.2 | 2.0 |
| Third | 27 | 1.3 | 1.5 | 2.9 |

TABLE 4
CLINICAL COURSE OF HPV LESIONS RELATED TO CIN

| Degree of HPV-CIN | No.of Cases | Regressed No. | Regressed % | Persistent No. | Persistent % | Progressed No. | Progressed % |
|---|---|---|---|---|---|---|---|
| HPV-NCIN | 149 | 39 | 26.2 | 92 | 61.7 | 18 | 12.1 |
| HPV-CIN I | 56 | 10 | 17.9 | 33 | 58.9 | 13 | 23.2 |
| HPV-CIN II | 31 | 4 | 12.9 | 24 | 77.4 | 3 | 9.7 |
| HPV-CIN III | 25 | 3 | 12.0 | 10 | 40.0 | 12 | 48.0 |
| Biopsy-series | 261 | 56 | 21.5 | 159 | 60.9 | 46 | 17.6 |
| Smear-series | 82 | 30 | 36.6 | 50 | 61.0 | 2 | 2.4 |
| Total series | 343 | 86 | 25.1 | 209 | 60.9 | 48 | 14.0 |

Table 4 summarizes the current follow-up results of the patients. As shown, a total of 261 patients have been followed up by biopsy, and 82 by PAP smear alone. The clinical course in these two series is different with regard to regression ( $p<0.05$ ) and progression ( $p<0.01$ ). The rate of regression was inversely related to the degree of HPV-associated CIN.

During the follow-up period, both increases and decreases in HSV titres were recorded, as summarized in Table 5. In a total of 21/216 women ( 9.7% ), the conversion in HSV titre was fourfold or greater.

TABLE 5
CONVERSION OF HSV TITRES DURING THE FOLLOW-UP

| Sample | No. of samples | Titre unchanged No. | Per cent | Change 4-fold or more No. | Per cent |
|---|---|---|---|---|---|
| I/II | 216/141 | 75 | 53.2 | 12 | 8.6 |
| II/III | 141/71 | 30 | 42.3 | 5 | 7.0 |
| III/IV | 71/24 | 10 | 41.7 | 4 | 16.7 |
| Total | 428/236 | 115 | 48.7 | 21 | 9.7 |

TABLE 6
HPV PARTICLES ON ELECTRON MICROSCOPY

| Type of HPV lesion | No. of cases | HPV particles discovered No. | Per cent |
|---|---|---|---|
| Flat | 74 | 46 | 62.1 |
| Inverted | 5 | 4 | 80.0 |
| Papillomatous | 1 | 1 | 100.0 |
| Lesion regressed | 22 | 14 | 63.6 |

Table 6 summarizes the detection rate of HPV particles on TEM. Viral particles are found in all three types of HPV lesions with an approximately equal frequency. Noteworthy is that also in 63.6% of the biopsies not containing an HPV lesion on light microscopy, i.e. in those regressed during the follow-up, viral particles can be found on TEM.

The results of HPV typing in the first 49 lesions by DNA hybridization as well as the HPV type changes during the follow-up are summarized in Table 7. A total of 29/49 (59%) of the lesions contained at least one HPV type, and in three of the patients, HPV type had changed from one to another in two subsequent biopsies.

TABLE 7
HPV TYPES AND THE FOLLOW-UP

| HPV type in second biopsy | HPV type in the first biopsy Negative | HPV 6 | HPV 11 | HPV 16 | HPV 18 |
|---|---|---|---|---|---|
| Negative | 2 | | 2 | | |
| HPV 6 | | | | | |
| HPV 11 | | | 2 | | |
| HPV 16 | | | 1 | 1 | |
| HPV 18 | 1 | | 1 | 1 | |
| Total series | 20/49(41%) | 4(8%) | 16(33%) | 5(10%) | 4(8%) |

DISCUSSION

In the prospective follow-up studies conducted so far for the classical CIN lesions, variable figures for regression, persistence and progression have been reported ( 10-15 ). As recently emphasized ( 11 ), in a follow-up of 894 females with CIN II from 50 to 78 months, the regression was 54%, persistence 16%, and progression 30%. Koss et al ( 15 ) followed-up women with CIN I and CIN II lesions for from seven months to ten years, and reported a 39% rate of RE, 46% PR, and 15% of PE. Figures of the same order of magnitude are to be found in a number of other reports ( 12,13,14 ). Thus, it is clear that CIN lesions are truly neoplastic in nature, as evidenced by the fact that they are potentially progressive to CIS and to invasive cancer if left untreated for a variable period of time ( 10-15 ). During the present average follow-up period of 18.7 months, 25% of the cervical HPV lesions regressed, 61% persisted, and 14% progressed into a more severe degree of HPV-CIN ( Table 4 ). This is in complete agreement with the data reported in a recent retrospective follow-up of 764 cervical HPV lesions for 18 months; 26.8% regressed, 52.9% persisted, and 20.3% progressed ( 9 ). Furthermore, the regression rate was shown to be inversely and the progression directly related to the degree of HPV-CIN, in both studies. Thus, these data substantiate the concept that HPV lesions in the uterine cervix behave clinically as do the classical CIN lesions ( 9,17 ). The only significant difference between the two is that the HPV lesions commonly occur in women more than 10 years younger than those presented with classical CIN ( 3-6,9,10,11,15 ). This has been interepreted to suggest that HPV infection accelerates the development of CIN in those women ( 5 ).

According to SALT/MALT concept ( 30 ), the local immune mechanisms are likely to resist and modify the course of HPV infections. Practically no data are available on the in situ immunological reactions in cervical HPV lesions, albeit a certain percentage of them seems to regress even within a short period of follow-up ( 8 ). Of the 163 lesions with the first biopsy available for immunophenotyping, 47 (28.8%) regressed, 85 (52.1%) persisted, and 31 (19.1%) progressed during the subsequent follow-up. Only minor fluctuations of the ICC levels were found in lesions with different clinical course ( Table 1 ). There seems to be, however, a relative increase in OKT-8$^+$ cells in regressed lesions. Thus, it seems that the shift in local immunoregulatory cell balance into favor of OKT-8$^+$ T cells might be associated with clinical progression of the lesions. This lowered OKT-4$^+$/OKT-8$^+$ ratio most probably is due to an increase of T suppressor cells inappropriately to the number of T helper cells. Until the means are available to distinguish between T suppressor and T cytotoxic cells ( both OKT-8$^+$ ), this interpretation is to be made with certain provisions, however.

In all types of HPV lesions, the local infiltrates proved to contain HNK-1$^+$ cells, i.e. LGLs with either a granular or a membrane staining with the HNK-1 antibody ( 29 ). There seems to be no statistically significant differences in the relative NK cell levels in the HPV lesions with different clinical course, however ( Table 2 ). Thus, the present study does not provide any evidence to support the concept that local NK cell function alone would significantly contribute to the clinical behaviour of cervical HPV lesions. The same seems to hold true with the relative levels of in situ OKT-6$^+$ Langerhans cells as well ( Table 3 ). Thus, it seems probable that the clinical course of cervical HPV lesions is not being conditioned by an increase or decrease of any single ICC type activity inappropriately to that of other cell types. This is in full agreement with the SALT/MALT concept, emphasizing the importance of a dynamic balance between the immunoregulatory cells for the mounting a proper immune response ( 30 ).

Recent data based on experimental evidence suggest a possible synergistic actions between HSV and HPV ( 36 ). Accordingly, HSV could act as an initiator and HPV as a promotor in cervical carcinogenesis ( 36 ). To gain clinical support to this hypothesis, HSV antibody levels are determined and also Chlamydia isolation performed in our follow-up patients. Evidence was obtained that some 10% of these women might have experienced a recent HSV infection ( Table 5 ). Similarly, Chlamydia cervicitis was detected in 10.4% of these patients by cultivation ( data not shown ). It will be of interest to find out, whether such double infections in the genital tract eventually influence the natural history of cervical HPV lesions.

In the ultrastructural studies reported so far, the detection rate of HPV particles has varied from 20% to 100% either in biopsies or in PAP smears ( 33,34,35 ). In the present series, some minor fluctuation was found in the detection rate of HPV particles in different types of lesions ( Table 6 ). Of special interest to understanding the biology of HPV infections is the discovery of HPV particles in 63.6% of the punch biopsies devoid of an HPV lesion on light microscopy ( Table 6 ). These biopsies represent the HPV lesions regressed during the follow-up period, and the presence of HPV particles in such biopsies is a strong argument in favor of the concept that HPV can persist in the squamous epithelium as a latent form ( 5 ). After a dormant period, the virus might be activated by some yet unknown factors, leading to either a permissive or a non-permissive infection ( or both ) ( 5 ). Such a future activation ( appearance of new HPV lesions ) of a currently latent infection remains to be shown by the continuous prospective follow-up.

The DNA hybridization disclosed four distinct HPV types in the present lesions ( HPV 6, 11, 16 and HPV 18 ). The latter two have been reported so far preferentially in cervical carcinomas ( 1,39,40 ), in contrast to HPV 6, 10 and 11, which are almost exclusively confined to benign genital warts. Since the most recent evidence suggests that HPV 16 and HPV 18 DNA can exist in integrated state in cervical cancer cells, an etiological relationship between HPV infection and the subsequent malignant conversion appears to gain increasing probability ( 1,5,7,38-40 ). This concept is strongly substantiated by the observations of the present study, where cervical HPV lesions are shown to possess a potential to progress into CIS. The present findings reveal moreover that simultaneous infections, even with two of the high risk HPV types (1) may occur simultaneously in an individual HPV lesion (data not shown). Of special interest are the present tentative data ( not reported before ) on the possibility of HPV type change during the infection ( Table 7 ). This further emphasizes the clinical importance of HPV typing by DNA hybridization in cervical HPV lesions, because according to current understanding, the virus type seems to be one of the most important factors to determine whether the lesion is prone to develop malignancy or not ( 1,2,38-40 ). Whether this concept on low risk ( HPV 6,10,11 ) and high risk ( HPV 16 and 18 ) HPV types holds true more generally, remains to be established by the further DNA hybridization experiments of our prospectively collected cervical biopsy material.

## ACKNOWLEDGMENTS

The skillful technical assistance of Mrs. Heli Eskelinen and Miss Ritva Savolainen is gratefully acknowledged.

## REFERENCES

1. Dürst M, Gissmann L, Ikenberg H, zur Hausen H ( 1983 ). A papillomavirus DNA from a cervical carcinoma and its prevalence in cancer biopsy samples from different geographic regions. Proc Natl Acad Sci USA 80: 3812.
2. Gissmann L, Wolnik L, Ikenberg H, Koldovsky U, Schnürch HG, zur Hausen H (1983). Human papillomavirus types 6 and 11 DNA sequences in genital and laryngeal papillomas and in some cervical cancers. Proc Natl Acad Sci USA 80: 560.
3. Syrjänen KJ (1979). Morphologic survey of the condylomatous lesions in dysplastic and neoplastic epithelium of the uterine cervix. Arch Gynaecol 227: 153.
4. Syrjänen KJ (1983). Human papillomavirus ( HPV ) lesions in association with cervical dysplasias and neoplasias. Obstet Gynecol 62: 617.
5. Syrjänen KJ (1984). Current concepts on Human papillomavirus (HPV) infections in the genital tract and their relationship to intraepithelial neoplasia

and squamous cell carcinoma. Obstet Gynecol Surv 39: 252.

6. Syrjänen KJ, Heinonen U-M, Kauraniemi T, (1981). Cytological evidence of the association of condylomatous lesions with the dysplastic and neoplastic changes in uterine cervix. Acta Cytol 25: 17.
7. zur Hausen H (1977). Human papillomaviruses and their possible role in squamous cell carcinomas. Curr Top Microbiol Immunol 78: 1.
8. Syrjänen K, Väyrynen M, Castrén O, Yliskoski M, Mäntyjärvi R, Pyrhönen S, Saarikoski S (1984). Sexual behaviour of the females with Human papillomavirus ( HPV ) lesions in the uterine cervix. Brit J Vener Dis 60: 243.
9. de Brux J, Orth G, Croissant O, Cochard B, Ionesco M (1983). Lesions condylomateuses du col uterin: evolution chez 2466 patientes. Bull Cancer 70:410.
10. Nasiell K, Auer G, Nasiell M, Zetterberg A (1979). Retrospective DNA analyses in cervical dysplasia as related to neoplastic progression or regression. Anal Quant Cytol 1: 103.
11. Nasiell K, Nasiell M, Vaclavinkova V (1983). Behavior of moderate cervical dysplasia during long-term follow-up. Obstet Gynecol 61: 609.
12. Richart RM Barron BA (1969). A follow-up study of patients with cervical dysplasia. Am J Obstet Gynec 105: 386.
13. Spriggs AI (1981). Natural history of cervical dysplasia. Clin Obstet Gynaecol 8: 65.
14. Starreveld AA, Romanowski B, Hill GB, Koch M, Pearce KI (1983). The latency period of carcinoma-in-situ of the cervix. Obstet Gynecol 62: 348.
15. Koss LG, Stewart FW, Foote FW, Jordan MJ, Bader GM, Day E (1963). Some histological aspects of behavior of epidermoid carcinoma in situ and related lesions of the uterine cervix. A long-term prospective study. Cancer 9: 1160.
16. Syrjänen K, Väyrynen M, Castrén O, Mäntyjärvi R, Yliskoski M (1984). The relation between the type of immunoreactive cells found in Human papillomavirus (HPV) lesions of the uterine cervix and the subsequent behaviour of these lesions. Arch Gynecol 234: 189.
17. Walker PG, Singer A, Dyson JL, Oriel JD (1983). Natural history of cervical epithelial abnormalities

in patients with vulvar warts. Brit J Vener Dis 59: 327.

18. Väyrynen M, Syrjänen K, Castrén O, Saarikoski S, Mäntyjärvi R (1985). Colposcopic findings in women followed-up for Human papillomavirus (HPV) lesions of the uterine cervix. Obstet Gynecol In press.
19. De Palo G, Stefanon D (1983). Colposcopic patterns of condylomatous lesions of the uterine cervix. Cervix & l.f.g.t. 1:17.
20. Jablonska S, Orth G, Lutzner MA (1982). Immunopathology of Papillomavirus-induced tumors in different tissues. Springer Semin Immunopathol 5: 33.
21. Kossard S, Xenias SJ, Palestine RF, Scheen SR, Winkelmann RK (1980). Inflammatory changes in verruca vulgaris. J Cutan Pathol 7: 217.
22. Tagami H, Oguchi M, Ofuji S (1980). The phenomenon of spontaneous regression of numerous flat warts: Immunohistological studies. Cancer 45: 2557.
23. Kienzler JL, Lemoine MTH, Orth G, Jibard N, Blanc D, Laurent R, Agache P (1983). Humoral and cell-mediated immunity to human papillomavirus type 1 ( HPV-1 ) in human warts. Br J Dermatol 108: 665.
24. Chardonnet Y, Beauve P, Viac J, Schmitt D (1983). T cell subsets and Langerhans cells in wart lesions. Immunol Lett 6: 191.
25. Morris HHB, Gatter KC, Sykes G, Casemore V, Mason DY (1983). Langerhans cells in human cervical epithelium: effects of wart virus infection and intraepithelial neoplasia. Br J Obstet Gynecol 90: 412.
26. Syrjänen KJ (1983). Immunocompetent cells in uterine cervical lesions of Human papillomavirus origin. Gynecol Obstet Invest 16: 327.
27. Herberman RB, Holden HT (1979). Natural cell-mediated immunity. Adv Cancer Res 27: 305.
28. Rola-Pleszczynski M, Lieu H (1984). Natural killer cell activity linked to time of recurrence of herpes labialis. Clin exp Immunol 55: 224.
29. Abo T Balch CM (1981). A differentiation antigen of human NK and K cells identified by a monoclonal antibody (HNK-1). J Immunol 127: 1024.
30. Streilein JW (1983). Skin-associated lymphoid tissue (SALT): origins and functions. Invest Dermatol 80: 012S.
31. Murphy E, Bhan AK, Sato S, Mihm MC, Harrist TC (1981). A new immunologic marker for human Langerhans'

cells. N Engl J Med 304: 791.

32. Fletcher S, Norval M (1983). On the nature of the deep cellular disturbances in human-papilloma-virus infection of the squamous cervical epithelium. Lancet ii: 546.
33. Casas-Cordero M, Morin C, Roy M, Fortier M, Meisels A (1981). Origin of the koilocyte in condylomata of the human cervix. Ultrastructural study. Acta Cytol 25: 383.
34. Della Torre G, Pilotti S, de Palo G Rilke F (1978). Viral particles in cervical condylomatous lesions. Tumori 64: 549.
35. Roy M, Morin C, Casas-Cordero M, Meisels A (1983). Human papillomavirus and cervical lesions. Clin Obstet Gynecol 26: 949.
36. zur Hausen H (1982). Human genital cancer: Synergism between two virus infections or synergism between a virus infection and initiating events? Lancet ii:1370.
37. Kung PC, Goldstein G, Reinherz EL, Schlossman SF (1979). Monoclonal antibodies defining distinctive human T-cell surface antigens. Science 206: 347.
38. Gissmann L, Diehl V, Schultz-Coulon HJ, zur Hausen H Molecular cloning and characterization of human papillomavirus DNA derived from a laryngeal papilloma. J Virol 1982; 44: 393-400.
39. zur Hausen H, Gissmann L, Schlehofer JR (1984). Viruses in the etiology of human genital cancer. Prog med Virol 30: 170.
40. Bochart M, Gissmann L, Ikenberg H, Kleinheinz A, Scheurlen W, zur Hausen H (1984). A new type of papillomavirus DNA, its presence in genital cancer biopsies and in cell lines derived from cervical cancer. EMBO J 3: 1151.

**Papillomaviruses: Molecular and Clinical Aspects, pages 47–56**


# PRESENCE OF PAPILLOMAVIRUS DNA SEQUENCES, AMPLIFICATION OF c-myc AND c-Ha-ras ONCOGENES AND ENHANCED EXPRESSION OF c-myc IN CARCINOMAS OF THE UTERINE CERVIX

G.F. Riou, M. Barrois, V. Dutronquay*, and G. Orth*

Laboratoire de Pharmacologie Clinique et Moleculaire
Institut Gustave Roussy, 94800 Villejuif and
* Unité des Papillomavirus (INSERM U 190)
Institut Pasteur, 75015 Paris (France)

ABSTRACT Invasive squamous cell carcinomas of the uterine cervix from 37 untreated patients were examined for the presence of human papillomavirus (HPV) genomes and for the state of the oncogenes c-myc and c-Ha-ras. The presence of HPV DNA sequences was demonstrated in 33 out of 37 tumors. HPV16 genomes at a high copy number were found in 16 tumors and HPV18 in only one. Integrated HPV16 DNA sequences at a low copy number, or additional as yet uncharacterized HPV types were detected in other tumors. A 3 to 30 fold amplification of c-myc (20/37) and of c-Ha-ras (14/35) was observed in tumors corresponding to advanced stages of the disease (stages 2, 3 and 4). A concomitant amplification of both oncogenes was found in 13 cancers. The c-myc or c-Ha-ras oncogenes were weakly amplified in only 4 of the 11 tumors restricted to the uterine cervix (stage 1). Neither HPV DNA sequences, nor oncogene amplification were detected in the lymphocytes of 12 patients. Furthermore, a high level of c-myc RNA was found in 11/11 tumors corresponding to stages 2, 3 and 4, while only in 1 out of 4 tumors of stage 1. Six of the advanced stage tumors showed enhanced transcription in the absence of detectable gene amplification. Thus, it seems likely that specific HPV types play a role in the development of cervical carcinomas and that activated cellular oncogenes are involved at least in some steps of tumor progression.

## INTRODUCTION

Uterine cervix carcinoma is one of the most frequent cancer in woman. This cancer involves a multistep process, where lesions of cervical intraepithelial neoplasia are the precursors of invasive carcinomas [1]. The cervical carcinoma thus is a good model to analyze the factors and mechanisms involved in human carcinogenesis. Epidemiological studies have suggested that an infectious agent, sexually transmitted, could be a risk factor for the development of cervical carcinomas [2]. It seems now likely that certain human papillomavirus (HPV) types constitute this risk factor [1, 3-6]. The genomes of HPV16 and HPV18 have been detected with a high frequency in cervical carcinomas. The precursor lesions could be flat condylomas associated with HPV16 and showing abnormal mitotic figures [1].

The mechanisms of progression of intraepithelial neoplasia into invasive carcinoma are as yet unknown. Among other hypothesis, it may be assumed that this progression involves a cooperation between viral genes and cellular oncogenes possibly activated by mutation, amplification, or gene rearrangement [6-11].

The data presented in this paper confirm the association of cervical carcinomas with specific HPVs, in particular HPV16. They show that the amplification of c-*myc* and c-Ha-*ras* oncogenes and the over-expression of c-*myc* gene characterize the most advanced tumors.

## METHODS

*DNA and RNA preparations*. Biopsies of squamous cell carcinomas at different clinical stages were obtained from 37 French or African patients and stored in liquid nitrogen. The lymphocytes of 12 of these patients were fractionated in a Ficoll Hypaque gradient. High molecular weight DNAs were prepared [6] from tumors, lymphocytes, human placenta, as well as from EJ and N417 cell lines originating from human bladder [12] and small cell lung [13] carcinomas, respectively. The DNA concentrations were evaluated by fluorometric assay [6]. Whenever the amount of tumor specimen available was sufficient, total RNA was also prepared [14].

*Analysis of oncogenes*. The DNA preparations were treated with *Eco* RI endonuclease or with a mixture of *Hpa*

II and Msp I enzymes and the DNA fragments were fractionated by agarose slab gel electrophoresis and analyzed by Southern blot hybridization [6, 14]. Probes were prepared from pBR322 plasmids containing the Eco RI-Cla I fragment (third exon) of the human c-myc oncogene (O. Brison et al., in preparation) and from pSV2-neo plasmids containing the 6.6 kb Bam HI fragment of the c-Ha-ras oncogene from EJ cells [12]. The probes were labeled by nick-translation with $^{32}$P dCTP (specific activity $3.5 \times 10^{8}$ cpm/µg). The hybridizations were performed under stringent conditions [6]. The blots were exposed to Kodak XAR5 or Fuji RX films. The copy number of the oncogenes was evaluated by scanning the autoradiograms with the laser microdensitometer Ultroscan (LKB) and compared with varying concentrations of DNA from N417 cells (47 copies of c-myc/cell) [13] and from EJ cells (1 copy of c-Ha-ras/cell) [12].

Analysis of the c-myc gene expression. The expression of the c-myc oncogene was analyzed by Northern blot and dot blot hybridization of total RNA [14] from neoplastic tissues, from the placenta of one patient, and from N417 cells which contain a high level of c-myc RNA [13]. After hybridization with the $^{32}$P-labeled c-myc probe, the radioactivity of the dot blots was evaluated by counting in a scintillation spectrometer.

Detection of HPV DNA sequences. Tumor and lymphocyte DNAs were treated with Bam HI or Pst I endonucleases, then analyzed by Southern blot hybridization [6]. Viral DNAs, purified from recombinant plasmids containing HPV6a, HPV11a, HPV16 or HPV18 genomes, were used to prepare $^{32}$P-labeled probes. The DNAs were hybridized under stringent conditions (1 M NaCl, 50 % formamide, 42°C) with HPV16 DNA or HPV18 DNA or under less stringent conditions (20 % formamide) with a mixture of HPV6 and HPV11 DNAs (specific activities ranging from $7.10^{7}$ to $2.10^{8}$ cpm/µg) [3-6, 15].

## RESULTS

HPV DNA sequences were detected in 33 out of 37 tumors (89 %) (Table 1). HPV16 genomes were found in 16 tumors, at a high copy number (20-200 per cell). After cleavage with Bam HI or Pst I endonucleases, typical HPV16 DNA patterns were observed for some tumors but, in most cases abnormal patterns were detected, suggesting that integration into the cell genome and/or rearrangements of

HPV16 genomes had occurred (Figure 1, lanes 1-4). For 14 tumors, the HPV16 DNA probe used under stringent conditions detected bands whose intensity corresponded to less than one to a few copies of HPV16 genome equivalent per cell. Usually no linear HPV DNA molecules were detected after cleavage with Bam HI. The Pst I cleavage patterns showed bands with mobilities close to only some Pst I HPV16 DNA fragments or were completely different from the HPV16 DNA pattern (Figure 1, lanes 5-10). In some cases, additional bands and higher signals were detected after hybridization under non stringent conditions, pointing to the existence of other cervical cancer-associated HPV(s). Finally, HPV18 genomes were detected in one cancer and sequences weakly related to HPV18 DNA in two others. No HPV DNA sequences were detected in the lymphocytes of 12 patients.

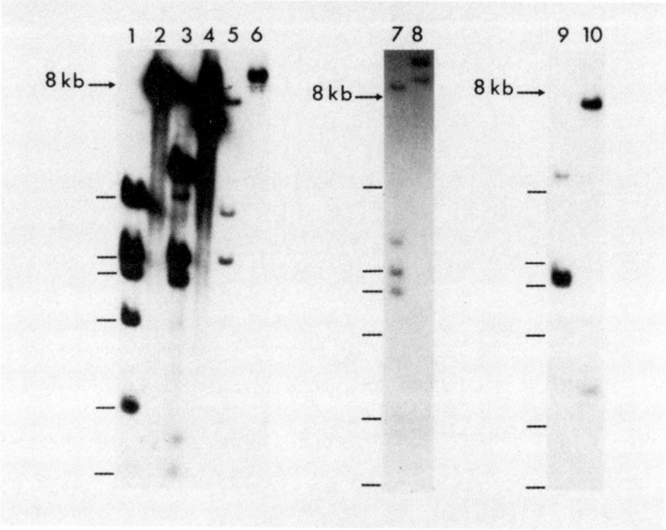


FIGURE 1. HPV16 or HPV16-related DNA sequences in cervical carcinomas. DNA preparations from tumors U12 (1,2), U17 (3,4), U7 (5,6), U14 (7,8), U15 (9,10) (5 μg) were cleaved with the endonucleases Pst I (1,3,5,7,9) or Bam HI (2,4,6,8,10) and analyzed by blot hybridization using a $^{32}$P-labeled HPV16 DNA probe under stringent conditions. The migrations of the linear HPV16 DNA fragments generated by Bam HI (8 kb) and of the six fragments generated by Pst I (bars) [6] are indicated. Exposure time, 16 hrs (1-6) or 1 week (7-10).

The analysis of oncogenes in carcinomas showed a frequent amplification of c-*myc* and c-Ha-*ras* oncogenes in the cervical tumors of more advanced clinical stages (2,3 and 4) (Table 1, Figure 2 A and B). After DNA cleavage by *Eco* RI endonuclease, a fragment of about 12.5 kb was detected by blot hybridization with the human c-*myc* oncogene (Figure 2A). The densitometric analysis revealed a 3 to 30 fold amplification of c-*myc* in 20 out of 37 tumors, taking N417 cells as a standard (Table 1) [6][13]. When the DNA preparations were cleaved with a mixture of *Hpa* II and *Msp* I endonucleases, a main fragment of about 1 kb was revealed by hybridization with the human c-Ha-*ras* probe (Figure 2B). The intensity of the bands was compared with that obtained with EJ cells [12]. A 3 to 30 fold amplification of c-Ha-*ras* oncogene was observed in 14 out of 35 tumors. An amplification of both oncogenes was revealed in 13 carcinomas. No amplification of either oncogene was observed in the 12 lymphocyte DNA preparations.

TABLE 1
HPV DNA SEQUENCES AND AMPLIFICATION OF c-*myc* AND c-Ha-*ras* ONCOGENES IN CERVICAL CARCINOMAS

| Clinical stage | HPV detection | Amplification of c-*myc* DNA | c-Ha-*ras* DNA |
|---|---|---|---|
| 1 | 10/11* | 2/11* (3-5 fold)** | 2/11* (3-4 fold)** |
| 2 | 3/3 | 2/3 (3 fold) | 1/2 (4 fold) |
| 3 | 13/15 | 12/15 (3 - 30 fold) | 8/14 (3 - 30 fold) |
| 4 | 7/8 | 4/8 (3 - 30 fold) | 3/8 (3 - 24 fold) |

*Number of positive tumors over total number of tumors analyzed. ** In brackets, extent of amplification.

Total RNAs prepared from 15 tumors and from the placenta of one patient, were analyzed by Northern blot and dot blot hybridization techniques (Figure 3 and Table 2). The human c-*myc* probe detected a 2.4 kb RNA band, as

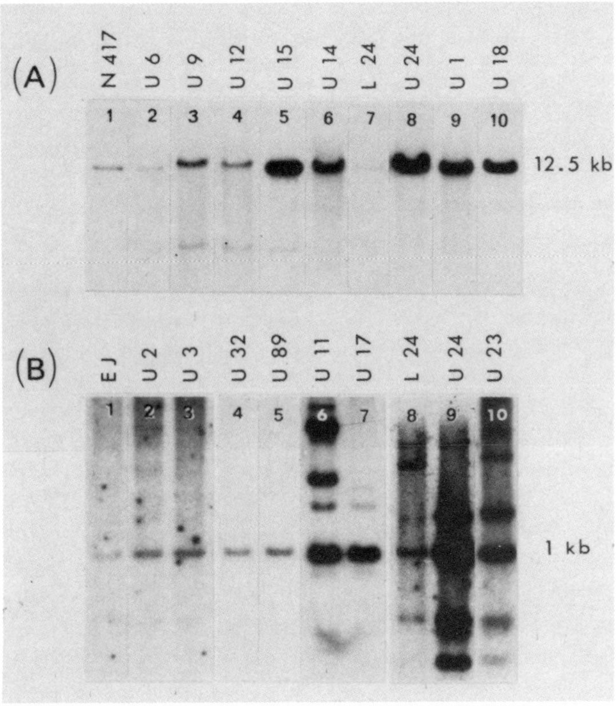


FIGURE 2. Analysis of c-myc and c-Ha-ras oncogenes in cervical carcinomas. (A) The DNA preparations from N417 cells (0.12 μg, 1), tumors (5 μg) designated U6 (2), U9 (3), U12 (4), U15 (5), U14 (6), U1 (9) and U18 (10), tumor U24 (8) and lymphocytes L24 (7) of the same patient were treated with Eco RI and analyzed by blot hybridization using a $^{32}$P-labeled DNA probe specific for the human oncogene c-myc. (B) The DNA preparations (5 μg) from EJ cells, tumors U2 (2), U3 (3), U32 (4), U89 (5), U11 (6), U17 (7), U23 (10), tumor U24 (9) and lymphocytes L24 (8) of the same patient were treated with a mixture of Hpa II and Msp I and analyzed by blot hybridization using a $^{32}$P-labeled DNA probe specific for the human oncogene c-Ha-ras1. The tumors belonged to stage 1 (U2, U3, U6, U9, U12, U32 and U89), stage 3 (U11, U14, U15, U17 and U24) or stage 4 (U1, U18 and U23).

TABLE 2
EXPRESSION OF c-*myc* ONCOGENE
IN INVASIVE CERVICAL CARCINOMAS

| Clinical stage | Tumors with high level of c-*myc* RNA* | Relative amounts of c-*myc* RNA*** |
|---|---|---|
| 1 | 1/4 ** | 0.4 |
| 2 | 2/2 | 0.4 and 0.6 |
| 3 | 6/6 | 0.4 to 0.9 |
| 4 | 3/3 | 0.4 to 0.6 |

* The tumors containing one-sixth of the c-*myc* RNA level found in N417 cells [13] by dot blot analysis are considered as tumors with high level of c-*myc* RNA. ** Number of positive tumors over total number analyzed. *** Relative amounts of c-*myc* RNA in tumors compared to that of N417 cells, as determined by the radioactivity of dot blots.

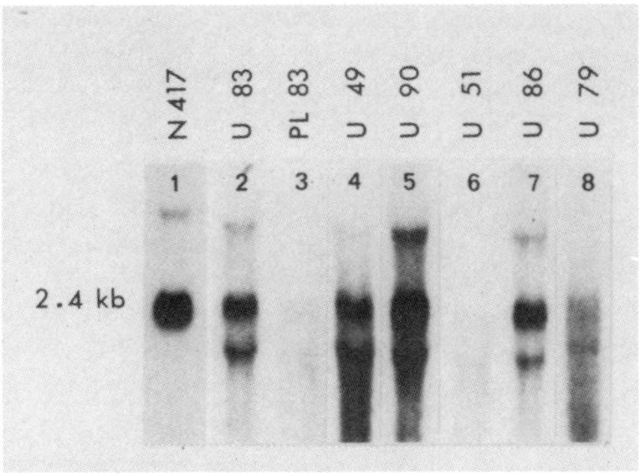


FIGURE 3. Northern blot hybridization analysis of c-*myc* RNA from cervical carcinomas. The total RNAs (10 µg) from N417 cells (1), tumors U83 (2), U49 (4), U90 (5), U51 (6), U86 (7), and U79 (8), and the placenta of patient 83 (Pl 83, 3) were analyzed by blot hybridization using a $^{32}P$-labeled DNA probe specific for the human oncogene c-*myc*. The tumors belonged to stage 1 (U83), stage 2 (U49 and U90), and stage 3 (U51, U86 and U79).

expected in human cells [16]. Two minor bands, with a migration close to that of 28 S and 18 S ribosomal RNAs, were also detected (Figure 3). Most carcinomas exhibited high levels of c-myc RNA (Figure 3 and Table 2).

## DISCUSSION

An association of HPV DNA sequences with invasive squamous cell carcinomas of the uterine cervix was found in 33 out of 37 tumors (89 %), and HPV16 was by far the most frequently encountered, as reported by other authors [4][5]. HPV16 genomes were found either at a high or at a low copy number, but there was no obvious correlation between the copy number and the clinical stage of the tumors. Abnormal HPV16 DNA cleavage patterns were frequently observed, suggesting that viral DNA sequences are integrated in the cellular genome and/or rearranged, as previously reported [5][16].

The amplification of c-myc or/and c-Ha-ras oncogenes was observed in 21 tumors (57 %) thus confirming and extending previous results [6]. A concomitant amplification of both oncogenes was found in 13 cancers. The amplification of c-Ha-ras and c-myc genes in fresh tumor material has so far seldom been reported [17] and there are only few examples of the amplification of other oncogenes [9-11][18]. The amplification of c-myc and c-Ha-ras was detected in the cervical cancers of more advanced stages (2 to 4). A similar observation has been reported for amplification of N-myc gene in neuroblastomas [10].

High levels of c-myc RNA were found in 12 out of the 15 cancers analyzed, as previously reported for fresh specimens of various tumor types [19][20]. An elevated expression of the c-myc gene was found in the 11 cancers having reached advanced stages. The only stage 1 tumor with a high level of c-myc RNA (Figure 3, lane 2) showed a moderate amplification of both c-myc and c-Ha-ras genes and evolved rapidly into stage 4. It is worth stressing that 6 cancers of the cervix showed a high level of c-myc transcription in the absence of detectable c-myc amplification. A similar phenomenon has been described in the case of hematopoietic malignancies in the absence of obvious genetic changes at the c-myc locus [19].

According to the data reported in this paper it seems likely that specific HPV types play a role in the development of cervical carcinomas and that activated cellular oncogenes are involved at least in the more advanced stages of tumor progression.

## ACKNOWLEDGMENTS

We thank Drs. H. zur Hausen and L. Gissmann for their kind gift of cloned HPV11, 16 and 18 DNAs, Drs. F. Dautry and O. Brison for helpful discussion, Drs. D. Castaigne, P. Charpentier, P. Duvillard, M. George, C. Haie and F. Rochard for providing us tumors and Dr. M. Tubiana for his constant support.

## REFERENCES

1. Crum CP, Ikenberg H, Richart RM, Gissmann L (1984). Human papillomavirus type 16 and early cervical neoplasia. N Eng J Med 310:880.
2. Rotkin ID (1973). A comparison review of key epidemiological studies in cervical cancer related to current searches for transmissible agents. Cancer Res 33:1353.
3. Gissmann L, Wolnik L, Ikenberg H, Koldovsky U, Schnürch HG, Zur Hausen H (1983). Human papillomavirus types 6 and 11 DNA sequences in genital and laryngeal papillomas and in some cervical cancers. Proc Natl Acad Sci USA 80:560.
4. Dürst M, Gissmann L, Ikenberg H, Zur Hausen H (1983) A papillomavirus DNA from a cervical carcinoma and its prevalence in cancer biopsy samples from different geographic regions. Proc Natl Acad Sci USA 80:3812.
5. Boshart M, Gissmann L, Ikenberg H, Kleinheinz A, Scheurlen W, Zur Hausen H (1984). A new type of papillomavirus DNA, its presence in genital cancer biopsies and in cell lines derived from cervical cancer. The Embo J 3:1151.
6. Riou G, Barrois M, Tordjman I, Dutronquay V, Orth G (1984). Présence de génomes de papillomavirus et amplification des oncogènes c-myc et c-Ha-ras dans des cancers envahissants du col de l'utérus. C R Acad Sc Paris 299:575.
7. Bishop JM (1983). Cellular oncogenes and retroviruses. Ann Rev Biochem 52:301.
8. Land H, Parada LF, Weinberg RA (1983). Cellular oncogenes and multistep carcinogenesis. Science 222:771.
9. Lee WH, Murphree AL, Benedict WF (1984). Expression and amplification of the N-myc gene in primary retino-

blastoma. Nature 309:458.
10. Brodeur GM, Seeger RC, Schwab M, Varmus HE, Bishop JM (1984). Amplification of N-myc in untreated human neuroblastomas correlates with advanced disease stage. Science 224:1121.
11. Pelicci PG, Lanfrancone L, Brathwaite MD, Wolman SR, Dalla-Favera R (1984). Amplification of the c-myb oncogene in a case of human acute myelogenous leukemia. Science 224:1117.
12. Shih C, Weinberg RA (1982). Isolation of a transforming sequence from a human bladder carcinoma cell line. Cell 29:161.
13. Little CD, Nau MM, Carney DN, Gazdar AF, Minna JD (1983). Amplification and expression of the c-myc oncogene in human lung cancer cell lines. Nature 306:194.
14. Maniatis T, Fritsch EF, Sambrook J (1982). In Molecular Cloning, A Laboratory Manual, Cold Spring Harbor Laboratory, New York.
15. Kremsdorf D, Favre M, Jablonska S, Obalek S, Rueda LA, Lutzner MA, Blanchet-Bardon C, Van Voorst Vader PC, Orth G (1984). Molecular cloning and characterization of the genomes of nine newly recognized human papillomavirus types associated with epidermodysplasia verruciformis. J Virol 52:1013.
16. Schwarz E, Freese UK, Gissmann L, Mayer W, Roggenbuck B, Stremlau A, Zur Hausen H (1985). Structure and transcription of human papillomavirus sequences in cervical carcinoma cells. Nature 314:111.
17. Hayashi K, Karizoe T, Sugimura T (1983). In vivo amplification and rearrangement of the c-Ha-ras-1 sequence in a human bladder carcinoma. Gann 74:798.
18. Libermann TA, Nusbaum HR, Razon N, Kris R, Lax I, Soreq H, Whittle N, Waterfield MD, Ullrich A, Schlessinger J (1985). Amplification, enhanced expression and possible rearrangement of EGF receptor gene in primary human brain tumours of glial origin. Nature 313:144.
19. Rothberg PG, Erisman MD, Diehl RE, Rovigatti UG, Astrin SM (1984). Structure and expression of the oncogene c-myc in fresh tumor material from patients with hematopoietic malignancies. Mol Cell Biol 4:1096.
20. Slamon DJ, deKernion JB, Verma IM, Cline MJ (1984). Expression of cellular oncogenes in human malignancies. Science 224:256.

Papillomaviruses: Molecular and Clinical Aspects, pages 57–65


# ORGANIZATION AND EXPRESSION OF HUMAN PAPILLOMAVIRUS TYPE 16 GENOMES IN HUMAN CERVICAL CARCINOMAS

Hermann Lehn and Gerhard Sauer

Institute for Virus Research, German Cancer Research Center, 6900 Heidelberg, FRG

ABSTRACT Six human cervical carcinomas were analyzed for the presence of HPV DNA and RNA. Four of the tumor specimens were shown to contain the DNA of HPV16 as a single copy per cell exclusively in an integrated state. There is compelling evidence for the monoclonal origin of the cervical carcinomas. HPV16 specific RNA sequences were revealed in only one out of the four tumors, while we consistently failed to detect such sequences in the three other specimens under conditions that permitted the detection of less than one mRNA molecule per cell. We conclude that continuous expression of the HPV16 genomes is not required for the maintenance of the malignant state.

## INTRODUCTION

The DNA of human papillomavirus (HPV) types 16 and 18 was detected in the majority of human cervical carcinoma biopsies (1, 2). The frequent presence of HPV16 and 18 DNAs in malignant genital tumors together with epidemiological data suggest that papillomaviruses play an important role in the development of genital cancer (3, for a review). Therefore, we have analyzed both organization and transcriptional activity of HPV genomes in human cervical tumor biopsies.

## METHODS

Biopsy material. Biopsy specimens of invasive cervical carcinomas were provided by the Universitätsfrauenklinik Heidelberg.

Extraction of DNA and RNA. DNA and RNA from tumor biopsies were prepared as described (4).

DNA and RNA Blot Hybridization. Southern blot and Northern blot analyses under stringent conditions to $^{32}P$-labeled nick-translated cloned HPV-DNAs were performed as described (5, 6).

Synthesis of cRNA. The HaeIII-fragments of 2091 bp (covering the E6/E7 and part of the El region) and the HaeIII B-fragment of 1068 bp (covering E4/E5 and part of the E2 region) of HPV16 were cloned into the SmaI-site of the plasmid pSP62-PL (NEN) and used for in vitro RNA synthesis as described (7). The resulting $^{32}P$-labeled cRNAs were employed in Northern blots according to Melton et al. (7).

## RESULTS

### Organization of HPV16 Genomes in Cervical Carcinomas.

Four out of six tumor biopsies contained the DNA of HPV16 under stringent hybridization conditions. The remaining two as well as normal cervical biopsy material from two of the HPV16-containing tumors lacked DNA sequences of HPV6, 11, 16 or 18. All four tumors (CC328, CC357, CC511, CC527) were shown to contain the HPV16 DNA covalently linked to the cellular DNA as single copies (8). There was no evidence for tandem integration or for the existence of extrachromosomal HPV16 genomes in the four tumors (8).

The detailed analysis of the integration sites of the HPV16 DNA into the cellular DNA was performed by digestion of the tumor DNAs with the multi-cut restriction enzymes PstI, AvaII and HaeIII (8; unpublished data). A synopsis of the regions within which the circular viral genomes were opened before integration is shown in Fig.1.

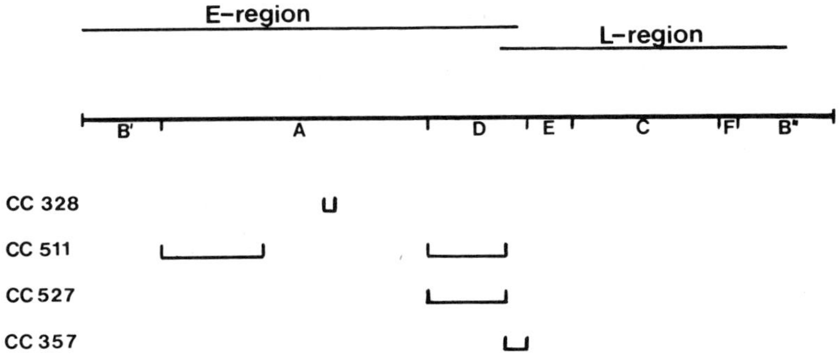


FIGURE 1. Organization of HPV16 in four human cervical carcinomas. Above, the putative early (E) and late (L) regions of HPV16. Middle, the linear map of HPV16 (7904 bp) with the six PstI-fragments A - F. Below, the organization of the HPV16 genomes in the four cervical tumors CC328, CC511, CC527 and CC357. The open boxes span the regions within which the HPV16 genomes were opened. The area in tumor CC511 between the two boxes in the PstI A-fragment represents a deletion of the HPV16 DNA.

It can be seen that only tumor CC357 contained an uninterrupted "early" region of HPV16, and that there existed a large deletion of at least 1900 bp in tumor CC511 affecting the "early" region.

## Monoclonal Origin of Human Cervical Carcinomas.

The question of whether human tumors are of monoclonal or polyclonal origin has important implications (9, for a review). If a tumor arises as the result of a rare event, a unicellular origin is anticipated. The method used to investigate whether human cervical carcinomas are of monoclonal origin consisted of the comparison of the restriction enzyme cleavage patterns of the integrated HPV16 DNA from different sections of a given tumor. Although the BamHI/ApaI-pattern varied from tumor to tumor, the pattern was identical in all sections from each tumor which was analyzed (CC328, CC357, CC511) (Fig. 2, one example). This observation demonstrated the monoclonal origin of the three cervical carcinomas.

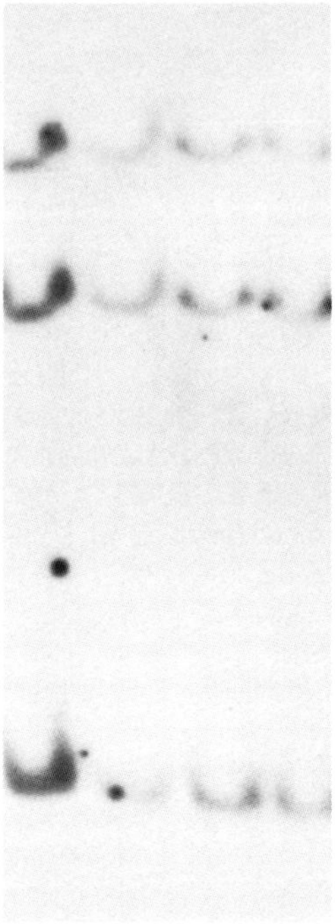

FIGURE 2. Monoclonal origin of tumor CC328. DNA was isolated from four different sections of tumor CC328, digested with BamHI/ApaI (both "single-cut" enzymes for HPV16) and separated on a 1.4 % agarose gel (10 μg/track). After transfer to nitrocellulose, the DNA was hybridized to 1 x $10^6$ cpm/ml $^{32}$P-labeled cloned pHPV16 DNA (3 x $10^8$ cpm/μg).

Transcriptional State of the Integrated HPV16 Genomes.

Northern blot analysis of the tumor RNAs revealed HPV16-specific mRNA species (1.4, 1.6, 1.8 kb) in tumor CC328 only, while we consistently failed to detect any HPV RNA sequences in tumors CC357, CC511 and CC527 (8). The integrity of the RNA was shown by the demonstration of the undegraded transcripts of the human oncogene c-myc in the tumor RNA preparations (8). The apparent absence of HPV16-transcripts from the three tumors cannot be accounted for by the failure to detect small amounts of transcripts, as we have shown that our method permitted the identification of one mRNA molecule per cell (8). Northern blots were performed using $^{32}$P-labeled cRNAs as hybridization probes (7); with this method, the sensivity of detection of specific DNA or RNA sequences is significantly increased (7). Employing 2 µg of the RNA of tumor CC328, the three HPV16-specific mRNA species of 1.4, 1.6, 1.8 kb were detectable (Fig. 3, lane b), while we were unable to reveal HPV16 RNA in tumors CC357, CC511 and CC527 employing 10 µg of the respective tumor RNA (Fig. 3, lanes c, d, e). With this method, however, we are able to detect 0.1 specific RNA molecule per cell.

## DISCUSSION

In this work, the functional analysis of HPV16 genomes in four human cervical tumors is described. While two biopsy specimens lacked any detectable HPV DNA sequences, four tumors contained HPV16 DNA as a single copy per cell exclusively in an integrated state. The monoclonal origin of three of the tumors (CC328, CC357, CC511) suggests that the development of cervical carcinomas in humans represents a very rare event. It is concluded from the different integration patterns of the HPV16 genomes that the integration of the viral genome into the cellular DNA had occurred in a random fashion.

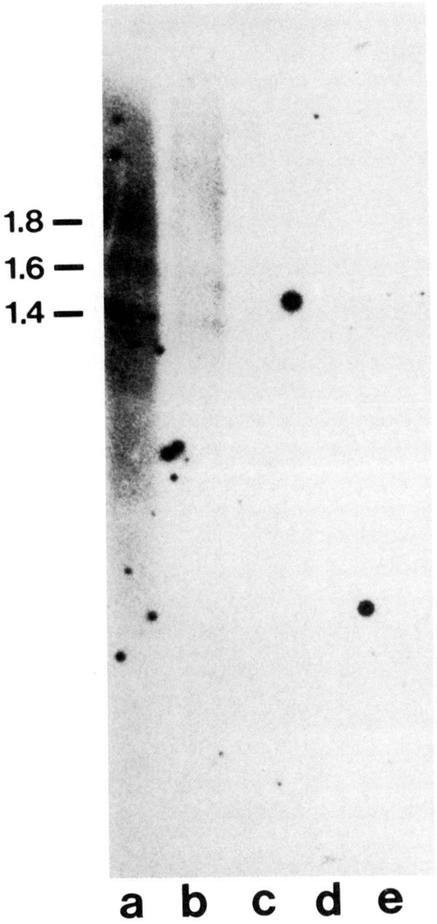


FIGURE 3. Northern blot analysis of RNA from cervical carcinomas. Total RNA from tumors CC328 (lane a: 10 µg; lane b: 2 µg), CC511 (lane c: 10 µg), CC527 (lane d: 10 µg) and CC357 (lane e: 10 µg) was fractionated on a 1.4 % agarose gel containing 10 mM methylmercury hydroxide and hybridized to a mixture of the $^{32}P$-labeled cRNAs of the HaeIII A-fragment and the HaeIII B-fragment of HPV16 ($10 \times 10^6$ cpm/ml, respectively). The autoradiogram was exposed for 3 days.

Mapping of the integration regions revealed that only tumor CC357 possessed a complete uninterrupted "early" region. In tumors CC328, CC511 and CC527, the putative "early" region of HPV16 was affected by the integration event (Fig. 1). A large deletion of at least 1900 bp within the "early" region was detected in tumor CC511. This deletion affected the open reading frames E2/E4/E5 (8). This region was shown to be essential for the transformation of rodent cells by bovine papillomavirus type 1 (BPV-1) (11), and the main bodies of the early mRNA species of BPV-1 (6, 12) and HPV6 (13) are transcribed from this region. Because of the close relationship of the genome organization of HPV16 with other papillomaviruses (10), one may assume that the E2/E4/E5 regions have similar biological properties. The absence of HPV16 transcripts in tumor CC511 was not surprising in view of the large deletion affecting the E2/E4/E5 region. In tumor CC527, viral transcripts were also absent. Most remarkably, tumor CC357 lacked HPV16 transcripts despite the presence of an intact "early" region. Tumor CC328 turned out to be the only one with HPV16 mRNA species. It is not known, however, whether these transcripts coded for biologically active proteins that might be involved in the malignant state of this tumor.

These data demonstrate that the continuous expression of the integrated HPV16 genomes is not required for the maintenance of the malignant state of at least three of the four cervical tumors studied. One can speculate that the HPV16 genomes may be involved as one prerequisite in the development of these squamous carcinomas, e.g., by inducing the flat condylomata with abnormal mitotic figures traditionally classified as mild dysplasia or cervical intraepithelial neoplasia 1 (CIN 1). This prerequisite event, acquisition of HPV16 genomes, may preceed the extremely rare event of malignant conversion of CIN to monoclonal cervical tumors.

ACKNOWLEDGEMENTS

We thank Dr. G. Leppien for the tumor biopsies, Dr. L. Gissmann for the cloned HPV DNAs and K. Seedorf for providing the DNA sequence of HPV16 before publication.

REFERENCES

1. Dürst M, Gissmann L, Ikenberg H, zur Hausen H (1983). A papillomavirus DNA from a cervical carcinoma and its prevalence in cancer biopsy samples from different geographic regions. Proc Natl Acad Sci USA 80: 3812.
2. Boshart M, Gissmann L, Ikenberg H, Kleinheinz A, Scheurlen W., zur Hausen H (1984). A new type of papillomavirus DNA: its presence in genital cancer biopsies and in cell lines derived from cervical cancer. EMBO J 3: 1151.
3. Zur Hausen H (1977). Human papillomaviruses and their possible role in squamous cell carcinomas. Curr Top Microbiol Immunol 78: 1.
4. Krieg P, Amtmann E, Sauer G (1983). The simultaneous extraction of high molecular weight DNA and of RNA from solid tumors. Analyt Biochem 134: 288.
5. Krieg P, Amtmann E, Jonas D, Fischer H, Zang K, Sauer, G (1981). Episomal simian virus 40 genomes in human brain tumors. Proc Natl Acad Sci USA 78: 6446.
6. Amtmann E, Sauer G (1982). Bovine papillomavirus transcription: polyadenylated RNA species and assessment of the direction of transcription. J Virol 43: 59.
7. Melton DA, Krieg PA, Rebagliati MR, Maniatis T, Zinn K, Green MR (1984). Efficient in vitro synthesis of biologically active RNA and RNA hybridization probes from plasmids containing a bacteriophage SP6 promoter. Nucl Ac Res 12: 7035.
8. Lehn H, Krieg P, Sauer G (1985). Papillomavirus genomes in human cervical tumors: analysis of their transcriptional activity. Proc Natl Acad Sci USA, in press.

9. Fialkow PJ (1979). Clonal origin of human tumors. Ann Rev Med 30: 135.
10. Seedorf K, Krämmer G, Dürst M, Suhai S, Röwekamp WG (1985). Human papillomavirus type 16 DNA sequence. Virol, in press.
11. Nakabayashi Y, Chattopadhay SK, Lowy DR (1983). The transforming function of bovine papillomavirus DNA. Proc Natl Acad Sci USA 80: 5832.
12. Engel LW, Heilmann CA, Howley PM (1983). Transcriptional organization of bovine papillomavirus type 1. J Virol 47: 516.
13. Lehn H, Ernst TM, Sauer G (1984). Transcription of episomal papillomavirus DNA in human condylomata acuminata and Buschke Löwenstein tumors. J gen Virol 65: 2003.

# II. PAPILLOMAVIRUSES AND HUMAN CUTANEOUS DISEASES

Papillomaviruses: Molecular and Clinical Aspects, pages 69–83


# THE CLINICAL MORPHOLOGY, PATHOLOGY AND IMMUNOLOGY OF PAPILLOMAVIRUS INFECTIONS OF THE SKIN AS RELATED TO THE VIRUS TYPE

Stefania Jablonska[a/], Gerard Orth[b/], Odile Croissant, Slavomir Obalek[a/]

[a/]Department of Dermatology, Warsaw School of Medicine, 02-008 Warsaw, Poland
[b/]Institut Pasteur, 75-724, Paris, France

ABSTRACT We are presenting our data on preferential association of various HPVs inducing cutaneous warts with distinct warts and wart-like lesions, and stress an almost perfect correlation between the histological patterns and the types of causative HPVs. The cytopathic effect, related to a viral DNA replication, as shown by molecular hybridization in vivo, is a specific marker for HPV infections. The intermediate warts and unusual morphological warts and/or wart-like lesions are described. The diverse types of warts in immunosuppressed patients and immune phenomena responsible for the persistence and regression of warts were studied. Malignant conversion of benign lesions of epidermodysplasia verruciformis appears to be related to special types of potentially oncogenic E.V.-specific HPVs. Two new HPVs were disclosed in cutaneous Bowen's disease and keratosis senilis.

This work was supported by grant 21-10 of the Polish National Cancer Program PR6

## DIVERSITY OF HPVs INDUCING CUTANEOUS WARTS

Plurality of HPVs disclosed in cutaneous warts /1-5/ and wart-like lesions /6, 7/ raised the problem of the relation of clinical and pathological morphology of the distinct types of HPVs

### Preferential Association of Various HPVs with Distinct Cutaneous Warts.

A specific or preferential association of HPV types with warts differing in morphology and location, remains still controversial. Our studies performed in 112 persons, including 54 butchers displaying diversity of warts, have shown a preferential association of various morphological types of warts with distinct HPVs, as identified by restriction enzyme analysis and/or blot hybridization experiments. Deep single plantar warts were found to be associated with HPV1, however in palmar and plantar location may also occur HPV2 and HPV4-induced warts. Common warts were found to be induced by HPV2, HPV4 and HPV7, plane warts by HPV3, HPV10 and HPV28. HPV7 was detected in common warts or papilloma-like hyperproliferative, hyperkeratotic, cauliflower lesions in butchers. However, the clinical morphology of warts does not only depend on the virus type, but also on the age of the lesions, the anatomical location and, to some extent, on the immune status of the host.

Presently recognized types of cutaneous warts: deep myrmecia warts, common and plane warts, do not allow to classify some unusual wart-like lesions, specifically those displaying features of both plane and common warts, small keratosis punctata-like endophytic warts, some papillomas and pigmented papillomas, plaque-like lesions, etc. A great diversity of cutaneous lesions is associated with epidermodysplasia verruciformis /EV/ induced by specific HPVs: very flat reddish or whitish plane wart-like lesions, red plaques, red-brownish, brownish and/or achromic plaques, pityriasis versicolor-like lesions. Although these changes are highly characteristic of EV the diagnostic significance has histological examination, as for other cutaneous HPV-induced lesions.

## Correlation Between the Histological Patterns and HPV Types

Applying histological criteria for the recognition of the type of causative HPVs in cutaneous warts described earlier /8/, we have performed studies on DNA extracted from 260 lesions. The virus types was identified by restriction enzyme analysis and/or blot hybridization experiments. These studies have shown an evident correlation between the histological patterns and the types of infecting virus, whereas the clinical recognition of the causative virus was not always possible.

The only type-specific marker of HPV infection was found to be the cytopathic effect related to DNA replication /9/. Distinctive features of the cytopathic effects induced by various HPVs enable classification of cutaneous warts in accordance with the causative viruses.

TABLE 1
HISTOLOGICAL PATTERNS OF WARTS AS RELATED TO THE HPV TYPE

| The HPV as determined by restriction enzyme analysis or blot hybridization | Number of warts with patterns characteristic of infection by HPV types | | | | | | Inconclusive |
|---|---|---|---|---|---|---|---|
| | 1 | 2 | 4 | 7 | 3 | 10 or 28 | |
| HPV 1 | 5 | | | | | | |
| HPV 2 | | 46 | | | | | 2 |
| HPV 4 | | | 14 | | | | |
| HPV 7 | | | | 39 | | | 2 |
| HPV 3 | | | | | 10 | 3 | 1 |
| HPV 10 or 28 | | | | | 7 | 15 | |

As shown in Table 1, there is an almost perfect correlation between the histological patterns and the types of infecting HPVs, if the specimens are properly chosen and cut in their centers, so that the cytopathic effect can be evaluated. If it is absent, the architecture of the wart itself, related to the arrangement of terminally differentiating non-permissive cells, is not a sufficient criterion and the findings are inconclusive.

## UNUSUAL TYPES OF WARTS

### Intermediate Warts

We have proposed the term intermediate warts for lesions displaying clinical features of both common and plane warts. They are more raised and hyperkeratotic than plane warts, but differ from common warts by a somewhat flatter surface and, not infrequently, by a linear arrangement /Koebner phenomenon/, characteristic of plane warts. These lesions are often recognized clinically as common warts /10/, but the cytopathic effect is highly characteristic of HPV3. Intermediate warts differ in histological pattern from verrucae planae by more pronounced hyperkeratosis and parakeratosis, and usually more prominent papillomatosis and branching of rete ridges. They were found to be associated with newly characterized HPVs 10 and 28, the viruses, that may also induce plane warts /11/. Although there are some characteristic clinical and histological features of intermediate warts induced by HPV10 and HPV28, differentiation between warts induced by these viruses and plane warts induced by HPV3 may be very difficult, if at all possible.

TABLE 2
CLINICALLY RECOGNIZED PLANE OR INTERMEDIATE WARTS AS RELATED TO THE HPV TYPE

| Number of DNA preparations studied by restriction enzyme analysis and/or blot hybridization | Number of DNA preparations containing HPV DNA | | | | | |
|---|---|---|---|---|---|---|
| | 1 | 2 | 4 | 7 | 3 | 10 or 28 |
| 58 | 1 | 10 | 1 | 1 | 19 | 22 |

As seen in Table 2, in a proportion of warts recognized as intermediate, we have found HPV2. Thus criteria of clinical differentiation of intermediate warts from common warts, especially young ones, are not always satisfactory. However, the cytopathic effect is in these cases characteristic of HPV2 infection, i.e. differs from that of HPV3, HPV10 and HPV28.

## Keratosis Punctata-Like Warts

These small warts, of a few mm in size, usually at skin level, with depression in the central part, are as a rule located on palms and soles. They are sometimes not recognized as warts, and overlooked by the patients and the doctors. A part of these warts were found to be induced by HPV4 /11/. However, HPV4 also induces common warts in palmar or dorsal localization /12/. On the other side, very young common or small plane warts, especially in palmar localization, may be indistinquishable from small lesions of keratosis punctata type. Warts due to HPV4 were found to have a very characteristic cytopathic effect, and HPV type can be easily recognized histologically /8, 11-14/.

## Papilloma-Like Warts

The hyperproliferative and hyperkeratotic warts on hands of butchers were found to be induced by HPV7. This virus is associated also with common warts that are usually intermingled with the characteristic papillomatous lesions. In our series, HPV7 was present exclusively in butchers warts. However, the molecular hybridization did not disclose any nucleotide homology to bovine papillomaviruses type 1, 2, 3 and 4 /8/. The histological pattern of HPV7 infection is diagnostic due to a highly characteristic cytopathic effect /8, 11, 14/.

Papillomatous lesions may also be induced by other viruses, especially by HPV2 on the face and neck.

Pigmented papillomas on the skin of the ano-genital region. They were found to be preferentially associated with HPV6. These papillomas differ from ano-genital condylomas on mucous membranes by absence of cytopathic effect, i.e. koilocytes. The histological features are analogous to papillomas in other locations with no detectable viral genomes. Interestingly, ano-genital cutaneous warts with somewhat unusual clinical features, intermediate between plane warts and flat condylomas /with smooth surface/, were also found to be associated with HPV6. Thus, the clinical and histological morphology of warts induced by HPV6 appears to depend on their location - on mucosa or the skin.

## Plaque-Like Lesions

Red and pigmented plaques are characteristic of epidermodysplasia verruciformis induced by diverse EV-specific HPVs /6, 14/. Single red plaques in renal transplant patients were found to be induced by HPV5, i.e. HPV associated with EV /15, 16/. However, this infection was transitional.

Somewhat elevated brownish plaques with irregular outlines found in patients with EV are usually induced by HPV3.

## WARTS AND IMMUNOSUPRESSION

Immunodepressed persons, allograft recipients and patients suffering from systemic diseases or immunosuppressive therapy are prone to infection with all types of HPVs /9, 10, 17, 18/.
The course of the infection in our series of 40 patients was very protracted due to a decreased cell mediated immunity /CMI/. Twenty six lesions in 23 patients were examined by molecular hybridization and restriction enzyme analysis.

TABLE 3
WARTS IN IMMUNOSUPPRESSED

| Clinical type | Type of HPVs[x] | | | | |
|---|---|---|---|---|---|
| | 1 | 2 | 4 | 3 | 10 |
| Common warts | | | | | |
| palmar or lateral | 3 | 2 | 1 | | |
| dorsal | | 4 | | | |
| periungueal | | 1 | | | |
| Plane or intermediate warts | | | | 5 | 8 |
| Brownish plaques | | | | | 1 |

x/ as determined by restriction enzyme analysis or blot hybridization

As seen in Table 3, the most frequent causative viruses were HPV2 and HPV10, although all cutaneous wart viruses, with the exception of HPV7, were detected. Common warts in palmar and lateral location were induced by HPV1, 2 or 4, dorsal and periungueal warts by HPV2, and plane warts by HPV3 or HPV10. HPV10 was also detected in intermediate warts, displaying some clinical features of common warts.
The histological picture was consistent with

infecting HPV. In 10 further patients, histological studies were sufficient to establish the type of virus: HPV1 in one patient with palmar and plantar warts, HPV4 in one palmar wart, HPV2 in two dorsal common warts, HPV10 or HPV3 in v. plana-like or intermediate warts in 5 patients. HPV1, HPV2 and HPV4 are easily recognizable, but distinction between histological features of HPV10 and HPV3-induced warts was difficult, and evaluation rather presumptive. It is to be stressed that, in a proportion of cases, clinical recognition of virus type was not possible. HPV10 was a frequent causative agent and the lesions had sometimes unusual features, such as plaques, dome-shaped tumors with smooth surface, etc.

## IMMUNE PHENOMENA IN HPV INFECTIONS

Immune phenomena are of basic importance for the development, persistence and regression of warts.

### Immune Phenomena as Related to the Type of Infecting Virus

Recognition of the type of infecting virus is of practical importance since HPV infections differ considerably in the immune responses of the host /18, 19/. Cell mediated immunity /CMI/ was found to be least decreased in infections by HPV1 /myrmecia warts/and HPV6 or HPV11 /condylomata acuminata/, and most depressed in infections by HPV3, HPV10 and HPV28. These viruses, not infrequently, were found in immunosuppressed persons. The patients with EV, induced both by EV-specific HPVs and HPV3 or HPV10, had in general a low CMI and were unable to reject their warts /20/. However, the majority of patients have been resistant to other infections, i.e. there was a specific, virus-related defect of immunity.

Regression of Warts as Related to the Virus Type.

The phenomenon of warts rejection differs for various HPVs. HPV-1 induced warts regress with macroscopically visible hemorrhagic reaction and prominent inflammatory infiltrates around the vessels. The histological features were of Arthus reaction type.

In 20 patients with warts induced by HPV3- -and HPV10 the regression was systemic and occured simultaneously on all lesions, with pronounced inflammatory reaction. The infiltrates consisting predominantly of lymphocytes and macrophages, destroyed rete ridges. The cytophatic effect was no more detectable, with simultaneous disappearance of the granular layer. In patients with decreased cell mediated immunity /CMI/, after warts were rejected, the non specific and specific CMI, as determined by migratory inhibition test with the use of purified HPV3 particles, became normal.
We could not detect any differences in the regression of warts induced by HPV3 vs those induced by HPV10. However, if plane or intermediate warts in heavily immunosuppressed patients regressed at all, the process was slow, with no visible inflammation in and around the warts. Interestingly, the regression of HPV-1 induced warts was in these patients comparable to that in normals.

We have not seen HPV2- and HPV7-induced lesions disappear simultaneously, and the inflammation was not recognizable macroscopically. However, the histological pattern of regressing warts due to HPV2 and HPV7 combined some features of mononuclear invasion into the rete ridges with their eventual destruction, characteristic of HPV3-and HPV10-induced warts, as well as perivascular infiltrations and extravasations characteristic of HPV1 infection.

We have never seen regression of EV cases induced by EV specific viruses, although some lesions disappeared and/or changed morphology. In a unique case of HPV3-induced EV in which the lesions regressed completely, after two deliveries, the process was slow and gradual within two years, with no inflammatory reaction both clinically and histologically. The regression was accompanied by restoration of CMI /18/.

## MALIGNANT TRANSFORMATION OF HPV-INDUCED TUMORS

### Epidermodysplasia Verruciformis

Malignant progression of HPV-induced tumors was studied extensively in patients with EV /21-26/. The causative viruses differ in their oncogenic potentials, HPV5 and related HPVs, 8 and 14 genomes, were found in carcinomas /21, 23, 24/, and patients infected with these viruses are in a group of high risk of malignant conversion. The cell mediated immunity was decreased in all patients with EV irrespective of the type of causative HPV. However, in 5 patients with no cutaneous malignancies natural killer cell activity was found to be normal /27/, and steadily increased in 4 patients with numerous carcinomas and precancerous lesions. Since these cells are responsible both for the resistance to viral infections and host surveillance against tumor development, they appear to play a significant role in preventing malignant cell spreading and metastases. Basides that, the increased activity of NK cells, which are known to exert a suppressor cell function, could contribute to the defect of CMI.
Also lymphocyte induced angiogenesis, as determined according to the method of Sidky and Auerbach /28/ was found to be increased in patients with cutaneous malignancies, and correlated with the increased natural killer cell activity /Majewski et al. - in preparation/. Increased angiogenic capability in cases with cutaneous malignancies may reflect activation of mononuclears.and proneness to to epidermal proliferation and malignant

transformation.

## Other Cutaneous Malignancies Associated with HPVs

Cutaneous Bowen's disease and keratosis senilis with histological features of Bowen's atypia are presently being studied, and two new HPVs, one from the lesions of keratosis senilis type and one from Bowen's disease of the finger, are being characterized /M. Kawashima et al. - in preparation/. In one patient in whom the new HPV was characterized Bowen's disease on the finger coexisted with long-lasting hand warts induced by HPV 4. In one patient having warts for several years, in a single lesion of Bowen's disease localized in the skin of inguinal region, without involvement of the vulva, HPV16 genome was detected.

In conclusion, infection of the skin with diverse HPVs is associated with distinct morphologic and pathologic lesions and various immune response of the host. Malignant conversion appears to depend on the HPV type. EV specific HPVs: 5, 8 and 14 were shown to be potentially oncogenic and their genomes were found in carcinomas developing from benign lesions of EV. Two new, not yet fully characterized HPVs were detected in lesions of Bowen's disease and keratosis senilis localized on the hands.

## REFERENCES

1. Gissmann L., Pfister H, Zur Hausen H /1977/. Human papilloma viruses /HPV/ Characterization of four different isolates. Virology 76:569.
2. Orth G, Favre M, Croissant O /1977/. Characterization of a new type of human papillomavirus that causes skin warts. J Virol 24:108.
3. Orth G, Jablonska S, Breitburd F, Favre M, Croissant O /1978/. The human papillomaviruses. Bull Cancer 65:151.
4. Ostrow R, Zachow KD, Watts S, Bender M, Pass F, Faras A /1983/. Characterization of two HPV-3 related papillomaviruses from common warts that are distinct clinically from flat warts or epidermodysplasia verruciformis. J Invest Dermatol 80:436.
5. Orth G, Favre M /1985/. Human papillomaviruses: Biochemical and biological properties in Human Papillomaviruses, Jablonska S, Orth G /eds/. Clinics in Dermatology, Lippincott Comp. Philadelphia - in press.
6. Orth G, Jablonska S, Favre M, Croissant O, Jarząbek-Chorzelska M, Rzęsa G /1978/. Characterization of two types of human papillomaviruses in lesions of epidermodysplasia verruciformis. Proc Natl Acad Sci USA 75:1537.
7. Gassenmaier A, Lammel M, Pfister H /1984/. Molecular cloning and characterization of five human papillomavirus DNA from an epidermodysplasia verruciformis patient. J Virol 52:1019.
8. Orth G, Jablonska S, Favre M, Croissant O, Obałek S, Jarząbek-Chorzelska M, Jibard N /1981/. Identification of papillomaviruses in butcher's warts. J Invest Dermatol 76:97.
9. Croissant O, Breitburd F, Orth G Specificity of the cytopathic effect of cutaneous human papillomaviruses. In Human Papillomaviruses, Clinics in Dermatology S Jablonska, G Orth /eds/, publ Lippincott

Comp, Philadelphia-in press.
10. Ostrow RS, Zachow KR, Thompson O, Faras AJ /1984/. Molecular cloning and characterization of a unique type of human papillomavirus from an immune deficient patient. J Invest Dermatol 82:362.
11. Jablonska S, Orth G, Obalek S, Croissant O /1985/. Cutaneous warts: Clinical, histological and virological correlations. In Human Papillomaviruses. Clinics in Dermatology. Jablonska S, Orth G /eds/, publ. Lippincott Comp. Philadelphia - in press.
12. Grussendorff EI /1980/. Lichtmikroskopische Untersuchungen an typisierten Virus-Warzen /HPV 1 and HPV 4/. Arch Dermatol 268:141.
13. Gross G, Pfister H, Hagedorn M, Gissmann L /1982/ Correlation between human papillomavirus /HPV/ type and histology of warts. J Invest Dermatol 78 /2/:160.
14. Jablonska S, Orth G /1983/. Human Papovaviruses. Recent Advances in Dermatology, vol. 6 /eds/ A. Rook, H. Maibach publ Churchill Livingstone, London, p. 1-36.
15. Lutzner M, Croissant O, Ducasse MF, Kreis H, Crosnier J, Orth G /1980/. A potentially oncogenic human papillomavirus /HPV-5/ found in two renal allograft recipients. J Invest Dermatol 75:353.
16. Lutzner M, Croissant O, Ducasse MF, Kreis H, Crosnier H, Orth G /1981/. An unusual wart-like skin lesions found in a renal allograft recipient. Arch Dermatol 117:43.
17. Pfister H, Gross G, Hagedorn M /1979/. Characterization of human papilloma virus 3 in warts of a renal allograft patient. J Invest Dermatol 73:349.
18. Jablonska S, Orth G, Lutzner MA /1982/. Immunopathology of papillomaviruses induced tumors in different tissues. Springer Seminars Immunopathology, 5:33.
19. Jablonska S, Orth G, Gliński W, Obalek S, Jarząbek-Chorzelska M, Croissant O, Favre M, Rzęsa G /1980/. Morphology and Immunology of human warts and familial warts.

Leukaemias, Lymphomas and Papillomas: Comparative Aspects. /ed/ PA Bachmann, publ. Taylor and Francis, London pp. 107-131.

20. Orth G, Jablonska S, Jarząbek-Chorzelska M, Obalek S, Rzęsa G, Favre M, Croissant O /1979/. Epidermodysplasia verruciformis: characteristics of the lesions and risk of malignant conversion as related to the type of human papillomavirus lesions. Cancer Research, 39:1074.

21. Orth G, Favre M, Breitburd F, Croissant O, Jablonska S, Obalek S /1980/. Epidermodysplasia verruciformis. A model for the role of papillomaviruses in human cancer. Cold Spring Harbor Conf Cell Proliferation 7:259.

22. Pfister H, Nurnberger F, Gissmann L, Zur Hausen H /1981/. Characterization of a human papillomavirus from epidermodysplasia verruciformis lesions of a patient from Upper-Volta. Int J Cancer 27:645.

23. Ostrow RS, Bender M, Niimura M, Seki T, Kawashima M, Pass F, Faras AJ /1982/. Human papillomavirus DNA in cutaneous primary and metastasized squamous cell carcinoma from patients with epidermodysplasia verruciformis. Proc Natl Acad Sci USA 79:1634.

24. Pfister H, Gassenmaier A, Nurnberger F, Stüttgen S /1983/. Human papilloma virus 5-DNA in carcinoma of an epidermodysplasia verruciformis patient infected with various human papillomavirus types. Cancer Res 43:1436.

25. Kremsdorf D, Jablonska S, Favre M, Orth G /1983/. Human papillomaviruses associated with epidermodysplasia verruciformis. II. Molecular cloning and biochemical characterization of HPV 3a, 8, 10 and 12 genomes. J Virol 99, 48:340.

26. Kremsdorf D, Favre M, Jablonska S, Obalek S, Rueda LA, Lutzner MA, Blanchet-Bardon C, Voorst PC, Orth G /1984/. Molecular cloning and characterization of

the genomes of nine newly recognized human papillomavirus types associated with epidermodysplasia verruciformis. J Virol, 52: 1013

27. Kamiński MJ, Pawińska M, Jablonska S, Szmurło A, Majewski S, Orth G /1985/. Increased natural killer cell activity in patients with epidermodysplasia verruciformis. Arch Dermatol 121: 84.

28. Sidky YA, Auerbach R /1975/, Lymphocyte-induced angiogenesis: a quantitative and sensitive assay of the graft-vs-host reaction. J Exp Med 141:1084.

**Papillomaviruses: Molecular and Clinical Aspects, pages 85–100**


# PAPILLOMAVIRUSES FROM EPIDERMODYSPLASIA VERRUCIFORMIS PATIENTS AND RENAL ALLOGRAFT RECIPIENTS[1]

Herbert Pfister, Thomas Iftner, and Pawel G. Fuchs

Institut für Klinische Virologie der Universität Erlangen-Nürnberg, D-8520 Erlangen, F.R. Germany

ABSTRACT Human papillomaviruses (HPV) from epidermodysplasia verruciformis (ev) patients show a complex relationship, which offers a chance to correlate DNA structure and biological functions such as oncogenic potential. The nucleotide sequence of HPV8, which is closely associated with skin cancers in ev, was analyzed and showed a number of special features. Of interest are promoter consensus sequences for RNA polymerase II and III within the putative transforming region and striking sequence homology with Epstein-Barr virus (EBV). On the protein level, the theoretical E4 protein of HPV8 turned out to be related with the EBV specific EBNA2, which is probably involved in immortalization. Apart from the ev syndrome, DNA of "ev viruses" was detected in two out of five keratoacanthomas and in a wart biopsy of one immunosuppressed patient among 17 patients tested. The latter indicates that "ev-viruses" are not prevalent in transplant recipients, who also harbored HPV2, 3, 4, 10, and 16. The presence of DNA of "ev viruses" in keratoacanthomas is noteworthy. It may point to an etiologic role and demonstrates infections with these viruses apart from ev.

[1]This work was supported by the Deutsche Forschungsgemeinschaft (SFB 118).

## INTRODUCTION

The disease epidermodysplasia verruciformis (ev) offers peculiar aspects, which are unique to the papillomavirus field. Some of these properties may be very helpful to study questions of general interest, e.g. the molecular basis of malignant conversion of papillomavirus induced tumors, the reservoir of papillomaviruses, and their evolution.

Ev-patients suffer from congenital defects in cell-mediated immunity, which make them prone to infection with a large number of papillomavirus types (1). Most of these viruses were never isolated from wart patients with a well preserved immune response. The DNAs of 14 "ev-specific" human papillomaviruses (HPV) were cloned and characterized during the past few years, namely HPV5, 8, 9, 12, 14, 15, 17, 19-25 (2-6). The viruses induce very flat warts and macular lesions, which arise first during childhood. They gradually spread over the skin of extremities, head and trunk and usually persist life-long (7). About a quarter of the ev patients develop squamous cell skin carcinomas on average 20 years after the onset of verrucosis. It was of special interest to note that only few HPV types persist in the malignant tumors, i.e. mainly HPV5 and 8 (for review, see 8). This may point to an increased cancerogenic potential of these viruses.

All "ev-specific" HPVs are more or less closely related. Some isolates show up to 30% DNA cross-hybridization under stringent conditions. The homology between two virus types may be very high within one DNA fragment and rather low for the rest of the genome and different viruses may share homology in different regions of their genomes (6). The close and complex relationship among "ev viruses" offers a chance to compare DNAs from viruses, which persist in carcinomas, with those, which were only observed in benign tumors, and to look for sequences, which might be relevant for the biological differences. In this paper we will discuss the nucleotide sequence of HPV8, which was of special interest due to its association with skin cancer.

The origin of the heterogeneity of "ev viruses" is not clear at the moment. Isolates from different countries, which are far apart, show very similar DNA cleavage patterns (3, 5, 6, 9), which suggests that individual types exist as defined entities around the world. The low number of ev cases thereby necessarily raises the question as to the reservoir of these viruses. The most likely explanation seems to be that "ev viruses" are spread by inapparent infections, and in doing so, infection of people with specific immune defects would lead to an apparent disease.

It has been repeatedly speculated that HPV types from ev patients play a role in wart and cancer developments in immunosuppressed transplant recipients. This is why immune defects play an important role in the pathogenesis of epidermodysplasia itself (1). Warts appear in 42% of renal allograft recipients after more than one year of immunosuppression (10). Squamous cell carcinomas are 60 times as frequent as in the normal population in contrast to basal cell carcinomas, which are not significantly elevated (11). The skin cancers were observed to appear in beds of epidermodysplasia like warts (10) and last not least HPV5 DNA was demonstrated in benign (12) and malignant (13) lesions from two renal allograft recipients. We looked for "ev-specific" papillomaviruses in a number of immunosuppressed patients and these data will be presented in the second part of this paper.

## RESULTS AND DISCUSSION

### 1. Genome Organization of HPV8

Cloned DNA of HPV8 (2) was sequenced according to Maxam and Gilbert (14). The sequence was evaluated by means of the program of the University of Wisconsin, Genetics Computer Group (15). The general organization turned out to be very similar to other papillomaviruses (16). Two large open reading frames L1 and L2 appear in the late region, which is supposed to code for structural proteins. The L1 frame of HPV8 showed a high degree of homology with the L1 frames of previously sequenced papillomaviruses. The L2 frames of HPV8 and cottontail rabbit papillomavirus (CRPV) also were surprisingly similar whereas gaps of increasing size had to be introduced to align the L2 frames of HPV1a, HPV6b, and bovine papillomavirus (BPV) 1. The L2 relationship correlates with the tissue tropism of the viruses as pointed out previously (17). HPV8, 1, and CRPV infect the skin, HPV6 induces papillomas on the mucosa, and BPV1 infects both fibroblasts and keratinocytes (8).

Within the early region of HPV8 the carboxy terminal

moiety of reading frame E1 revealed the highest degree of homology with other papillomaviruses. Two overlapping reading frames (E2 and E4) were disclosed between E1 and L2 as usual (Fig. 1). Regarding the oncogenic potential

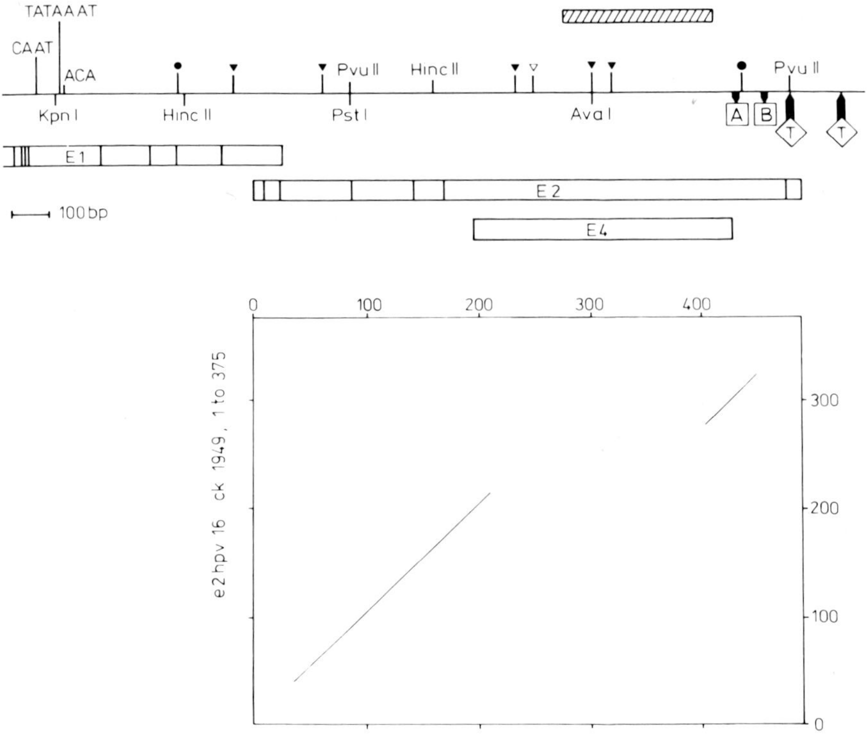


FIGURE 1. Organization of a putative transforming region of HPV8. The open reading frames E2 and E4 and part of E1 are depicted beneath the physical map. Black lines in the open bars indicate the positions of the translational initiation codon ATG. Transcription control elements are indicated by the following symbols: (CAAT) CAT-box, (TATAAAT) Tata-box, (ACA) cap site, (▽) splice donor sequence, (▼) splice acceptor sequence, (●) polyadenylation signal, ( A B ) RNA polymerase III promoter ( T ) RNA polymerase III terminator sequence. The region, which is displayed by the hatched bar, is rich in repeat elements. A comparison of the amino acid sequences of E2 of HPV8 and HPV16 (20) by dot plot analysis is shown in the lower part.

of HPV8 this genome region is of special interest. The corresponding segment of BPV1 DNA was shown to harbor transforming activity and the E2/E4 area is actively transcribed in BPV1 and HPV6 induced tumors (18, 19). We translated reading frame E2 of HPV8 into a theoretical protein, which was then compared with translations from DNA sequences of HPV1, 6, 16, CRPV, and BPV1. The amino-terminal moieties and the carboxytermini are highly conserved, which is clearly indicative of a common biological function of E2 proteins. The homology is entirely lost, however, in that area, which overlaps with reading frame E4 (Fig. 1). The theoretical E4 proteins of the different papillomaviruses also show hardly any relationship, which points to a virus type specific role.

HPV8 showed a number of special features in and around the E2/E4 region. They concerned DNA structure, transcription control signals, and the information of reading frame E4 and are dealt with in the following.

## 2. Direct and Inverted Repeats in HPV8 DNA Coding for E4

An unusual cluster of repeat elements was observed in the DNA sequences coding for reading frame E4 (Fig. 2). Three inverted repeats appear close together, which may form three stems of considerable length with relatively small non-homologous loops. The sequences are not reminiscent of insertion elements; for example there are no

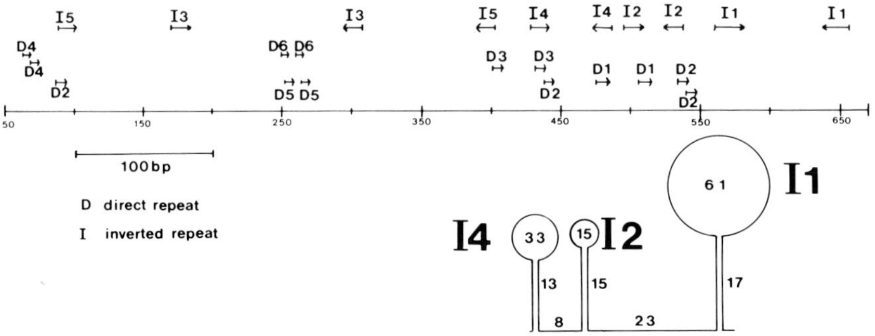


FIGURE 2. Localization of direct and inverted repeats within the DNA sequence of reading frame E4. The repeats are numbered according to size. The number of nucleotides in loops, stems, and intervals is indicated in the schematic drawing.

direct repeats flanking the stems. The structures may serve as signals but their function cannot be evaluated at the moment. A 9 base pair direct repeat (CCCCCACCA = D2 of Fig. 2), which was found five times in HPV8 (four times in E4 and once in L2) appears 14times within the BamHI Y fragment of Epstein-Barr Virus B95-8 (21). These common direct repeats are part of an extensive sequence homology between both viruses, which amounts to 38% within 650 bp. The DNA relationship is also reflected on the protein level (see below).

3. Transcription Control Signals Close to E2

A TATAAAT sequence, which is diagnostic of a RNA-polymerase II promoter, is located 513 nucleotides in front of reading frame E2. It is preceded by a CAAT box 55 nucleotides upstream and a potential cap site ACA follows 6 nucleotides downstream. There is evidence for a functional promoter in BPV1 at a comparable position (22) although the nucleotide sequence does not perfectly correspond to the consensus sequence. It may be of interest that HPV16, which is closely associated with cervical carcinomas, reveals a classical polymerase II promoter in front of E2 like HPV8 (20). An analysis of RNA transcripts must decide whether these sequences represent active promoters, which trigger the gene expression of the putative transforming regions.

Potential polyadenylation recognition signals defining the 3'-ends of m-RNAs were observed downstream of HPV8 reading frames E4 and E2.

The 3'-end of the early region of HPV8 revealed sequences, which may be transcribed by RNA polymerase III (Fig. 1). Promoters of that enzyme were well characterized within t-RNA genes and were shown to consist of two blocks being 29 to 68 bp apart (23). Fig. 3 shows the striking similarity between HPV8 sequences and the t-RNA promoter consensus sequence. Potential terminators of RNA polymerase III transcription are located 70 bp and 224 bp downstream from the second promoter block. Only HPV1 among the sequenced papillomaviruses has comparable signals, which point to a gene transcribed by polymerase III, and they are located in a homologous region of the genome. Preliminary experiments with DNAs of HPV8, 1, 6 16, 18, and BPV1 failed to obtain polymerase III transcripts in a cell-free system derived from Hela cells

```
                 29-68bp
TRRYNNARYGGNAG --------- GTTCGA ---------- oligo (dT)
                  53bp                70bp                 146bp
TGGTTCGAGGGGAG --------- GTTCAA ---------- TTCTGTTT ----------- TTTTT
```

FIGURE 3. Consensus sequence of t-RNA (RNA polymerase III) promoters (23) and below homologous sequences of HPV8 (for localization, see Figure 1). The oligo (dT) stretches are likely to represent transcription terminators. R = Purine, Y = Pyrimidine

(Fuchs and Dingermann, unpublished) but this may well be due to cell-type specific restrictions.

## 4. HPV8 Reading Frame E4 is Related to Epstein-Barr Virus EBNA2

Comprising 687 nucleotides, reading frame E4 of HPV8 is larger than those of other papillomaviruses sequenced so far. Over the entire length, there is no ATG start codon for protein translation, however. Whereas most papillomaviruses have start codons right at the beginning of E4, HPV16 also lacks an ATG (20). Expression could be achieved in case of HPV8 and 16 by splicing ATG containing exons to the 5'-ends of the reading frames E4. In this regard, it is interesting to note that the most abundant RNA from BPV1 transformed cells is composed of two exons; one very short exon is derived from the beginning of E2, and the second one starts at a splice acceptor site in the middle of E4 (22). Potential splice acceptor sites at comparable positions could also be disclosed within E4 of HPV8 (Fig. 1).

To get an idea if E4 of HPV8 may be coding indeed, the codon usage within the three possible translation frames was analyzed, using the L1 gene of HPV8 as a standard (24). The E4 frame codon usage was very similar to L1 except for the amino terminus (Fig. 4). The position where the codon usage method suggests the beginning of a coding region coincides with a potential splice acceptor site, which might serve as the start point of an exon covering the rest of E4. These data are very much in line with the above-mentioned hypothesis on the expression of E4. The E2 frame codon usage was also similar to L1 for

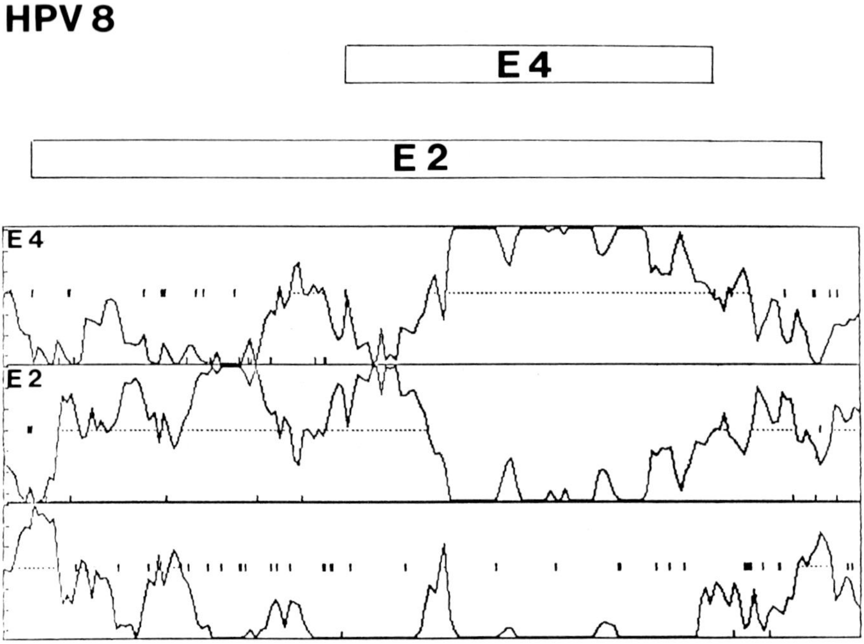


FIGURE 4. Test for coding genes in the E2/E4 region of HPV8 by the codon usage method (24) using the HPV8 L1 gene as a standard. The three tested reading frames harbor E4, E2, or no major open reading frame. If the curve is above the dotted lines, the respective reading frame is likely to be coding.

the amino terminal moiety and for the carboxy terminus (Fig. 4). The drop in the correlation in the central part may be partially explained by the computer program's tendency to exaggerate in favor of one reading frame. In summary, the codon usage analysis suggests that both E2 and E4 might code, E4 at least downstream from an internal splice acceptor signal.

The E4 protein of HPV8 has a remarkably high content of proline (37%), which implies a hydrophobic character, a bizarre tertiary structure, and an anomalous electrophoretic migration in SDS-polyacrylamide gels. Looking for related proteins we compared E4 with the translation product from the open reading frame within the Epstein-Barr Virus (EBV) BamHI Y DNA fragment, which showed extensive sequence homology with HPV8 DNA (see above). This reading frame is very likely to code for the EBV-specific nuclear antigen EBNA2. Size differences between reading frames of various EBV strains correlate with the size of the respective EBNA2 proteins and expression of the reading frame in bacterial vectors leads to proteins reacting with EBNA2 specific antisera (25, 26). Fig. 5 shows a comparison between E4 of HPV8 and EBNA2 of EBV B95-8 and AG876. There are basically three areas of significant homology where the sequences can be aligned without introduction of major gaps. In the first segment homology is mainly based on proline repeats, whereas in the second and third segments the three proteins share unique sequences. A number of residues are common to E4 and both EBNA2 proteins. In some positions there is only homology between HPV8 and B95-8 and in others between HPV8 and AG876. The relationship is more obvious between HPV8 and B95-8. The sequence homologies in addition to common proline clusters are important in terms of common antigenic determinants, and increase the significance of the over-all relationship.

We checked the NBRF data bank for further proteins related to HPV8 E4. A degree of homology comparable to that with EBNA2 was only observed with a proline-rich phosphoprotein, which was isolated from human saliva (27). The stretch of homology was shorter, however, than with EBNA2.

## 5. Perspectives from the HPV8 DNA Sequence

Some aspects of the nucleotide sequence of HPV8 should be examined in more detail. Possible RNA polymerase III transcripts might play a regulatory role in viral and cellular protein synthesis as demonstrated recently for adenovirus-associated $RNA_I$ (28). A classical promoter consensus sequence in front of E2 and the lack of an initiation codon for translation within reading frame E4 are common features of HPV8 and HPV16, which are both closely associated with malignant tumors. The significance of these properties should be evaluated.

The relationship between HPV8 and EBV is of special interest. EBV is pathogenic in humans, it immortalizes B-lymphocytes and is regularly associated with anaplastic nasopharyngeal carcinomas (29). The EBNA2 protein seems to play an important role in EBV induced transformation.

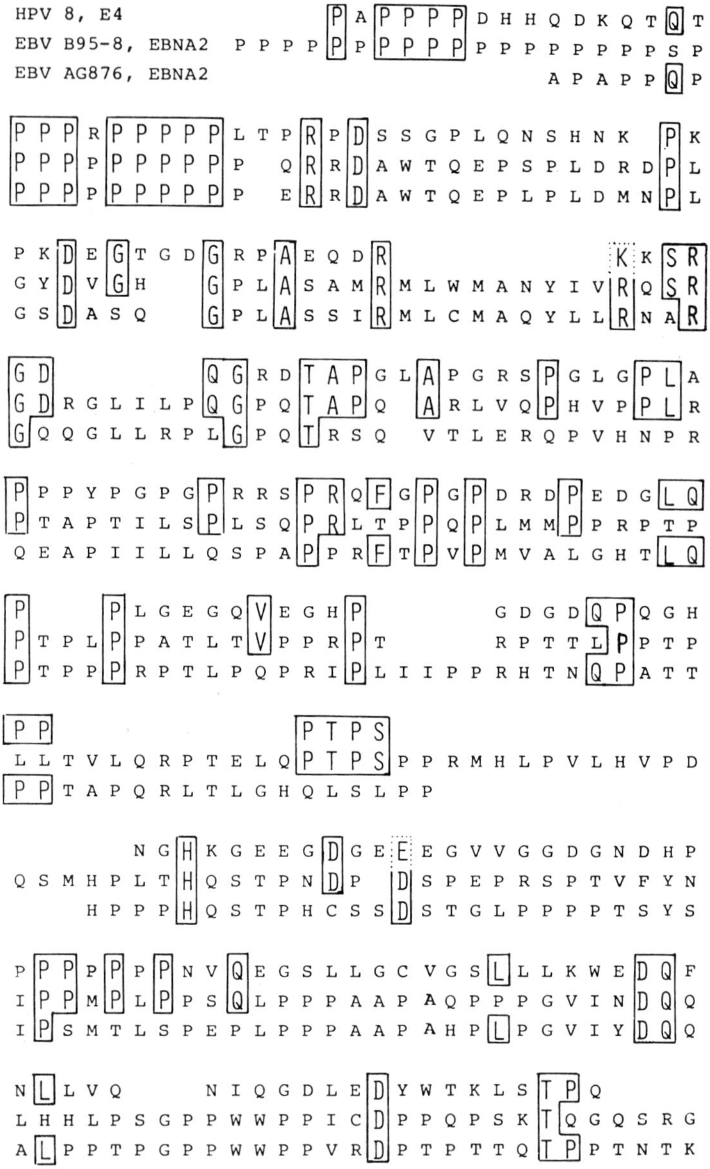


FIGURE 5. Comparison of translation products of reading frames E4 of HPV8 and U2 (EBNA2) of EBV B95-8 and AG 876 (25). Amino acids are given in the standard one-letter code. Boxes indicate identical residues. Chemically similar amino acids are framed by dotted lines.

It is expressed in latently infected cells (30). The non-transforming EBV isolate P3HR1 has undergone a deletion affecting the EBNA2 gene (31) and there is no EBNA2 protein detectable in virus-producing P3HR1 cells as would be expected (25). Finally, superinfection of Raji cells with P3HR1 leads to transformation competent recombinants (32), which have regained the sequence deleted in P3HR1. It remains to be established if the homologies between EBV and HPV8 reflect a common transforming principle.

## 6. Papillomaviruses from Renal Allograft Recipients and Occurrence of "EV Viruses"

We examined wart biopsies from 17 patients, who were immunosuppressed for at least three months and up to 8 years by systemic application of corticoids and immurec or endoxan. Total DNA was isolated from the biopsies and HPV-DNA was disclosed and characterized by Southern blot hybridization with radioactively labelled reference DNAs for HPV1 to HPV26. In the case of tiny biopsies, total wart DNA was labelled by nick translation and hybridized to HPV reference DNAs, which were blotted to a nitrocellulose filter. HPV2 was detected twice, HPV3 once, HPV4 and HPV10 twice, respectively, and HPV16 once. Labelled DNA from a common wart reacted strongly with DNAs of HPV2, 3, 10, and 26 and a group of "ev viruses", namely HPV14, 19, 20, 21, and 25 (Fig. 6). The biopsy is likely to harbor more than one HPV type; probably at least one virus related to HPV3 and 10, which do cross-hybridize themselves (8), and one member of the familiy of "ev viruses". A more precise classification was impossible because of the lack of DNA.

We tested for papillomavirus-specific sequences in DNA from 10 squamous cell skin carcinomas and five keratoacanthomas of immunologically inconspicuous patients. HPV16 DNA was detected in two patients in a carcinoma from the skin and from the mucosa of the lower lip, respectively. HPV-DNA was furthermore revealed in keratoacanthomas of two patients by hybridization with labelled HPV20 DNA. One of these cases was followed further. Labelled biopsy DNA hybridized with reference DNAs of HPV12, 14, 19, 20, 21, and 25. The restriction enzyme cleavage pattern of the viral DNA was revealed by Southern blot hybridization with HPV25 DNA (Fig. 7). BamHI cut once,

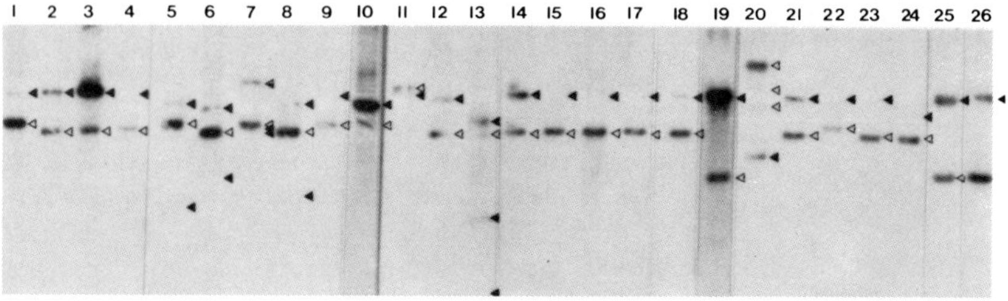


FIGURE 6. Southern blot hybridization of reference DNAs for HPV1 to 26 with $^{32}P$-labelled DNA from a common wart of an immunosuppressed transplant recipient. Reference DNAs were cleaved with appropriate restriction enzymes to separate viral (◀) from vector (◁) DNA. Hybridization was carried out in 40% formamide and 5 x SSC at 37°C.

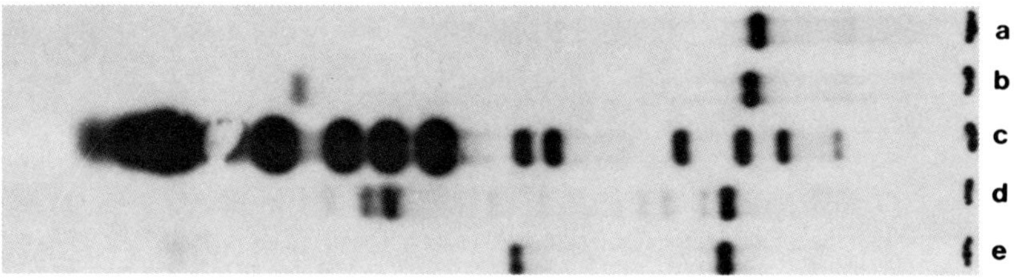


FIGURE 7. Cleavage patterns of papillomavirus-specific DNA from a human keratoacanthoma after digest with BamHI (a), EcoRI (b), BglII (d), and HindIII (e) as revealed by hybridization with $^{32}P$-labelled HPV25 DNA under stringent conditions (40% formamide, 5 x SSC, 37°C). Lane c shows labelled length standards: Lambda DNA cut with HindIII and ØX174 DNA cut with HaeIII.

EcoRI twice, HindIII three times, and BglII four times. The cleavage patterns are different from those of known "ev viruses", although the close relationship with HPV19 is obvious from DNA-DNA hybridization.

The above data suggest that "ev-specific" papillomaviruses are not prevalent in transplant recipients. Only one among 17 lesions tested harbored a virus, which seemed to be closely related to HPV19. This result may not be too surprising, for the absolute incidence of skin carcinomas in immunosuppressed patients is still very low when compared with the ev-situation. Other HPV types like HPV2 and 16 might also play a role in malignant conversion. HPV2 was demonstrated in cases of Bowen's disease of the skin (33, de Villiers EM, pers. comm.). HPV16 DNA was detected in Bowen's disease (34, Pfister H, unpublished), and in cancers of the skin as well as the genital and oral mucosa (35, this paper).

The association between an "ev-specific" HPV and keratoacanthomas was observed for the first time. More biopsies must be examined to see if this indicates an etiologic relationship, or by the chance persistence of HPV DNA in these tumor tissues. Irrespective of the answer to this question, it must be noted that HPV types from ev patients do occur in immunologically competent persons. This is a first step to prove the assumed widespread distribution of these viruses.

## ACKNOWLEDGMENTS

We are indebted to P. Farrell for running the codon usage program, to A. Gassenmaier and H. Schell for providing tumor biopsies, to K. Seedorf and O. Danos for sending the HPV16 and CRPV sequences prior to publication, and to J. Stoerker for a critical reading of the manuscript.

## REFERENCES

1. Jablonska S, Orth G, and Lutzner MA (1982). Immunopathology of papillomavirus-induced tumors in different tissues. Springer Semin Immunopathol 5:33.
2. Pfister H, Nürnberger F, Gissmann L, and zur Hausen H (1981). Characterization of a human papillomavirus from epidermodysplasia verruciformis lesions of a patient from Upper Volta, Int J Cancer 27:645.
3. Kremsdorf D, Jablonska S, Favre M, and Orth G (1982). Biochemical characterization of two types of human papilloma viruses associated with epidermodysplasia verruciformis. J Virol 43:436.
4. Kremsdorf D, Jablonska S, Favre M, and Orth G (1983). Human papillomaviruses associated with epidermodysplasia verruciformis: II. Molecular cloning and bio-

chemical characterization of human papillomavirus 3a, 8, 10, and 12 genomes. J Virol 48:340.
5. Kremsdorf D, Favre M, Jablonska S, Obalek S, Rueda LA, Lutzner MA, Blanchet-Bardon C, van Voorst Vader PC, and Orth G (1984). Molecular cloning and characterization of the genomes of nine newly recognized human papillomavirus types associated with epidermodysplasia verruciformis. J Virol 52:1013.
6. Gassenmaier A, Lammel M, and Pfister H (1984). Molecular cloning and characterization of the DNAs of human papillomaviruses 19, 20, and 25 from a patient with epidermodysplasia verruciformis. J Virol 52:1019.
7. Lutzner MA (1978). Epidermodysplasia verruciformis. Bull Cancer 65:169.
8. Pfister H (1984). Biology and biochemistry of papillomaviruses. Rev Physiol Biochem Pharmacol 99:111.
9. Pfister H, Gassenmaier A, Nürnberger F, Stüttgen G (1983). HPV5 DNA in a carcinoma of epidermodysplasia verruciformis patient infected with various human papillomavirus types. Cancer Res 43:1436.
10. Koranda FC, Dehmel EM, Kahn G, and Penn I (1974). Cutaneous complications in immunosuppressed renal homograft recipients. JAMA 229:419.
11. Hoxtell EO, Mandel JS, Murray SS, Schuman LM, Goltz RW (1977). Incidence of skin carcinoma after renal transplantation. Arch Dermatol 113:436.
12. Lutzner M, Croissant O, Ducase M-F, Kreis H, Crosnier J, and Orth G (1980). A potentially oncogenic human papillomavirus (HPV-5) found in two renal allograft recipients. J Invest Dermatol 75:353.
13. Lutzner MA, Orth G, Dutronquay V, Ducase M-F, Kreis H, and Crosnier J (1983). Detection of human papillomavirus type 5 DNA in skin cancers of an immunosuppressed renal allograft recipient. Lancet 2:422.
14. Maxam AM, and Gilbert W (1980). Sequencing end-labelled DNA with base-specific chemical cleavages. Methods in Enzymology 65:499.
15. Devereux J, Haeberli P, and Smithies O (1984). A comprehensive set of sequence analysis programs for the VAX. Nucl Acids Res 12:387.
16. Pettersson U, Ahola H, Stenlund A, and Moreno-Lopez J (1985). Organization and expression of papillomavirus genomes. In Salzman NP, Howley P (eds): "The Papovaviridae: The Papillomaviruses", New York: Plenum Press, in press.

17. Danos O, Giri I, Thierry F, and Yaniv M (1984). Papillomavirus genomes: Sequences and consequences. J Invest Dermatol 83:7s.
18. Freese UK, Schulte P, and Pfister H (1982). Papilloma virus-induced tumors contain a virus-specific transcript. Virology 117:257.
19. Lehn H, Ernst T-M, and Sauer G (1984). Transcription of episomal papillomavirus DNA in human condylomata acuminata and Buschke-Löwenstein tumours. J gen Virol 65:2003.
20. Seedorf K, Krämer G, Dürst M, Suhai S, and Röwekamp WG (1985). Human papillomavirus type 16 DNA sequence. Virology, in press.
21. Baer R, Bankier AT, Biggin MD, Deininger PL, Farrell PJ, Gibson TJ, Hatfull G, Hudson GS, Satchwell SC, Sèguin C, Tuffnell PS, and Barrell G (1984). DNA sequence and expression of the B95-8 Epstein-Barr virus genome. Nature 310:207.
22. Stenlund A, Zabielski J, Ahola H, Moreno-Lopez J, and Pettersson U (1985). The messenger RNAs from the transforming region of bovine papilloma virus type 1. J Mol Biol, in press.
23. Sharp S, Schaack J, Cooley L, Johnson-Burke D, and Söll D (1985). Structure and transcription of eucaryotic tRNA genes. Crit Rev Biochem, in press.
24. Staden R (1984). Measurements of the effects that coding for a protein has on a DNA sequence and their use for finding genes. Nucl Acids Res 12:551.
25. Dambaugh T, Hennessy K, Chamnankit L, and Kieff E (1984). U2-region of Epstein Barr Virus DNA may encode EB-nuclear antigen 2. Proc Natl Acad Sci USA 81:7632.
26. Hennessy K, and Kieff E (1985). A second nuclear protein is encoded by Epstein-Barr virus in latent infection. Science 227:1238.
27. Wong RSC, and Bennick A (1980). The primary structure of a salivary calcium-binding proline-rich phosphoprotein (protein C), a possible precursor of a related salivary protein A. J Biol Chem 255:5943.
28. Reichel PA, Merrick WC, Siekierka J, and Mathews MB (1985). Regulation of a protein synthesis initiation factor by adenovirus virus-associated RNA. Nature 313:196.
29. zur Hausen H (1980). The role of Epstein-Barr virus in Burkitt's lymphoma and nasopharyngeal carcinoma. In

Rapp F (ed): "Oncogenic herpesviruses", Cleveland, CRC press, Vol. II, p 13.
30. Hennessy K, and Kieff E (1983). One of two Epstein-Barr virus nuclear antigens contains a glycine-alanine copolymer domain. Proc Natl Acad Sci USA 80:5665.
31. Heller M, Dambaugh T, and Kieff E (1981). Epstein-Barr virus DNA. IX. Variation among viral DNAs from producer and nonproducer infected cells. J Virol 38: 632.
32. Fresen KO, Cho M-S, and zur Hausen H (1980). Recombination between Epstein-Barr virus genomes. Viruses in naturally occuring cancers. Cold Spring Harbor Conf Cell Proliferation 7:35.
33. Pfister H, and Haneke E (1984). Demonstration of human papilloma virus type 2 DNA in Bowen's disease. Arch Dermatol Res 276:123.
34. Ikenberg H, Gissmann L, Gross G, Grussendorf-Conen E-I, and zur Hausen H (1983). Human papillomavirus type-16-related DNA in genital Bowen's disease and in bowenoid papulosis. Int J Cancer 32:563.
35. Dürst M, Gissmann L, Ikenberg H, and zur Hausen H (1983). A papillomavirus DNA from a cervical carcinoma and its prevalence in cancer biopsy samples from different geographic regions. Proc Natl Acad Sci USA 80: 3812.

Papillomaviruses: Molecular and Clinical Aspects, pages 101–122


# PRESENCE AND POSSIBLE INVOLVEMENT OF HPV DNA IN PREMALIGNANT AND MALIGNANT TUMORS[1]

Ronald S. Ostrow, Karen Zachow, Dawn Weber, Takashi Okagaki[2], Michio Fukushima[2], Barbara A. Clark[2], Leo B. Twiggs[2], and Anthony J. Faras

Department of Microbiology, University of Minnesota
Minneapolis, Minnesota 55455

ABSTRACT We have recently completed a survey of over 400 neoplasias from a wide variety of anatomical sites for the presence of HPV-related nucleotide sequences employing Southern blot and in situ hybridization procedures. Two groups of neoplasias consistently exhibited the presence of HPV-related nucleotide sequences: 1) squamous cell carcinomas from patients with the chronic flat wart disease syndrome epidermodysplasia verruciformis (EV), and 2) premalignant and malignant tumors of the anogenital tract. In the former group of neoplasias, all of the primary and metastic carcinomas tested contained HPV DNA, indicating the association of HPV DNA with 100% of the tumors. In the latter neoplasias, the presence of HPV-related sequences has been established in a variety of premalignant and malignant tumors to varying degrees. Of the 250 cases of cervical, vaginal and vulvar premalignant and invasive lesions analyzed for the present of HPV DNA, the presence of these sequences could be identified in 40-80% of biopsies from patients exhibiting mild, moderate and severe dysplasia of the uterine cervix, Bowen's disease and Bowenoid atypia,

[1]This work was supported by grants from the NIH (CA 25462) and the Leukemia Research Fund of the University of Minnesota.
[2]Departments of Obstetrics and Gynecology and Laboratory Medicine and Pathology, University of Minnesota, Minneapolis, Minnesota 55455

condylomatous carcinoma of the vulva, vaginal dysplasia and carcinoma in situ, invasive carcinoma of the uterine cervix and frank invasive squamous cell carcinoma of the vulva. Although this strong association of HPV with these malignancies makes a compelling case for HPV as a causative agent, this data alone does not establish an unequivocal role of the virus in the development of these malignancies. DNA transfection studies using molecularly cloned HPV-5 DNA obtained from a carcinoma from a patient with EV indicated that HPV DNA exhibited oncogenic potential and therefore the capacity to facilitate malignant progression.
Epidemiological studies have indicated high risk of HPV infection of the genitalia among the sexually promiscuous and sexual partners of infected patients, suggesting that sexual contact may reflect one mode of transmission. We have obtained data supporting this contention by demonstrating the presence of HPV DNA in semen from patients in high risk groups exhibiting debilitating chronic wart disease.

## INTRODUCTION

One of our primary objectives in papillomavirus (PV) research has been to determine the association of human papillomavirus (HPV) DNA with various human cancers, particularly those in which there is a high correlation with chronic or recurring wart disease. Our ultimate goal is to demonstrate the possible involvement of HPV in human malignancies. Several disease syndromes that involve wart disease and associated neoplasia have expedited the studies of papillomaviruses and their oncogenic potential.

The study of patients with a rare, chronic flat wart disease known as epidermodysplasia verruciformis (EV) has been particularly interesting. Approximately 30% of these patients develop skin carcinomas (1). In some cases, this disease appears to be an autosomal recessive trait that often runs in families, particularly where parental consanguinity exists (1). Although two types of HPV, HPV-5 and HPV-3, are predominantly associated with EV, there are about a dozen HPV types that have been found only in connection with this disease syndrome (2-8). Due to their presence in malignant tissues, some of these types (HPV-5, 8 and 14) are thought to have a higher oncogenic potential than the others (9,10). These patients seem to be susceptible to more than a single HPV type as well, perhaps due to their lowered immune competence (11,12).

Genital neoplasias offer a unique opportunity to examine the relationship of HPV to the entire spectrum of benign, premalignant and malignant tumors. The epidemiology of cervical cancer has long indicated the venereal nature of this disease (13). The suggestion that an infectious agent is involved is further supported by the high correlation of penile condylomata in male sexual partners of women with cervical premalignant lesions (14). Although many different types of HPV have been observed in genital tumors, HPV-16 and 18 are most often associated with high grade neoplasias (15-18). This implies that these types may have a high oncogenic potential. The most dramatic fact is that HPV nucleic acids have been found in an overwhelming majority of all genital neoplasias studied throughout the world (15,16,19-21). While one cannot rule out the possibility that HPV may simply be a passenger virus in an immunologically impaired host, these correlations along with the known oncogenic potential of papillomaviruses in vitro (22) and in animal systems (23-26) make a strong case for a direct role of HPV in human oncogenesis.

Two animal systems demonstrate the oncogenic potential of papillomaviruses. In cottontail rabbits, naturally occuring PV induced warts progress to carcinomas in 25% of the animals studied, while warts induced in domestic rabbits (not natural hosts) progress to malignancies in 3 out of 4 cases (23,24). This indicates that an important co-factor is host response. Also, the use of carcinogenic hydrocarbons dramatically increases the rate of malignant progression in both hosts (27,28). Similar evidence for the effect of co-carcinogens is observed in cattle where alimentary tract papillomas progress to malignancy when brakenfern is consumed (29). BPV-4 is usually associated with these lesions indicating that various bovine papillomavirus types may have different oncogenic potentials (30).

Co-carcinogens involved in HPV associated cancers include ultraviolet light with EV patients (31) and smoking with genital neoplasias (32). The host immune response probably plays a key role in human wart formation and neoplastic progression (33,34). EV patients usually have impaired immune responses (1) and immunosuppressed renal transplant patients have a high incidence of both wart disease and skin cancer (35-37). Some renal transplant recipients also appear susceptible to HPV-5 (38,39). Host response, or perhaps even occupational influences, may be responsible for the chronic and recurring nature of the wart disease seen in meathandlers (40,41) and HPV-7 has thus far only been observed in this group of patients (42,43).

The oncogenic potential of PVs also have been implicated by active in vitro manipulations of viral genomes. For example, many in vitro studies have been completed on the well characterized BPV-1 genome. Functional areas have been localized in the genome that can induce, in cultured mouse cells, characteristics indicative of a malignant transformation (44). Here we summarize our studies on the association of HPVs with various malignant conditions and discuss the potential for future treatment based upon current molecular biological techniques.

## RESULTS

The most dramatic case for the oncogenic potential of a human papillomavirus was seen in the studies of EV patients. HPV-5 has repeatedly been found in most primary and metastatic malignancies of these patients (9). In DNA transfection studies, where the HPV genome was inserted into cultured mouse cells, the resultant cells exhibited many of the characteristics of malignantly transformed cells as listed below (Table 1) (22).

TABLE 1
HPV-5 DNA TRANSFECTION STUDIES

1. HPV-5 DNA transforms cells in culture
2. HPV-5 DNA transfected cells grow in soft agar
3. HPV-5 DNA transfected cells cause carcinomas in mice
4. Transformed cells in culture maintain 5-50 copies of HPV DNA
5. Tumors induced by single-cell clones contain HPV DNA

HPV-3, while also found in EV lesions, was rarely asso-

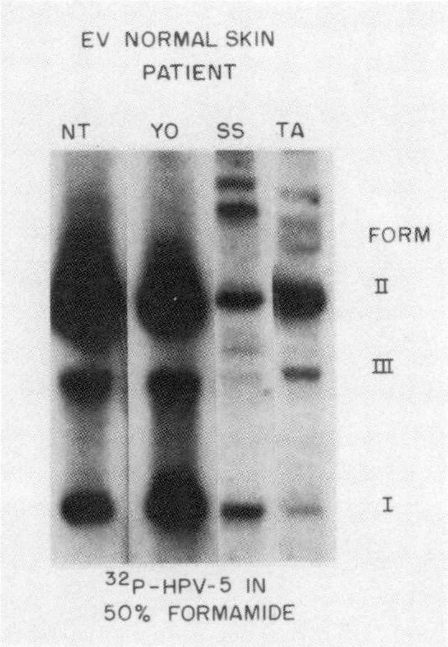


FIGURE 1. HPV-5 DNA in clinically normal skin of EV patients.

ciated with malignancies indicating that the oncogenic potential of HPVs may be type specific. The recurring and chronic nature of the disease may be explained in part by subclinical or latent infections. Similar to previous reports of HPV nucleic acids being detected in clinically normal tissue of laryngeal papilloma patients with active disease and patients in remission (45), we have found HPV-5 DNA in clinically normal skin of EV patients (Fig. 1). Other tissues may also harbor hidden HPV infections. In the cases of an EV patient and a meathandler with severe wart disease and chronic myelogenous leukemia, HPV-5 and HPV-2, respectively, were detected in semen samples (Fig. 2A, B, respectively). Interestingly, a clinically normal son of the EV patient also had evidence of HPV-5 in his semen. Our studies revealed that most of the HPV DNA in these samples could be localized in the seminal fluid. A sampling of semen from eleven clincally normal donors revealed no evidence of HPV DNA. The study of semen from potential high risk donors, such as sexual partners of women with genital neoplasias, is currently in progress.

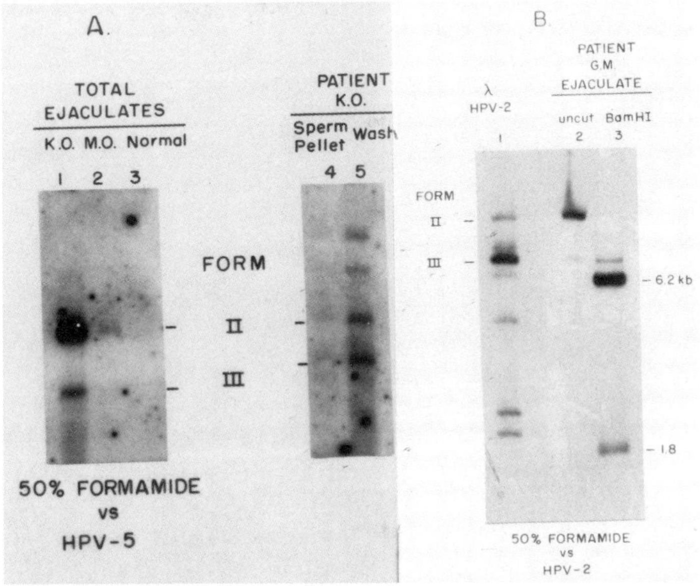


FIGURE 2. Presence of HPV DNA in human semen of high risk patients. A. EV patients, father (K.O.) and son (M.O.). B. Meathandler (G.M.)

Occasionally, Southern blot analysis reveals HPV genomes that are smaller than the wild type size of 8000 base pairs. Most often these are found in malignant tissues (9) but they have also been found in benign tumors. Three of these subgenomic forms of HPV-5 have been molecularly cloned and analyzed by various techniques including restriction endonuclease mapping and DNA sequencing (Fig. 3). By comparison of the HPV-5 genome with the completely sequenced HPV-1a genome (46), it is clear that all deletions map in the L1 or L2 transcriptional open reading frames know to code for the viral structural proteins. Despite the relatively high DNA and amino acid conservation of the L1 and L2 regions among papillomaviruses (47), this region may be genetically more active that it appears. HPV-27, a virus closely related to HPV-2, has been found to have a small section of the late region closely related to HPV-6 by hybridization analysis and thus may represent evidence for a recombinational event (Fig. 4).

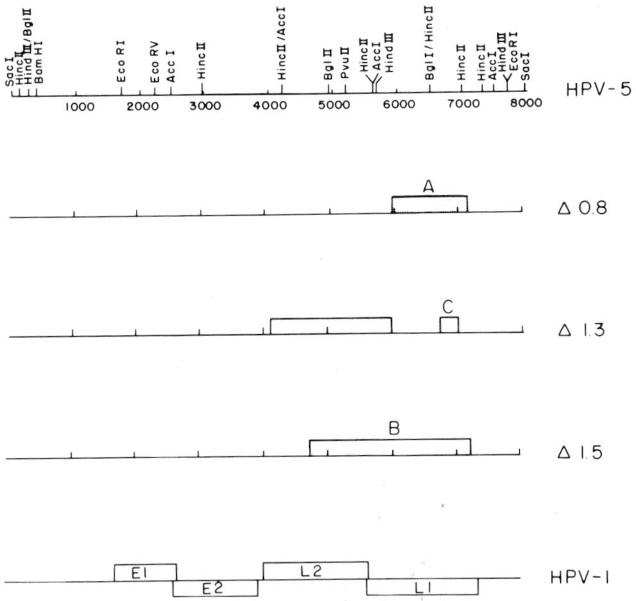


FIGURE 3. Restriction endonuclease map of HPV-5 and localization of deletions in molecularly cloned mutant genomes.

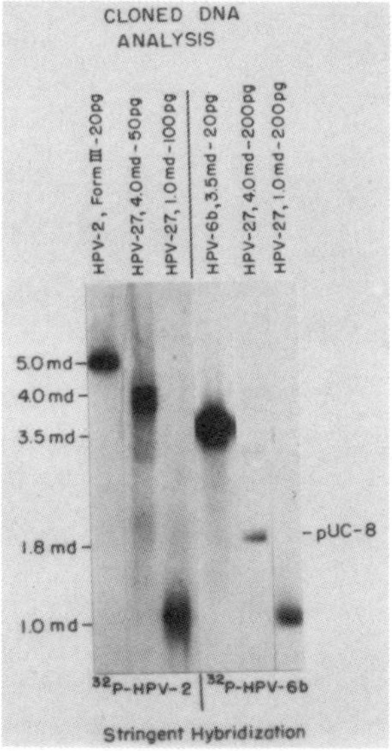


FIGURE 4. Hybridization of small Bam HI fragment of HPV-27 with both HPV-2 and HPV-6.

The study of the association of HPV nucleic acids with genital neoplasias has been greatly facilitated by the use of two highly sensitive detection techniques: Southern blot hybridization and in situ hybridization (48-51).

An example of the sensitivity of the former procedure is shown in Figure 5. Under stringent hybridization conditions, only HPV nucleic acids of a type similar to that of the probe will hybridize (e.g., both probe and sample are HPV-6). As few as 1 viral genome in 30 cells can be detected (0.03 copy/diploid cell equivalent). Under low stringency conditions of hybridization, other types of PV having as much as 30% base pair mismatch may also be detected (e.g., probe is HPV-6 and sample is HPV-1) (52). While the sensitivity of the low stringency conditions is about ten fold lower than the stringent conditions, the ability to detect any HPV type present at 1 copy/cell or greater using a single probe represents a very powerful tool. Using these techniques, we have examined various genital neoplasias ranging from benign to premalignant and malignant tumors (Table 2) (19-21,53,54). HPV nucleic acids were detected in 70-80% of all non-malignant tumors.

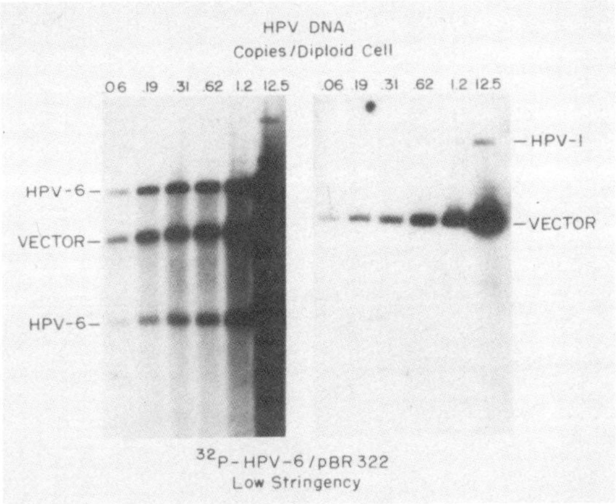


FIGURE 5. Hybridization of a homologous (HPV-6) or heterologous (HPV-1) DNA with radiolabelled HPV-6 under conditions of low stringency: A sensitivity test.

TABLE 2
ASSOCIATION OF HPV DNA WITH VARIOUS ANOGENITAL TUMORS

| | Benign | Dysplasia | CIS* | Verrucous Carcinoma | Invasion Associated with wart-like Pattern or CIS | Invasive Carcinoma |
|---|---|---|---|---|---|---|
| Vagina | 2/5 | 20/21 | 1/1 | 2/3 | | 2/4 |
| Cervix | 4/4 | 13/16 | 2/3 | | 1/1 | 3/17 |
| Vulva | 12/18 | | 16/22 | | 6/8 | 2/12 |
| Perineum | 15/17 | | 2/2 | | | |
| Penis | 3/5 | | | 1/1 | | |
| | 36/49 (73%) | 33/37 (89%) | 21/28 (75%) | 3/4 (75%) | 7/9 (78%) | 7/33 (21%) |

*This category in vulva, perineum and skin includes Bowen's disease, Bowenoid atypia, Bowenoid papullosis and Bowenoid dysplasia.

While our detection of HPV DNA in only about 20% of frank invasive carcinomas of the cervix by Southern blot hybridization is lower than that found in other laboratories (15,16), the correlation of HPV with the entire spectrum of genital neoplasia is quite compelling.

The technique of in situ hybridization involves conducting the nucleic acid hybridization directly on formalin-fixed paraffin embedded tisses that have been sectioned and placed on microscope slides. The cells are made permeable to the probe and, following hybridization and washing, the slides are coated with a photographic emulsion. Some examples of the results are shown in Figure 6. With relatively little effort, HPV DNA may be detected in sections of tissue (Fig. 6). Since this technique permits the detection of individually infected cells, it can, in fact, be a more sensitive technique than Southern blot hybridization where large amounts of normal cellular DNA may dilute a small amount of HPV DNA to below the level of detection. Using this technique, we have shown HPV positive cells in benign tumors, carcinoma in situ and invasive carcinomas of vulva and cervix (Fig. 7). We have begun to use this technique to examine a large number of invasive carcinomas

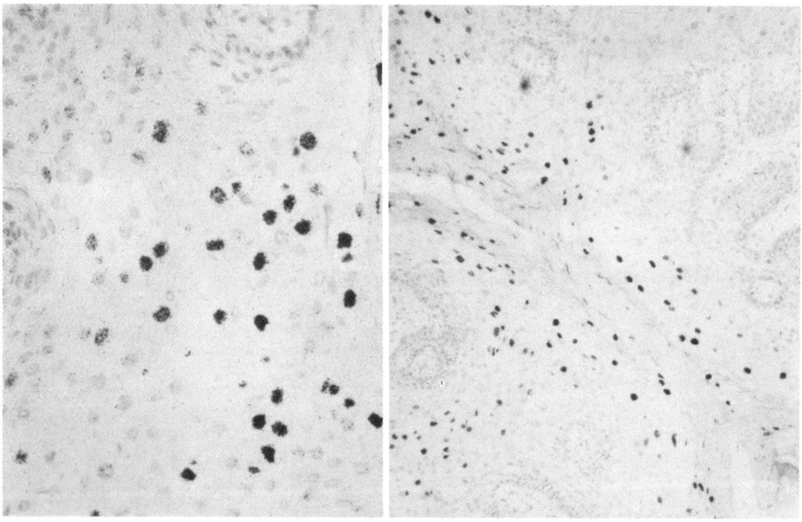

FIGURE 6. In situ hybridization with HPV-6 in condyloma accuminatum of vulva. 223x left, 93x right.

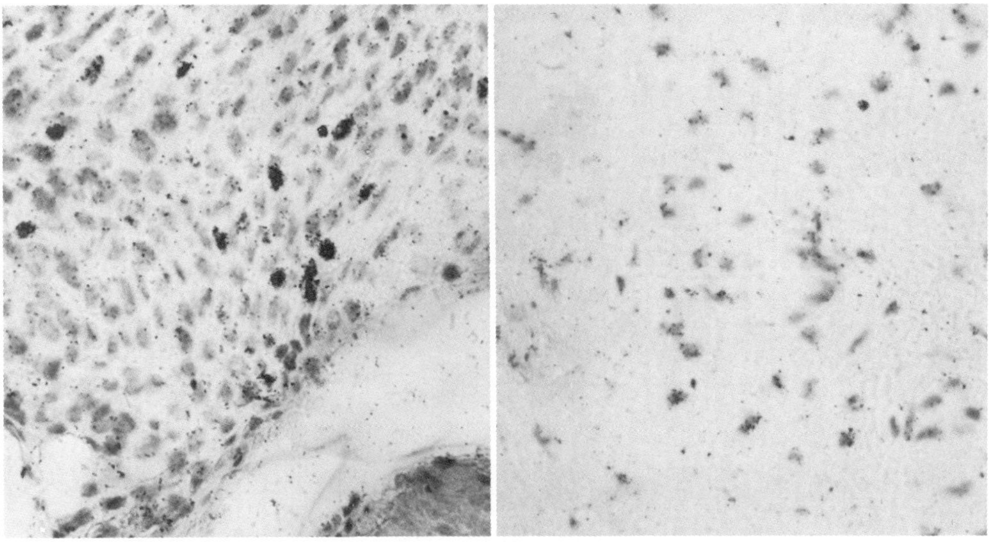

FIGURE 7. *In situ* hybridization with mixed probe in Bowen's disease (left) and connnective tissue in biopsy of cervical cancer (right).

(Table 3). The preliminary results of a comparison of the findings by *in situ* and by Southern blot analysis of the same tissue samples showed that HPV infected cells were detected by the former technique that had been missed by the latter. At this time, approximately 40% of invasive cervical cancers and 80% of invasive vulvar cancers appear to be positive for HPV. This increases the number of HPV-positive cervical cancers approximately two-fold when compared to the Southern blot hybridization procedure. Moreover, using this technique, we have detected positive cells not only in the squamous epithelium of invasive carcinomas, but also in connective tissue (Fig. 7). The significance of this preliminary finding is not clear but may be important in the surgical removal and possible reoccurrence of the lesions.

The strong association of HPV with the cancers decribed above facilitated a similar study of the possible association of HPV with other human cancers. Using Southern blot analysis in conjunction with a restriction enzyme that

TABLE 3
INVASIVE CARCINOMAS

| Sample | Tissue | Preliminary Results In situ | Preliminary Results Southern |
|---|---|---|---|
| 5774 | vulva | + | + HPV-6 |
| 1253 | vulva | + | - |
| 3169 | vulva | + | - |
| 454 | vulva | + | - |
| 5252 | vulva | + | ND |
| 4671 | vulva | + | ND |
| 1888 | vulva | - | - |
| 440 | vulva | + | - |
| 4761 | vulva | + | - |
| 4501 | vulva | - | ND |
| 833 | cervix | + | - |
| 6114 | cervix | - | - |
| 4292 | cervix | + | - |
| 4544 | cervix | +/- | - |
| 3313 | cervix | - | - |
| 373 | cervix | - | - |
| 2438 | cervix | - | - |
| 1015 | cervix | + | - |
| 3747 | cervix | + | - |
| 1866 | cervix | - | - |
| 214 | cervix | - | - |
| 1685 | cervix | + | - |
| 4507 | cervix | + | ND |
| 67A | cervix | +/- | ND |
| 4614 | cervix | + | ND |
| 3149 | cervix | - | - |
| 1050 | cervix | - | - |
| 4830 | cervix | - | ND |
| 67B | lymph node | + | ND |
| 133 | vagina | + | + |
| 441 | vagina | + | ND |

cleaves most HPV genomes only a few times, we have scanned extracts of more than 200 normal and tumor biopsies obtained from patients with malignancies (Table 4). We used a probe consisting of HPV-2, 6, 16 and 18 and low stringent hybridization conditions. Preliminary results indicate that a small proportion of these samples (about 1.8%) seem to be positive for HPV DNA (Fig. 8, Table 5). At least some of these appear to contain HPV-16 related nucleotide sequences under conditions of high stringency. The significance of this is not yet clear, but may be related to HPV susceptible tissues similar to the laryngeal and genital regions which are known to be HPV targets.

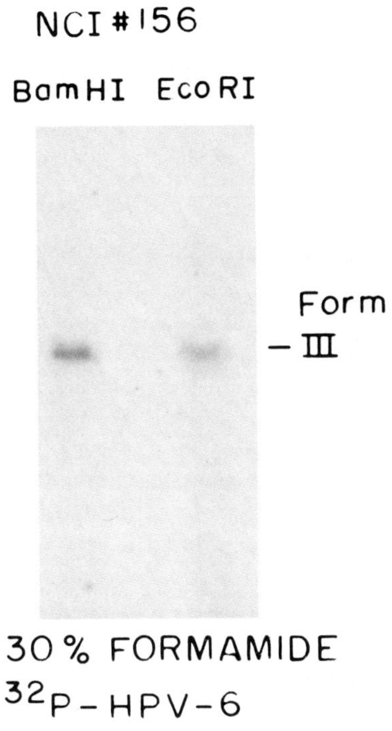


FIGURE 8. HPV DNA in a malignant connective tissue tumor of head and neck.

TABLE 4
SURVEY OF HUMAN MALIGNANCIES

| Type of Material | Total Number | Malignant | Metastatic | Normal | Normal/ Malignant |
|---|---|---|---|---|---|
| Base of tongue | 1 | 1 | | | |
| Bladder | 5 | 5 | | | |
| Breast | 25 | 15 | | | 10 |
| Cecum | 6 | 6 | | | |
| Connective Head/Face | 2 | 1* | 1 | | |
| Corpus uteri | 2 | 2 | | | |
| Esophagus | 5 | 5 | | | |
| Floor of mouth | 1 | 1 | | | |
| Gall bladder | 1 | 1 | | | |
| Gastronintestinal tract | 1 | 1 | | | |
| Kidney | 8 | 3 | 3 | | 2 |
| Large intestine | 28 | 15 | 2 | 1 | 10 |
| Larynx | 3 | 3 | | | |
| Liver | 21 | 2 | 16 | | 3 |
| Lung & bronchus | 37 | 20 | 4 | 3 | 10 |
| Maxillary sinus | 1 | 1 | | | |
| Mesentary | 2 | | 2 | | |
| Muscle | 1 | | 1 | | |
| Omentum | 2 | | 2 | | |
| Ovary | 14 | 10 | 4 | | |
| Pancreas | 6 | 5 | | | 1 |
| Pharynx | 1 | 1 | | | |
| Pleura | 1 | | 1 | | |
| Retromolar area | 1 | 1 | | | |
| Rib, sternum & clavicle | 1 | | 1 | | |
| Sigmoid colon | 5 | 5 | | | |
| SMall intestine | 6 | 4 | 2 | | |
| Spleen | 6 | | 2 | | 4 |
| Stomach | 13 | 9 | | | 4 |
| Testes | 6 | 4 | | | 2 |
| Trachea | 1 | | 1 | | |
| Transverse colon | 1 | 1 | | | |
| Uterus | 2 | 2 | | | |
| Vertebral column | 1 | | | | 1 |
| | 217 | | | | |

TABLE 5
PRELIMINARY RESULTS OF HPV-POSITIVE TISSUES - NCI

| Tissue # | Type of tissue examined | Primary patient diagnosis |
|---|---|---|
| 1 | Malignant cecum | Carcinoma of cecum with metastasis |
| 67 | Malignant lung and bronchus | Carcinoma of the left lung |
| 154 | Carcinoma of base of tongue | Carcinoma of base of tongue |
| 156 | Malignant connective tissue of head & neck | Epidermoid carcinoma of tongue |

## DISCUSSION

The great sensitivity and versatility of blot hybridization has been invaluable in determining the role that papillomaviruses may play in the etiology of some human malignancies. Hybridization has proved the most effective technique for detecting HPV infections in all grades of neoplasias. These findings have been further extended using in situ hybridization techniques capable of detecting HPV DNA or RNA within individual cells. Using subgenomic probes, RNA transcription patterns can now be examined in various tissues for various HPVs. A slight alteration of the technique permits simultaneous detection of HPV antigens as well as nucleic acids in the same cell (50). With the nucleotide sequence known, it should be possible to generate peptides of putative transforming regions of oncogenic HPVs to identify these previously undetected gene products and to localize them in HPV DNA positive cells of neoplastic tissues.

The high correlation between the presence of HPV-5 and malignancies in EV patients speaks strongly to its causative role. In addition, in vitro studies on HPV-5 indicate that it exhibits oncogenic potential. Similarly, the association of HPV-16 and 18 with high grade genital neoplasia and perhaps even some unrelated cancers strongly implies an oncogenic potential for these types. However, since HPV-6 and 11 have been found in some genital malignancies (19,55) and HPV-2 has been found in carcinoma in situ in one laboratory (56), definitive statements concerning the lack of oncogenicity of some common HPV types should be made with caution.

The ultimate case for the oncogenic potential of HPVs will be demonstrated in two kinds of studies. First, biosynthetic vaccines which reduce the incidence of wart disease should concommitantly reduce the incidence of malignancies in these patients if HPV plays a role in the development of this disease. Preliminary experiments involving such a vaccine in cattle have already been conducted (57). Biosynthetic viral structural proteins of BPV-1 have elicited neutralizing antibodies in both rabbits and cattle. In addition, this vaccine has protected cattle in virus challenge studies and has been efficacious in reducing the size of existing warts. Similar technology is applicable to HPV as well.

Second, a reduction of cancer as a result of identification and control of co-factors and biological control mechanisms such as RNA transcription or mutational events or host response to viral gene products would add additional confirming evidence to this important issue.

ACKNOWLEDGEMENTS

We thank Yvonne Guptill for valuable secretarial assistance in preparing this manuscript.

REFERENCES

1. Lutzner MA (1978). Epidermodysplasia verruciformis. An autosomal recessive disease characterized by viral warts and skin cancer. Bull Cancer (Paris) 65:169.
2. Orth G, Jablonska S, Favre M, Croissant O, Jarzabek-Chorzelska M, Rzesa G (1978). Characterization of two types of human papillomaviruses in lesions of epidermodysplasia verruciformis. Proc Natl Acad Sci USA 75:1537.
3. Pfister H, Nurnberg F, Gissmann L, zur Hausen H (1981). Characterization of a human papillomavirus from epidermodysplasia verruciformis lesions of a patient from Upper-Volta. Int J Cancer 27:645.
4. Yutsudo M, Tanigak T, Tsumori T, Watanabe S, Hakura A (1982). New human papillomavirus isolted from epidermodysplasia verruciformis lesions. Cancer Res 42:2440.
5. Kremsdorf D, Jablonska S, Favre M, Orth G (1982). Biochemical characterization of two types of human papillomaviruses associated with epidermodysplasia verruciformis. J Virol 43:436.
6. Kremsdorf D, Jablonska S, Favre M, Orth G (1983). Human papillomaviruses associated with epidermodysplasia verruciformis. J Virol 48:340.
7. Kremsdorf D, Favre M, Jablonska S, Obalek S, Rueda LA, Lutzner MA, Blanchet-Bardon C, Van Voost Vader PC, Orth G (1984). Molecular cloning and characterization of the genomes of nine newly recognized huyman papillomavirus types associated with epidermodysplasia verruciformis. J Virol 52:1013.

8. Gassenmaier A, Lammel M, Pfister H (1984). Molecular cloning and characterization of the DNAs of human papillomviruses 19, 20 and 25 from a patient with epidermodysplasia verruciformis. J Virol 52:1019.
9. Ostrow RS, Bender M, Niimura M, Seki T, Kawashima M, Pass F, Faras AJ (1982). Identification and characterization of human papillomavirus type 5 in cutaneous and metastasized carcinomas of patients exhibiting epidermodysplaisa verruciformis. Proc Natl Acad Sci USA 79:1634.
10. Lutzner MA, Blanchet-Bardon C, Orth G (1984). Clinical observations, virologic studies and treatment trials in patients with epidermodysplasia verruciformis, a disease induced by specific human papillomaviruses. J Invest Dermatol 83:185.
11. Ostrow RS, Watts S, Bender M, Niimura M, Seki T, Kawashima M, Pass F, Faras AJ (1983). Identification of three distinct papillomavirus genomes in a single patient with epidermodysplasia verruciformis. J Am Acad Dermatol 8:398.
12. Pfister H, Gassenmaier A, Nurnberger F, Stuttgen G (1983). Human papillomavirus 5 DNA in a carcinoma of an epidermodysplasia verruciformis patient infected with various human papillomavirus types. Cancer Res 43:1436.
13. Okagaki T (1984). Female genital tumors associated with human papillomavirus infection, and the concept of genital neoplasia-papilloma syndrome (GENPs). in Sommers SC, Rosen PP (eds): "Pathology Annual", Part 2, Volume 19. Connecticut: Appliton-Century-Crofts, p 31.
14. Levine RU, Crum CP, Herman E, Silvers D, Ferenczy A, Richart RM 91984). Cervical papillomavirus infection and intraepithelial neoplasia: A study of male sexual partners. Obstet Gynecol 64:16.
15. Durst M, Gissmann L, Ikenberg H, zur Hausen H (1983). A papillomavirus DNA from a cervical carcinoma and its prevalence in cancer biopsy samples from different geographic regions. Proc Natl Acad Sci USA 80:3812.
16. Boshart M, Gissmann L, Ikenberg H, Kleinheinz A, Scheurlen W, zur Hausen H (1984). A new type of papillomavirus DNA, its presence in genital cancer biopsies and in cell lines derived from cervical cancer. EMBO J 3:1151.
17. Gissmann L, Boshart M, Durst M, Ikenberg H, Wagner D, zur Hausen H (1984). Presence of human papillomavirus in genital tumors. J Invest Dermatol 83:265.

18. Wagner D, Ikenberg H, Boehm N, Gissmann L (1984). Identification of human papillomavirus in cervical swabs by deoxyribonucleic acid in situ hybridization. Obstet Gynecol 64:767.
19. Zachow KR, Ostrow RS, Bender M, Watts S, Okagaki T, Pass F, Faras AJ (1982). Detection of human papillomavirus DNA in anogenital neoplasias. Nature 300:771.
20. Okagaki T, Twiggs LB, Zachow KR, Clark BA, Ostrow RS, Faras AJ (1983). Identification of human papillomavirus DNA in cervical and vaginal intraepithelial neoplasia with molecularly cloned virus-specific DNA probes. Int J Gynecol Pathol 2:153.
21. Fukushima M, Okagaki T, Twiggs LB, Clark BA, Zachow KR, Ostrow RS, Faras AJ (1985). Histological types of carcinoma of the uterine cervix and the detectability of human papillomavirus (HPV) DNA. Cancer Res, in press.
22. Watts SL, Phelps WC, Ostrow RS, Zachow KR, Faras AJ (1984). Cellular transformation by human papillomavirus DNA in vitro. Science 225:634.
23. Rous P, Beard JW (1935). The progression to carcinoma of virus-induced rabbit papillomas (Shope). J Exp Med 62:523.
24. Syverton JT (1952). The pathogenesis of the rabbit papilloma-to-carcinoma sequence. Ann NY Acad Sci 54:1126.
25. Watts SL, Ostrow RS, Phelps WC, Prince JT, Faras AJ (1983). Free cottontail rabbit papillomavirus DNA persists in warts and carcinomas of infected rabbits and in cells in culture transformed with virus or viral DNA. Virology 125:127.
26. Lancaster WD, Olson C (1982). Animal papillomaviruses. Microbiol Rev 46:191.
27. Rous P, Kidd JG (1938). The carcinogenic effect of a papillomavirus on the tarred skin of rabbits. I. Description of the phenomenon. J. Exp Med 67:399.
28. Rous P, Kidd JG (1940). The activating transforming and carcinogenic effects of the rabbit papillomavirus (Shope) upon implanted tar tumors. J Exp Med 71:787.
29. Jarrett WFH, McNeil PE, Grimshaw WTR, Selman IE, McIntyre WIM (1978). High incidence area of cattle cancer with a possible interaction between an environmental carcinogen and a papillomavirus. Nature 274:215.
30. Campo MS, Moar MH, Jarrett WFH, Laird HM (1980). A new papillomavirus associated with alimentary cancer in cattle. nature 286:180.

31. Jabalonska S, Dabrowski J, Jakvbowicz K (1972). Epidermodysplasia verruciformis as a model in studies on the role of papovaviruses in oncogensis. Cancer Res 32:583.
32. Vonka V, Kanka J, Jelinek J, Subrt I, Suchanek A, Havrankova A, Vachal M, Hirsch I, Domorazkova E, Zavadova H, Richterova V, Naprstkova J, Dvorakova V, Svoboda B (1984). Prospective study on the relationship between cervical neoplasia and herpes simplex type-2 virus. Int J Cancer 33:49.
33. Barnett N, Mak H, Winkelstein JA (1983). Extensive verrucosis in primary immunodeficienty diseases. Arch Dermatol 119:5.
34. Rastkar G, Okagaki R, Twiggs L, Clark B (1982). Early invasive and in situ warty carcinoma of the vulva: Clinical, histologic and electron microscopic study with particular reference to viral association. Am J Obstet Gynecol 143:814.
34. 35encer ES, Andersen HK (1979). Viral infections in renal allograft recipients treated with long-term immunosuppression. Br Med J 2:829.
35. 36llen DL, Silverberg SG, Penn I, Hammond WS (1976). Squamous cell carcinoma of the skin and lip in renal homograft recipients. Cancer 37:729.
37. Koranda FC, Dehmel EM, Kahn G, Penn I (1974). Cutaneous complications in immuosuppressed renal homograft recipients. JAMA 229:419.
38. Lutzner M, Croissant O, Ducasse M-F, Kreis H, Crosnier J, Orth G (1980). A potentially oncogenic human papillomavirus (HPV-5) found in two renal allograft recipients. J Invest Dermatol 75:353.
39. Lutzner MA, Orth G, Dutronquay V, Ducasse M-F, Keris H, Crosnier J (1983). Detection of human papillomavirus type 5 DNA in skin cancers of an immunosuppressed renal allograft recipient. Lancet ii:422.
40. DePeuter M, DeClercq B, Minnette A (1977). An epidemiological survey of virus warts of the hands among butchers. Br J Dermatol 96:427.
41. Bosse K, Christophers B (1964). Beitrag zur epidemiologie der warzen. Hautartz 15:80.
42. Ostrow RS, Krzyzek R, Pass F, Faras AJ (1981). Identification of a novel human papillomavirus in cutaneous warts of meathandlers. Virology 108:21.

43. Orth G, Jablonsak S, Favre M, Croissant O, Obalek S, Jarzabek-Chorzelska M, Jibard N (1981). Identification of papillomaviruses in butcher's warts. J Invest Dermatol 76:97.
44. Lowy, DR, Dvoretzky I, Shober R, Law M-F, Engel L, Howley PM (1980). In vitro transformation by a defined subgenomic fragment of bovine papillomavirus DNA. Nature 287:72.
45. Steinberg BM, Topp WC, Schneider PS, Abramson AL (1983). Laryngeal papillomavirus infection during clinical remission. N Engl J Med 308:1261.
46. Danos O, Katinka M, Yaniv M (1982). Human papillomavirus 1a DNA sequence: A novel type of genome organization among papovaviridae. EMBO J 1:231.
47. Danos O, Engel LW, Chen EY, Yaniv M, Howley PM (1983). Comparative analysis of human type 1a and bovine type 1 papillomavirus genomes. J Virol 46:557.
48. Southern EM (1975). Detection of specific sequences among DNA fragments separated by gel electrophoresis. J Mol Biol 98:503.
49. Haase A, Brahic M, Stowring L (1984). Detection of viral nucleic acids by in situ hybridization. In Haramorsch L, Koprovoski H (eds): "Methods in Virology", Vol. 7, New York: Academic Press, p 189.
50. Blum H, Haase A, Byas G (1984). Molecular pathogenesis of hepatitis B virus infection: Simultaneous detection of viral DNA and antigens in paraffin imbedded liver sections. Proc Natl Acad Sci USA, in press.
51. Maniatis T, Jeffrey A, Kleid DG (1975). Nucleotide sequence of the right forward operator of phage lambda. Proc Natl Acad Sci USA 72:1184.
52. Law M-F, Lancaster WD, Howley PM (1979). Conserved polynucleotide sequences among the genomes of papillomaviruses. J Virol 32:199.
53. Okagaki T, Clark BA, Zachow KR, Twiggs LV, Ostrow RS, Pass F, Faras AJ (1984). Presence of human papillomavirus in verrucous carcinoma (Ackerman) of the vagina. Arch Pathol Lab Med 108:567.
54. Sato S, Okagaki T, Clark BA, Twiggs LB, Ostrow RS, Faras AJ (1985). Sensitivity of koilocytosis, immunocytochemistry and electron microscopy in detecting human papillomavirus (HPV) in the cervical and vaginal condyloma and intraepithelial neoplasia as compared to DNA hybridization. Int J. Gynecol Pathol, submitted for publication.

55. Gissmann L, Wolnik L, Ikenberg H, Koldovsky U, Schnurch HG, zur Hausen H (1983). Human papillomavirus types 6 and 11 DNA sequences in genital and laryngeal papillomas and in some cervical cancers. Proc Natl Acad Sci USA 80:560.
56. Pfister H, Haneke E (1984). Demonstration of human papillomavirus type 2 DNA in Bowen's disease. Arch Dermatol Res 276:123.
57. Pilacinski WP, Glassman DL, Krzyzek RA, Sadowski PL, Robbins AK (1984). Cloning and expression in Escherichia coli of the bovine papillomavirus L1 and L2 open reading frames. Biotechnology April:356.

# III. PAPILLOMAVIRUSES AND HUMAN ORAL AND LARYNGEAL DISEASES

**Papillomaviruses: Molecular and Clinical Aspects, pages 125–135**


# SCORING SYSTEM TO ASSESS SEVERITY AND COURSE IN RECURRENT RESPIRATORY PAPILLOMATOSIS

Haskins Kashima, M.D.,[1] Brigid Leventhal, M.D.,[2]
Phoebe Mounts, Ph.D.,[3] and Papilloma Study Group

[1]Department of Otolaryngology-Head and Neck Surgery
[2]Department of Pediatric Oncology
[3]Department of Immunology and Infectious Disease
Johns Hopkins Medical Institutions, Baltimore, MD

ABSTRACT Recent information regarding the etiology and some clinical and epidemiologic quest regarding recurrent respiratory papillomatosis are reviewed. A multi-institutional randomized study to evaluate interferon efficacy necessitated a system of objective scoring of disease severity. Analysis of 28 patients during a 6-month observation (no interferon) period disclosed that 23 patients exhibited no change in extent of disease, 4 showed an increase and one patient a decrease in disease extent. No complete remission or decannulations were achieved. The composite score from the observation period will be compared with findings during 6 months adjuvant interferon.

## INTRODUCTION

Papilloma in the respiratory tract occurs as a solitary growth of minimal clinical consequence or as widespread disease with life-threatening potential. In its most flagrant form the disease terrorizes the patient and his family and frustrates the surgeon charged with his care. The kinship between these disparate clinical forms and intermediate variations has long been suspected and is being verified in some recent studies. The determinants of clinical course, whether mild or severe, await identification.

The relative paucity of these cases, and their

prolonged and complicated clinical course, have created scattered concentrations of clinical experience, largely in universities and major medical centers. Papilloma in the respiratory tract is a histologically benign growth occurring in the larynx and the predominant victim is of pediatric age, hence the earlier designation of juvenile laryngeal papillomatosis. An alternate term, recurrent respiratory papillomatosis coined, by Stuart Strong,[1] emphasizes that the growths recur and have propensity to spread throughout the respiratory tract. It is recognized that there is a bimodal age distribution, namely those with childhood onset and those of adult onset; a conspicuously silent period occurs in late adolescence between ages 15 to 20 years.

The viral etiologic agent has been localized to the superficial-most layers of the papilloma, and the relationship of HPV subtype to clinical features has been described.[2]

The presence of condyloma in mothers of patients with juvenile onset disease has been recognized and HPV viruses have been identified as etiologic agents of condyloma and respiratory papillomatosis. A 2 - 5 percent prevalence of condyloma among women of child-bearing age in the U.S.A. translates to 60,000 to 150,000 pregnancies occurring in mothers with condyloma accuminatum. The number of new cases of clinically apparent recurrent laryngeal papillomatosis has been estimated to be 1500 new cases per year.[1] These figures suggest a risk of 1:40 to 1:100 for papilloma to occur in the child resulting from pregnancy in the mother with condyloma.

Review of histories in our department discloses that juvenile-onset papilloma patients are most frequently first born and a disproportionately high percentage (in excess of 10 percent) are adopted. Maternal condyloma was present in approximately a third of the cases. The mothers are young, frequently in the teens, and papillomatosis has not been identified among the siblings.

The clinical features of the recurrent respiratory papillomatosis are well known. The lesions occur most frequently at laryngeal sites, predominantly at the true and false cords. The lateral spread into contiguous and distant sites may result from mucosal trauma. Additional sites for papilloma growth are of tracheotomy, the carina, and the nasal vestibule. Search for an "occult focus" from which viral shedding could occur led to the detection of papilloma on the naso-pharyngeal surface of the soft palate. Among patients with tracheotomy, the level of trachea corresponding to the distal tip of the tracheotomy tube was regularly diseased with papilloma. Each of the foregoing sites represent transitional zones from ciliated to non-ciliated epithelium. Infectious particles accumulating at these lines of transition may predispose to development of new lesions at these locations. Bronchopulmonary papilloma occurs in the peripheral lung fields where the transition lines from cilated to non-ciliated epithelium are present.

Endoscopic excision has been the foundation for treatment of papillomatosis. Improved illumination, development of microsurgical instrumentation and ability to perform the operations under magnification have been extraordinarily helpful. The introduction of the Carbon Dioxide Laser has improved the surgeon's ability to ablate diseased tissue with maximum preservation and safety to the underlying stroma. In spite of these improvements. Long-term disease-free state has not been achieved by endoscopic treatment alone, and attention has been directed to adjuvant agents,[3] most recently to Interferon.

Beginning with the reports of Haglund and colleagues,[4] and additional pilot studies from Scandinavia and The United States, of complete remission under Interferon have been reported in a variable proportion of patients.[5,6,7,8] Lesser degrees of improvement, variously defined, have been achieved in the majority of patients reported. The duration of improvement has varied but is dependent on continued interferon administration. Relapsed cases respond to reinstitution of Interferon.

## MATERIALS AND METHODS

A controlled study was developed to evaluate interferon (Human Lymphoblastoid Interferon, ALFA-Nl. Burroughs-Wellcome Company) efficacy.[9] Patients with juvenile-onset RRP were enrolled in a 12-month randomized cross-over study during which each patient received Interferon for 6 months and received no Interferon for 6 months. Eligibility for entry into study was that the patient have histologically verified juvenile-onset papillomatosis and a minimum of 3 operations having been performed in the immediately preceding 6 months. $CO_2$ Laser endoscopic operations were performed at 2-monthly intervals at each of which the disease status was recorded.

Figure 1

| Months | 0 | 2 | 4 | 6 | 9 | 10 | 12 |
|---|---|---|---|---|---|---|---|
| Schedule I: | Inteferon (0–6) | | | | No Drug | | |
| Schedule II: | No Drug | | | | Inteferon (6–12) | | |
| Endoscopy | ↑ | ↑ | ↑ | ↑ | ↑ | ↑ | ↑ |

A standard system of objective scoring was designed to accurately evaluate disease severity at any single observation and to assess the course of disease. The objectives of the scoring system are (1) that the scoring reflect the disease status accurately, (2) the system of scoring be simple to assure accurate data collection, (3) the data be suitable for analysis and, finally, (4) the scoring system have sensitivity to detect subtle change.

A scoring system has been developed utilizing three criteria--numbers of diseased anatomic sites, and sites with surface area and lumen encroachment of advanced degree. The scoring system takes into account lesions occurring in the laryngo-tracheal regions only and does not consider papillomata in the nose, oral cavity or lungs. In the laryngotracheal region, 9 anatomic sites were identified, 5 of which were in the larynx (epiglottis, false cords, ventricle, true cords and subglottis) and 4 in the tracheobronchial region (tracheotomy site, trachea, carina and mainstem bronchus). The presence or absence of papilloma at each anatomic site was scored and the total number of anatomic sites involved was designated the AS score.

Surface area involvement was scored on basis of estimated surface area diseased at each of the 9 anatomic sites. Four degrees of involvement were recognized and scored as follows: 0, no disease present; 1, less than 1/3 surface area with disease; 2, 1/3 to 2/3 surface area with disease; 3, more than 2/3 surface area with disease. The number of anatomic sites with greater than 1/3 surface area of disease (SA scores of 2 or 3) is designated as the SA score.

The extent of lumen encroachment was scored on basis of degree of airway infringement at each of nine designated anatomic sites. Four degrees of involvement were specified and scored as follows: 0, no lumen encroachment; 1, less than 1/3 airway infringement, 2, 1/3 to 2/3 airway infringement; and 3, greater than 2/3 airway infringement. The number of anatomic sites with more than 1/3 lumen encroachment is designated the LE score.

Composite score was derived by totalling the number of diseased anatomic sites (maximum AS score of 9), the number of sites with greater than 1/3 surface area diseased (maximum SA score of 9) and the number of sites with greater than 1/3 lumen encroachment (maximum LE score of 9). The overall determination of improvement or progression of papilloma is based on change in composite score but scores for AS, SA and LE are also recorded for each operation. A composite score of 1-5 was rated mild, 6-11 as moderate and over 12 as severe.

The foregoing scoring system has been utilized in a 12 institution collaborative study in which 66 patients have been enrolled. Of 33 patients randomized to initial observation, 28 records were complete at the time of this review. The evaluation scores from 3 operations are reviewed in all patients.

## RESULTS

None of the 28 patients achieved complete clinical remission during the observation and none of the 8 patients with tracheotomy was decannulated. 8 patients were allowed to cross-over to Interferon after 3 endoscopies when operations failed to control symptoms for at least two months.

### Anatomic sites

A total of 337 diseased anatomic sites were recorded in 98 operations performed on 27 patients. Of this number, 282 were in the larynx (ASL) and 55 in the tracheobronchial region (AST).

In 98 operations laryngeal anatomic sites were diseased with papilloma in the following manner: true cord (76), false cord (65), ventricle (45), subglottis (41), and epiglottis (38). The true cord was papilloma positive in at least one operative observation in all but one patient. In the tracheobronchial region the tracheotomy site was the most frequently diseased (15), followed by trachea (14), mainstem bronchus (6) and carina (5). A tracheotomy was present in 8 patients and the trachea was diseased in all 8 and in one additional patient.

8 anatomical sites, disease-free at entry, developed papilloma during the course of observation; 10 anatomical sites, papillomapositive at entry, were papilloma-free at 6 months. The false cord (4) and epiglottis (4) were the sites most frequently involved in these changes.

Surface area

One hundred and eighty- four sites had greater than 1/3 surface area disease; of these 158 were in the laryngeal region (SAL) and 26 were in the tracheobronchial region (SAT). The highest frequency of positive SA scores were observed at the tracheotomy site (73%), and the trachea (71%).

Lumen encroachment

One hundred and thirty-three sites had greater than 1/3 lumen encroachment. Of these 105 were at laryngeal sites (LEL) and 28 at tracheobronchial sites (LET). The true cords (67%) and false cords (63%) had the highest proportion of lumen encroachment scores.

## CONSISTENCY OF SEQUENTIAL OBSERVATIONS

Anatomic sites

The mean AS score (± 1 S.D.) for the first operation was 3.8 ± 2.8; for the second operation was 3.3 ± 2.0, and for the third (early crossover) or final operation was 3.6 ± 1.8. Nine patients had the same number of sites involved at each operation; 10 showed an increase of one or more sites and 8 showed a decrease of 1 or more sites while under study. The mean change in AS per operation was 1.4 (range from -4 to +2).
Thus the AS score from operation to operation was relatively constant and by the paired T-test these differences are not significant.

Surface area

The mean SA score (±1 S.D.) at the first operation was 2.4 ± 1.7, at the second operation it was 1.8 ± 1.9 and at the third or final was 1.7 ± 1.9. Comparison of the SA scores from the first and the final operations revealed that 12 patients had no change in SA score, 11 showed a decrease and 4 showed an increase in SA score. By the Wilcoxon ranked sign test the SA score for the first operation show a borderline difference from the SA score for the second (p = 0.05) and last operations (p = 0.07); however the second operation is not different from the last, demonstrating that under uniform surgical conditions (skill and technique) surface area recurrence occurs at a constant rate.

Lumen encroachment

The mean ±1 S.D for LE score at each operation was 1.7 ± 1.9 for the first operation, 1.2 ± 1.7 for the second and 1.3 ± 1.6 for the last. When the first operation is compared with the last, 12 patients had no change in LE score, 10 showed a decrease and 5 an increase in LE score. The LE score difference between the first and second operation and between the first and third or last were or borderline significance (p more than 0.05 and less than 0.10) but the findings at the second and last operation were identical.

Composite Score

The mean ±1 SD for composite score was 8.5 ± 5.6 for the first operation, 7.2 ± 5.5 for the second operation 9.4 ± 5.0 for the last operation. When the first operation is compared to the last, 23 patients showed no change in category, 4 patients showed an increase in extent of disease and one had decrease in extent of disease.

Nine patients had composite score consistently in the mild range; six patients had consistently severe extent of disease. Of 13 patients with scores in the moderate range, 7 were consistently moderate, 2 were moderate-to-severe and 4 were mild-to-moderate. 22 of 27 patients exhibited constant extent of disease for the duration of the observation.

Figure 2
RRP: SEVERITY SCORING, MEAN S.D.
INITIAL OBSERVATION (N = 28)

| | Operation | | |
|---|---|---|---|
| | I | II | III |
| Anatomic sites | 3.8 ± 2.8 | 3.3 ± 2.0 | 3.6 ± 1.8 |
| Surface area | 2.4±1.7 | 1.8±1.9 | 1.7±1.9 |
| Lumen encroachment | 1.7 ± 1.9 | 1.2 ± 1.7 | 1.3 ± 1.6 |
| Composite score | 8.5 ± 5.6 | 7.2 ± 5.5 | 9.4 ± 5.0 |

## DISCUSSION

The objective of this study has been to assess papilloma severity and disease course at successive operative observations performed at regular intervals. Rationale for the three designated criteria is that AS score assesses distribution of disease, SA score, extent of disease, and LE score, bulk of disease at each operation. The observations reported herein demonstrate that evaluations on these bases, by individual examiners each performing consecutive operations on a given patient, can be compared. Of the three criteria considered, anatomical site (AS) score is the most precise but does not take lesion numbers or nature of growth into account. SA and LE scores are intended to account for the differences of narrow versus broad-based and sessile versus exophytic lesions. The composite score was designed account for these possible variations in growth features.

Laryngeal sites were more frequently diseased than tracheobronchial sites - 2.9 ASL and 0.6 AST per operation. More extensive lumen encroachment occurred at laryngeal sites with the true and false cords exhibiting the highest proportion of this feature. Severe surface area involvement was most frequently observed at the tracheotomy site and trachea.

The well-defined laryngeal sites lend themselves to accurate assessment whereas tracheal disease was more difficult to describe and quantitate. Tracheal involvement with papilloma occurred at the tracheostome and the level of the distal tip of the tracheotomy tube. The trachea above the carina was invariably papillomafree.

All 27 patients had papilloma positive sites in the larynx; nine had papilloma-positive sites in the tracheobronchial region. 8 ofthe 9 patients with tracheal involvement entered the study having had tracheotomy performed previously; it was not determined whether the trachea had been diseased with papilloma prior to tracheotomy. The tracheobronchial sites, notably the tracheostomal tract tends to have extensive SA involvement and was extraordinarily difficult to render papilloma-free; none of the papilloma-positive tracheobronchial sites became papilloma-free during the observation period. These findings reinforce the policy of avoiding tracheotomy unless the trachea is papilloma-positive.

Disease severity encompasses factors related to papillomatous growth (location, lesion numbers, nature of and rapidity of re-growth), symptomatic disturbance of airway, voice and swallowing, consequences of treatment (webs, scars, vocal cord motion impairment) and outcome (tracheotomy, malignant transformation, death). This report proposes a comprehensive and uniform anatomical scoring system. The concept of disease severity is critical to patient management and for assessment of treatment alternatives. The extent of disease is based on the quantitative estimate of the amount of papilloma disease present at each operation. Although all patients were regarded as "clinically severe" on basis of requiring frequent operations, the composite score derived to assess extent of disease at a single operation designates 6 patients as severe, 2 moderate-severe, 7 moderate, 4 mild-moderate, and 9, mild.

A consistent pattern of regrowth is seen for each patient during a conterolled period of observation with operations at regular intervals.

Our understanding of recurrent respiratory papillomatosis has been advanced by recent findings: notably, establishing the viral etiology, including the possible relevance of HPV subtypes to clinical course. Detailed documentation of disease status and systematic study is essential to understand the natural history of this disease and to evaluate efficacy of treatment alternatives.

## CONCLUSIONS

1. Clinical severity of recurrent respiratory papillomatosis has been designated mild, moderate or severe on the basis of a composite score summing the number of diseased anatomic sites (AS), sites with significant surface area involvement by disease (SA), and lumen encroachment (LE).

2. Disease severity remained constant at successive 2-monthly evaluations during the 6-months of observation, irrespective of disease severity at study entry.

3. No complete remissions were observed in this subset analysis of 27 subjects during the control observation.

4. The findings from the 6-month observation period will be compared with findings during 6 months adjuvant interferon administration. Each patient will act as his own control.

## ACKNOWLEDGEMENTS

The authors gratefully acknowledge the active collaboration of the co-investigators in the 12-institution randomized study of Interferon efficacy in RRP. Members of the study group are:

Keith Clark (Oklahoma), Seymour Cohen (Los Angeles), Herb Dedo (Univ. Calif.), Don Donovan (Baylor), B. Fearon (Toronto), L. Gardiner (Yale), H. Goepfert (M.D. Anderson), R. Lusk (Iowa), H. Muntz (Washington Univ.), M. Richardson (U. Washington), G. Singleton (U. Florida), J. Whisnant and P. Weck, Ph.D. (Research Triangle, N.C.), A. Yonkers (U. Nebraska).

BIBLIOGRAPHY


1. Strong, M.S., Vaughn, C.W., Healy, G.B. Recurrent Respiratory Papillomatosis in Laryngo-tracheal Problems in the Pediatric Patient. Healy, McGill, C. Thomas, Springfield, Illinois, 1979.

2. Mounts, P., Kashima, H. Association of humanpapillomavirus subtype and clinical course in respiratory papillomatosis. Laryngoscope 94:28-33, 1984.

3. Leventhal, B., Kashima, H., Levine, A., Levy, H. Treatment of recurrent laryngeal papillomatosis with an artificial interferon inducer (poly IC-LC) J. Pediatrics 99: 614-616, 1981.

4. Haglund, S., Lundquist, P.G., Cantell, K., Strander, H. Interferon therapy in juvenile laryngeal papillomatosis. Arch. Otolaryng. 107: 327-332, 1981.

5. Goepfert, H., Sessions, R., Gutterman. Leucocyte Interferon in patients with juvenile laryngeal papillomatosis. Ann. Otol. Rhinol. Laryng. 91: 432-4436, 1982.

6. McCabe, B.F., Clark, K.F. Interferon and laryngeal papillomatosis. The Iowa Experience. Ann. Otol. Rhin. Laryng. 92: 2-7, 1983.

7. Bomholt, A. Interferon therapy for laryngeal papillomatosis in adults. Arch. Otolaryng. 109: 550-552, 1983.

8. Lundquist, P.G., Haglund, S., Carlson, B., Strander, H., Lundgren, E. Interferon therapy in juvenile laryngeal papillomatosis. Otolaryngology-Head and Neck Surgery 92: 386-391, 1984.

9. Whisnant, John K., Kashima, H., Leventhal, B., et. al. Interferon Treatment of Juvenile Laryngeal Papillomatosis: The Design of a Cooperative Trial with Wellferon in The Biology of the Interferon System 1984. H. Kirchner and H. Schellekens. Elsevier Science Publishers, 1985.

**Papillomaviruses: Molecular and Clinical Aspects, pages 137–154**


# ANALYSIS OF HUMAN PAPILLOMAVIRUS TYPE 6 IN THE RESPIRATORY AND GENITAL TRACTS DURING INTERFERON THERAPY*

Phoebe Mounts,[1] Tzyy-Choou Wu,[1] Brigid Leventhal,[2] Haskins Kashima,[3] Herbert Dedo,[4] George Singleton,[5] Stanley Gall,[6] Phillip Weck,[7] and John Whisnant[7]

[1]Department of Immunology and Infectious Diseases, School of Public Health, The Johns Hopkins University, Baltimore, Maryland, 21205
[2]Division of Pediatric Oncology, The Johns Hopkins Hospital, Baltimore, Maryland, 21205
[3]Department of Laryngology and Otology, The Johns Hopkins Hospital, Baltimore, Maryland, 21205
[4]Department of Otolaryngology, School of Medicine, University of California, San Francisco, California, 94143
[5]Division of Otolaryngology, College of Medicine, University of Florida, Gainesville, Florida, 32610
[6]Department of Obstetrics and Gynecology, Duke University Medical Center, Durham, North Carolina, 27710
[7]Department of Clinical Investigation, Burroughs Wellcome Company, Research Triangle Park, North Carolina, 27709

ABSTRACT We are analyzing human papillomavirus type 6 in biopsy specimens from patients registered in multi-institutional clinical trials evaluating the efficacy of human lymphoblastoid interferon (Wellferon®) for condyloma acuminata and juvenile-onset respiratory papillomatosis. Using the Southern transfer technology we have determined the subtypes of HPV-6, which are distinguishable by restriction endonuclease digestion, in papillomata from fifty-three patients with respiratory papillomatosis and thirteen women with condyloma. We have examined the

*This work was supported by Public Health Service grant CA-35535 from the National Cancer Institute and by the Burroughs Wellcome Company.

relationship of HPV-6 subtypes to the clinical manifestations of disease in these patients and we have investigated the association between viral subtype and patient response to interferon. In addition, the impact of interferon therapy on the papillomavirus in three patients with respiratory tract lesions was analyzed by comparing levels of the viral genome and capsid antigen in relation to clinical assessment of disease during the course of drug therapy.

## INTRODUCTION

We have been investigating the role of human papillomavirus type 6 (HPV-6) in the etiology, pathogenesis, and clinical manifestations of condyloma acuminata (genital warts) and respiratory papillomatosis. Multiple subtypes of HPV-6 exist that hybridize under stringent conditions but are distinguishable on the basis of restriction endonuclease digestion patterns (1,2,3). To investigate the biological significance of the subtypes, we previously examined the relationship of HPV-6 subtypes to the clinical manifestations of respiratory papillomatosis in twenty-one patients, and found that patients infected with one subtype, HPV-6c, were characterized by extensive anatomical spread of disease and a need for a increased frequency of operations (4). To extend our findings, we are analyzing the papillomavirus in biopsy specimens from patients registered in multi-institutional clinical trials evaluating the efficacy of human lymphoblastoid interferon (Wellferon®) for condyloma and juvenile-onset respiratory papillomatosis. We report here the distribution of HPV-6 subtypes in 53 patients with respiratory tract lesions and 13 women with genital tract lesions. The relationship of viral subtype to sex and race of the patient, to the age of onset of disease, to the duration of disease, to the frequency of surgical excisions, and to the extension of disease, is reported for these patients. We also report our preliminary results on the association between viral subtype and patient response to interferon, including a comparison of the viral genome and capsid antigen in relation to clinical assessment of respiratory tract disease in three patients who are receiving interferon.

## METHODS

### Case Analysis.

Relevant clinical data were obtained from patient registration forms that were completed at the time of entry to the trials studying the efficacy of interferon for respiratory or genital tract papillomatosis. For purposes of the present study, the following information was tabulated: sex, race, age at first diagnosis of disease, duration of clinically active disease to the present time and, for respiratory papillomatosis patients, the presence of a tracheostomy, evidence of pulmonary disease, and the number of endoscopic excisions in the six months prior to entry.

### Clinical Trial Designs.

Patients analyzed for this study were entered in clinical trials to evaluate the efficacy of Wellferon®, which is a highly purified preparation of alpha interferons derived from viral induction of the human lymphoblastoid cell lane Namalwa (5).

Resistent, persistent condyloma acuminata. Women who had condyloma acuminata for at least six months and who had received at least ten podophyllin applications or equivalent treatments were eligible for this trial conducted at Duke University Medical Center. Wellferon® was injected intramuscularly at 5 mega units per meter squared ($Mu/m^2$) of body surface area, daily for 28 days followed by the same dose three times per week for two additional weeks. Dose modifications were made if patients encountered severe side effects or toxicities. Genital warts were documented by photographs and by recording bidimensional measurements of each wart on a divided grid of the external genital tract. Measurements were made at entry, after two weeks of treatment, and every two weeks thereafter for disease assessment.

Recurrent juvenile-onset respiratory papillomatosis. Patients who were more than 12 months and less than 35 years of age with the onset of disease prior to the age of 16 were eligible for this randomized cross-over trial. Clinical disease of more than 6 months duration and at least three surgical excisions in the 6 months prior to entry were required for admission at one of the twelve participating centers. At entry, patients were randomized to either surgical management and observation or surgical management with adjuvant interferon and were crossed-over to the alternative protocol after 6 months. Wellferon® was injected intramuscularly at 5 Mu/$m^2$ on a daily schedule for 28 days followed by the same dose given 3 times per week for a total of 6 months. Disease severity was assessed by endoscopic examination at two month intervals, as described by Kashima et al. (6). Briefly, a composite score was developed for disease in the airway with 9 sites scored. These were epiglottis, false cords, ventricle, true cords, subglottis, tracheostomy site, trachea, carina, and main stem bronchus. Involvement of a site was scored as 1 or 0. If the surface area of that site was involved by more than 1/3, then this was scored a 1, and if the lumen was occluded by more than 1/3, then this was scored an additional 1. Thus the maximum score for any involved site was 3 and the maximum total score was 27. Extra airway disease, such as nasopharynx and lung involvement, was not included in this composite score.

Papillomavirus Analysis.

DNA was extracted from biopsy specimens removed from patients at the time of entry to the clinical trial and the papillomavirus genome analyzed using the Southern transfer and hybridization (1). Papillomavirus subtypes were determined on the basis of hybridization patterns obtained under moderately stringent hybridization conditions ($T_m$ - 28°C) with radioactively labelled HPV-6 DNA when the DNA samples were digested with the restriction endonucleases HindIII, HpaI, EcoRI or PstI.

The presence of papillomavirus capsid antigen in paraffin sections of tissue processed for histopathological examination was determined using the avidin-biotin modification of the immunoperoxidase assay as described previously (1). The primary rabbit antibody was generated against detergent disrupted bovine papillomavirus particles and purchased from Accurate Chemical and Scientific Corporation (Westbury, NY). For comparative purposes, the distribution and number of antigen containing cells in all of the tissue fragments present on the slide were determined and a score of 0 to +3 was assigned: 0 was no positively staining cells; +1 was a single focus of positive cells or fewer than 10 positively staining cells that were scattered throughout the tissue fragments; +2 was two foci or fewer than 50 positively staining cells; and +3 was more than two foci or more than 50 positively staining cells.

## RESULTS

### Distribution of HPV-6 Subtypes in Patients with Respiratory Papillomatosis.

Demographic information. Shown in Table 1 is the distribution of HPV-6 subtypes in 53 of the 66 patients registered for the randomized, cross-over trial evaluating the efficacy of interferon for juvenile-onset respiratory papillomatosis, which is described in METHODS. Since there were incomplete data sets available for 13 of the patients at the time of this report, they are not included in the analysis.

TABLE 1
THE DISTRIBUTION OF HPV-6 SUBTYPES IN 53 PATIENTS WITH JUVENILE ONSET RESPIRATORY PAPILLOMATOSIS

| | Number of Patients (% of total) | | Sex[a] M | Sex[a] F | Race[b] B | Race[b] C | Race[b] O | Average Age at Onset (years) |
|---|---|---|---|---|---|---|---|---|
| HPV-6c | 29 | (55%) | 13 | 16 | 6 | 21 | 2 | 2.5 |
| HPV-6d | 2 | (4%) | 1 | 1 | 1 | 1 | 0 | 5.6 |
| HPV-6e | 13 | (24%) | 7 | 6 | 2 | 11 | 0 | 2.5 |
| HPV-6f | 9 | (17%) | 5 | 4 | 0 | 7 | 2 | 2.8 |
| | 53 | | 26 | 27 | 9 | 40 | 4 | 2.7 |

[a]M = male; F = female
[b]B = Black; C = Caucasian; O = other

The viral DNA in 29 patients (55%) was identified as HPV-6c, a frequency comparable to the 62% observed in 21 patients previously examined that included both juvenile and adult onset disease (4). The ratio of males to females infected with each of the four viral subtypes identified reflects the equal sex distribution in the study population. The racial composition of patients infected with HPV-6c and HPV-6e reflects the racial composition of the study population as a whole, where Hispanics and Asians were classified as Other in Table 1. It may be significant that the racial composition of the 2 patients (4%) infected with HPV-6d and of the 9 patients (17%) infected with HPV-6f does not reflect the distribution in the study group. We had previously found HPV-6d only in 4 black juveniles and HPV-6f in 2 white adults in a group of 21 patients examined (4). However, a larger number of patients must be examined before conclusions can be drawn.

There was no discernible geographical localization of the viral subtypes. The patients are registered at study centers across the United States and Canada and include individuals from other countries. When the viral subtypes in patients at individual centers registering 10% or more of the patients included in the analysis were examined, the distribution reflected the distribution of the study population as a whole.

The average age of the patients analyzed in Table 1 is 6.3 years with a range of 1.1 to 27.3 years. The average age at the first diagnosis of disease is 2.7 years with a range of 0.5 to 9.1 years even though patients were eligible with disease onset up to the age of 16. This is in agreement with data in the literature that indicate that individuals at 5 years of age or less are at the highest risk of developing disease (for review, see 7). The age at onset for patients infected with HPV-6c, -6e, and -6f is the same, around 2.7 years, but for patients infected with HPV-6d it is higher at 5.6 years. Since there are only two patients infected with HPV-6d it is not possible to attribute any significance to the difference.

Disease characteristics. Presented in Table 2 is a summary of some of the disease characteristics for 51 patients for whom a complete set of data was available at the time of this analysis. The average duration of disease in this study group was 1.7 years but was higher in patients infected with HPV-6c (2.3 years). The average number of excisions reflects the eligibility requirement of at least 3 excisions in the previous 6 months to select a group of patients with severe disease for therapy with an experimental drug. Additional indicators of severe disease are the high percentage of patients with a tracheostomy (31%), and pulmonary disease (5.8%) in this population. The extension of lesions into the lungs is not common but is frequently the cause of death (for review, see 7). The presence of HPV-6c in a higher percentage of patients in this population and the association of pulmonary disease with this subtype, support our previous observation that this subtype is associated with more severe disease in the respiratory tract (4).

Distribution of HPV-6 Subtypes in Patients with Condyloma Acuminata.

The papillomavirus DNA present in biopsy specimens collected from 13 women with persistent condyloma acuminata at entry to the interferon trial was analyzed as described in METHODS. The results of the viral subtype determination are presented in Table 3. The most frequent subtypes in

TABLE 2
HPV-6 SUBTYPE AND SEVERITY OF DISEASE IN 51 PATIENTS WITH JUVENILE ONSET RESPIRATORY PAPILLOMATOSIS

| | Average Duration (years) | Average Excisions in previous 6 mos. | Number of Patients with Tracheostomy | Number of Patients with Pulmonary Disease |
|---|---|---|---|---|
| HPV-6c | 2.3 | 4.3 | 9 | 3 |
| HPV-6d | 1.4 | 3.0 | 0 | 0 |
| HPV-6e | 1.6 | 4.6 | 6 | 0 |
| HPV-6f | 0.7 | 3.9 | 1 | 0 |
| | 1.7 | 4.2 | 16 | 3 |

this group of patients with severe disease were HPV-6e (30.8%) and HPV-6f (30.8%). This distribution is in contrast to the association of HPV-6c with more severe respiratory tract disease. HPV-6c and HPV-6d were also present in the genital tract lesions in addition to 2 other variants HPV-6h and HPV-6j that were not seen in the respiratory tract lesions. Because of the small number of patients in this trial for genital tract disease, it is not possible to look for demographic associations but the data for age at onset and duration of disease at the time of entry to the study are presented to characterize this patient population.

TABLE 3
THE DISTRIBUTION OF HPV-6 SUBTYPE IN THIRTEEN WOMEN WITH RESISTANT CONDYLOMA ACUMINATA

| | Number (% of total) | Race[a] B | Race[a] C | Average Age at Onset (years) | Average Disease Duration (years) |
|---|---|---|---|---|---|
| HPV-6c | 1 (7.7%) | 1 | 0 | 19 | 1 |
| HPV-6d | 1 (7.7%) | 0 | 1 | 42 | 1 |
| HPV-6e | 4 (30.8%) | 0 | 4 | 24.3 | 5.8 |
| HPV-6f | 4 (30.8%) | 0 | 4 | 24.5 | 4 |
| HPV-6h | 2 (15.4%) | 1 | 1 | 27.5 | 2.5 |
| HPV-6j | 1 (7.7%) | 0 | 1 | 36 | 6 |
| | 13 | 2 | 11 | | |

[a]B = Black; C = Caucasian

HPV-6 Subtype and Response of Condyloma Acuminata to Interferon.

To investigate the role of virus relative to the effects of interferon, the reduction of total condylomata lesion size (sum of products of bidimensional measurements) after 6 weeks from the initiation of interferon therapy as described in METHODS was compared to the HPV-6 subtype present in the lesions (Table 4). The lesions in only one patient (#7) failed to show a reduction of greater than 68%

and the virus in this patient was HPV-6c. However, since HPV-6c was present in only one patient in this group, it is not possible to conclude that this virus may be resistant to interferon. The 3 patients infected with HPV-6e exhibited an average clearance or reduction of 84%. The 4 patients with HPV-6f exhibited an average clearance of 95%. The 2 patients with HPV-6h exhibited an average clearance of 77%. These results suggest that systemic human lymphoblastoid interferon is effective in reducing those papilloma in the genital tract induced by human papillomavirus type 6.

TABLE 4
PAPILLOMAVIRUS SUBTYPE AND RESPONSE TO INTERFERON IN TWELVE WOMEN WITH RESISTANT CONDYLOMA ACUMINATA

| HPV-6 Subtype | Patient Number | Percent Clearance After 6 Weeks |
|---|---|---|
| HPV-6c | 07 | 27 |
| HPV-6d | 11 | 97 |
| HPV-6e | 05 | 100 |
| HPV-6e | 14 | 86 |
| HPV-6e | 15 | 68 |
| HPV-6f | 03 | 92 |
| HPV-6f | 08 | 96 |
| HPV-6f | 09 | 95 |
| HPV-6f | 10 | 99 |
| HPV-6h | 12 | 70 |
| HPV-6h | 13 | 84 |
| HPV-6j | 06 | 99 |

Analysis of HPV-6 DNA and Capsid Antigen in Respiratory Tract Papillomata from Three Patients Receiving Interferon.

To examine in detail the response of virus in respiratory tract lesions during systemic administration of interferon, three patients were selected for analysis from the patients registered on the multi-institutional clinical trial evaluating the efficacy of Wellferon®.

Analysis of Patient 01-202. Figure 1 presents the data obtained for patient 01-202 during a 3 year period including: 9 months prior to entry to the trial; 6 months of surgical management and observation on the trial; 6 months of interferon at 5 $Mu/m^2$ per day for 28 days and the same dose 3 times a week for 5 months; and 14 months on an addendum protocol randomized to 2 $Mu/m^2$ daily. The crossover points in this schedule are indicated at the top of Figure 1 above the calendar dates at which times the clinical evaluations were made. The clinical evaluation is presented as the total composite score with a higher number indicating more severe disease. The relative levels of papillomavirus capsid antigen are indicated by the score from 0 to +3 given below the date at which the biopsy was taken. Similarly, the relative levels of HPV-6c DNA are shown in the autoradiogram. The letters on the autoradiogram correspond to the dates indicated by the same letters at the top of the figure. Two micrograms of DNA extracted from the biopsy specimen was digested with the restriction endonuclease HindIII, size fractionated by agarose gel electrophoresis, transferred to nitrocellulose and hybridized with radioactively labelled HPV-6 DNA to compare relative quantities of viral DNA over a long period of time before and during interferon therapy.

It is apparent that there was a significant reduction in the amount of airway disease in this patient, as indicated by the declining value of the composite score representing the clinical evaluation. The scores from 1.27.82 to 3.11.83, the period before interferon therapy, range from 6 to 11 with an average of 8.7. The scores after 3.11.83, when interferon therapy was initiated, to 12.13.84 range from 2 to 10 with an average of 4.3. The change from 8.7 to 4.3 represents a 50% reduction in the amount and distribution of airway disease.

There was also a significant decrease in the amount of detectable papillomavirus capsid antigen during interferon therapy. This patient has an unusually high number of papillomavirus capsid antigen containing cells in his lesions and the 5 biopsies examined prior to interferon were all scored as +3. In contrast, the 3 biopsies examined during interferon therapy showed a marked reduction in the scores. After 2 months of interferon treatment, the score was +1 and after 4 months and 9 months there was no detectable antigen in the biopsy specimens. Since the presence of virions has been demonstrated in positively staining regions that have been reprocessed for electron microscopic examination (8,9), these results suggest that there has been a reduction in the quantity of virus produced during interferon therapy.

A comparison of the levels of papillomavirus DNA before (lanes a-f) and during (lanes g-l) interferon administration shows a reduction on average of the levels of viral DNA during drug therapy. However, the absolute levels during interferon therapy (lanes g-l) are never lower than the quantity observed in a biopsy collected on 1.27.82 (lane a) when the patient was being managed by laser excisions.

Thus, based on the data presented in Figure 1, this patient, 01-202, appears to have improved clinically on interferon therapy and this improvement is correlated at the molecular level with a reduction in the level of virus in the papillomata.

FIGURE 1

| 01-202 BF | | | OBS | | | IFN | | | IFN | | | |
|---|---|---|---|---|---|---|---|---|---|---|---|---|
| | a 1.27.82 | b 6.14.82 | c 9.16.82 | d 11.18.82 | e 1.31.83 | f 3.11.83 | g 5.9.83 | h 7.11.83 | i 12.9.83 | j 2.6.84 | k 9.13.84 | l 12.13.84 |
| Clinical Evaluation | 11 | 11 | 7 | 6 | 6 | 11 | 10 | 2 | 3 | 7 | 2 | 2 |
| Capsid Antigen | | +3 | +3 | +3 | +3 | +3 | +1 | 0 | 0 | | | |
| HPV-6c DNA | | | | | | | | | | | | |

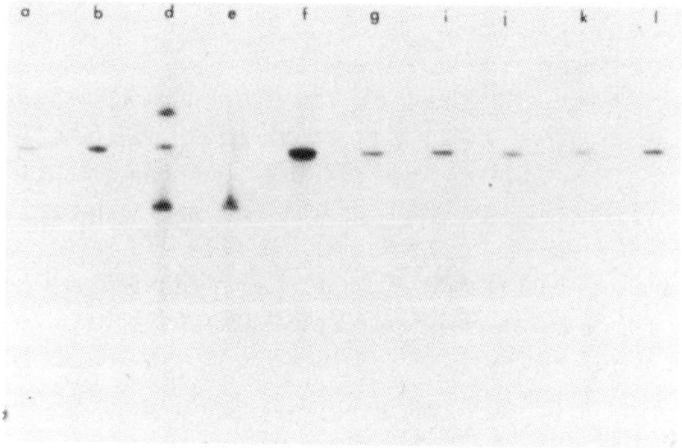


Analysis of patient 01-101. The results of the analysis of patient 01-101 during interferon therapy are presented in Fig. 2. This patient was randomized to interferon as described in METHODS on 8.9.82, crossed-over to observation 6 months later, and 9 months later on 11.3.83 was randomized on the addendum protocol to receive 2 $Mu/m^2$ daily. Examining patients who receive interferon first will allow us to determine if there is a rebound effect, i.e., if the virus is suppressed by interferon, does it rapidly increase to higher levels when drug therapy is discontinued?

A review of the composite scores derived from endoscopic examinations during interferon administration shows a reduction from 8 to 2 after approximately 14 weeks of interferon. Ten weeks later the composite score has increased to 6 but again drops to 3 on observation.

The fluctuations seen in the composite scores are also seen in the number of cells containing papillomavirus capsid antigen. It is interesting to note that an increase in the quantity of antigen-containing cells precedes an increase in airway disease as evidenced by an increase in the composite score. For example, a large number of antigen containing cells (+3) was seen in the biopsy removed on 11.29.82 and at the next endoscopic examination the severity of disease had increased from 2 to 6. Similarly, on 4.28.83 the capsid antigen evaluation had a score of +2 and airway disease increased from 3 to 5 at the next clinical examination. The fluctuations in levels of capsid antigen seen in this patient are characteristic of many respiratory papillomatosis patients, and in this patient the fluctuations did not appear to be different on drug therapy or observation.

The levels of viral DNA in the biopsy specimens analyzed over this 17 month period are also shown in Fig. 2. Two microgram samples of DNA were analyzed for each time point except lanes e and h where the yield of DNA was too low to quantify and the total DNA isolated from the small biopsies was analyzed. There is no apparent reduction in the level of viral DNA during interferon therapy for this patient. The level of viral DNA after 2 months (lane b) or after 14 weeks (lane c) of interferon is indistinguishable from the level of viral DNA at entry (lane a). There is also no evidence for a rebound effect when interferon therapy has been discontinued for one month (lane e) or 9 weeks (lane f).

FIGURE 2

01-101 NW

| | IFN | | | OBS | | | | IFN | |
|---|---|---|---|---|---|---|---|---|---|
| | a | b | c | d | e | f | g | h | i |
| | 8.9.82 | 10.12.82 | 11.29.82 | 2.11.83 | 3.17.83 | 4.28.83 | 6.13.83 | 11.3.83 | 1.10.84 |
| Clinical Evaluation | 8 | 4 | 2 | 6 | 3 | 3 | 5 | 5 | 7 |
| Capsid Antigen | 0 | | +3 | | 0 | +2 | 0 | | |
| HPV-6f DNA | | | | | | | | | |

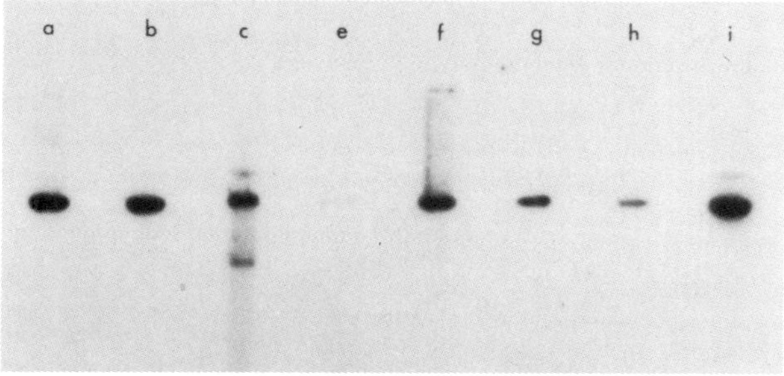


Analysis of patient 01-110. The results of the analysis of patient 01-110 during interferon therapy are presented in Fig. 3. It presents the data obtained during a 14 month period that includes 2 months prior to entry to the trial, 6 months of interferon and 6 months of observation. Because the disease in this patient was not primarily in the laryngotracheal region, the scoring system was not appropriate for evaluating disease in this patient. Therefore, the presence (indicated by +) or absence of disease (indicated by 0) primarily in the hypopharynx is presented. The sites involved included the nasopharynx, tonsils, uvula, and false cords. After 6 months of interferon followed by 4 months of observation there were no visible lesions at any of the 4 previously involved sites for 2 consecutive clinical evaluations.

The level of papillomavirus capsid antigen was stable at +2 for a 2 month period prior to interferon and dropped to +1 after 2 months of the drug. The only other biopsy examined immunocytochemically for virus was at 2 months after the patient crossed-over from interferon to observation and the score had returned to +2.

The level of HPV-6 DNA varied but showed no obvious correlation with the clinical evaluation. Shown in lanes a, b and c is the DNA during the 2 months before interferon, in lanes d and e during interferon therapy, and in lane g at 2 months after the patient crossed-over to observation. The level of viral DNA (lane g) is as high as at any time during the ten month period but the patient shows no evidence of clinical disease 2 months later.

FIGURE 3

**01-110 JS**

| | | | IFN | | | OBS | | | |
|---|---|---|---|---|---|---|---|---|---|
| | a | b | c | d | e | f | g | h | i |
| | 2.25.83 | 3.28.83 | 4.21.83 | 6.20.83 | 8.12.83 | 10.13.83 | 12.12.83 | 2.13.84 | 4.9.84 |
| Clinical Evaluation | | | | | | | | | |
| Nasopharynx | + | 0 | + | 0 | + | + | + | 0 | 0 |
| Tonsils | + | + | + | 0 | 0 | + | + | 0 | 0 |
| Uvula | + | + | + | + | 0 | + | 0 | 0 | 0 |
| False cords | + | 0 | 0 | 0 | 0 | 0 | 0 | 0 | 0 |
| Capsid Antigen | +2 | +2 | +2 | +1 | | | +2 | | |
| HPV-6f DNA | | | | | | | | | |

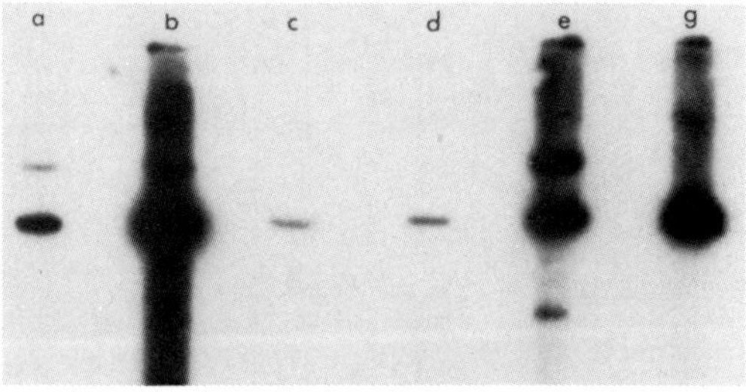

Preliminary Analysis of HPV-6 Subtype in Respiratory Papillomatosis Patients and Response to Interferon During the Six Months Prior to Cross-Over.

Table 5 presents the results of our preliminary analysis of 43 patients from the 66 patients who were registered in our clinical trial and who were randomized either to observation and surgical management for 6 months (20 patients) or to interferon and surgical management for 6 months (23 patients). The patients are grouped according to HPV-6 subtype present in biopsy specimens analyzed at entry to the trial. For each group, the averages of the composite scores, i.e., the quantitative assessment of airway disease, were calculated at entry and at 6 months on study.

TABLE 5
PAPILLOMAVIRUS SUBTYPE AND RESPONSE TO INTERFERON IN PATIENTS WITH JUVENILE ONSET RESPIRATORY PAPILLOMATOSIS

| Papillomavirus Subtype | Composite Score | | | | | | |
|---|---|---|---|---|---|---|---|
| | Observation | | | Interferon | | | |
| | N | Entry | 6 months | N | Entry | 6 months | |
| HPV-6c | 10 | 8.5 | 7.9 | 11 | 8.8 | 5.5 | mean |
| | | 4-15 | 1-15 | | 1-21 | 1-16 | range |
| | | | -7.1% | | | -35.3% | change |
| HPV-6d | 1 | 3 | 1 | 1 | 1 | 0 | |
| HPV-6e | 3 | 6.7 | 7.7 | 8 | 7.1 | 4.5 | mean |
| | | 2-12 | 1-11 | | 1-17 | 1-11 | range |
| | | | +14.9% | | | -36.6% | change |
| HPV-6f | 6 | 7.8 | 5.8 | 3 | 6 | 4.5 | mean |
| | | 1-24 | 1-9 | | 4-8 | 3-6 | range |
| | | | -25.6% | | | -25.5% | change |

The number of patients infected with HPV-6c and randomized to observation was 10. The average composite score at entry was 8.5 out of a maximum possible score of 27 with a range of 4 to 15. After 6 months of surgical management, the average composite score was 7.9 with a range of 1 to 15. This is a reduction in the composite score of 7.1% which indicates a reduction in respiratory tract disease visible at endoscopic examination.

The number of patients infected with HPV-6c and randomized to interferon was 11. The average composite score at entry was 8.8 with a range of 1 to 21 which is comparable to the observation control group. However, after 6 months of interferon there was a reduction of 35.3% in the average composite score to 5.5. This is a larger reduction than in the control group.

Only 2 patients were infected with HPV-6d with 1 randomized to observation and 1 randomized to interferon and both showed improvement.

Of the 11 patients infected with HPV-6e, 3 were randomized to observation and 8 were randomized to interferon. For the observation group, the average composite score was 6.7 at entry and 7.7 after 6 months with a similar range (2-12 vs. 1-11). This was an increase in the severity of disease of 14.9%. After 6 months of interferon there was a reduction in the average score of 36.6% and a reduction in the range from 1-17 to 1-11 within this group. This improvement in severity of disease is comparable to the improvement seen in the interferon treated patients infected with HPV-6c.

Of the nine patients infected with HPV-6f, 6 were randomized to observation and 3 were randomized to interferon with both groups showing similar levels of improvement. The mean composite score for the observation group was 7.8 at entry and 5.8 at 6 months for a decrease of 25.6%. The range at entry, 1-24, also decreased to 1-9. In the interferon group at entry, the mean composite score was 6 which decreased by 25.5% to 4.5 after 6 months of the drug. The range also decreased from 4-8 to 3-6.

This preliminary analysis of approximately two-thirds of the patients during the 6 months prior to cross-over suggests that at least two of the viruses in the respiratory tract may respond to interferon therapy. However, because of the small numbers of patients analyzed to date, it is not possible to make conclusions. It is necessary to evaluate the response data for the whole study group and in particular to evaluate the response data after cross-over where the patient serves as his/her own control.

## DISCUSSION

We have examined the relationship of HPV-6 subtypes to the clinical manifestations of disease in patients with recurrent respiratory papillomatosis and persistent condyloma acuminata. The course of a disease can be influenced by host-related and virus-related factors. An understanding of the role of viral subtypes in establishing the severity of disease will improve our knowledge of the virus and may provide a prognostic indicator as to the course and management of patients with papillomatosis. The biological significance of the genetic heterogeneity of papillomaviruses is unknown because *in vitro* systems are not available for the propagation and detailed examination of the behavior of these viruses. Therefore, we must examine the behavior of the virus in patients and attempt to correlate molecular analyses of the virus with clinical manifestations of disease.

The results presented identify HPV-6c as the most frequent subtype (55%) in 53 patients with recurrent respiratory papillomatosis. In contrast, HPV-6e and HPV-6f which were identified in 24% and 17%, respectively, of the respiratory papillomata, were the most frequent subtypes (30.8% for each) identified in 13 women with condyloma that were resistant to treatment with podophyllin or other conventional therapies. However, since the number of patients with genital tract infections was low, we are currently examining biopsy specimens from seventy women with persistent condyloma to extend these observations.

We also have presented the results of our preliminary investigations on the association between viral subtype and patient response to interferon therapy. There was significant reduction ($\geq$68% in 6 weeks) in the condylomatous growth in 11 of 12 women who were treated with systemic interferon. These 11 women were infected with HPV-6d, HPV-6e, HPV-6f, HPV-6h or HPV-6j. The only woman who failed to respond was infected with HPV-6c but with only one patient with this subtype tested, it is too early to determine if this virus is more resistant to interferon. We are currently analyzing a greater number of women who are being treated with interferon to continue our investigations.

The results of our preliminary analysis of 43 juveniles with recurrent respiratory papillomatosis who were randomized to interferon therapy or no drug evaluation in the precross-over period suggested that infections with HPV-6c as well as HPV-6e may respond to systemic administration of alpha interferon. There was an improvement in the clinical evaluation of disease in two groups of patients infected with HPV-6c (11 patients) or HPV-6e (8 patients) who were treated with interferon when compared to the no drug control groups infected with the same virus subtype (HPV-6c, 10 patients; HPV-6e, 3 patients). The 3 interferon treated patients infected with HPV-6f showed no improvement relative to their control group of 6 patients. We are continuing our analysis of the 66 juveniles registered for this trial. Therefore, conclusions cannot be made until all of the data are examined.

Previous pilot studies have reported that the majority of patients with recurrent respiratory papillomatosis show some response to alpha interferon (10-13). We and others have ongoing collaborative clinical trials evaluating the efficacy of interferon for papillomavirus infections that will provide response data on large numbers of patients and that may result in an effective therapy for these infections. However, there is variation among patients in the clinical behavior of these infections and it is of value to examine the response patterns of individuals and the response of the virus at the molecular level. The results of such an analysis on 3 patients with respiratory tract lesions are presented. These analyses demonstrate that there are differences between patients in the quantities of viral DNA and virus particles, as measured immunocytochemically for capsid antigen containing cells, even when they are infected with the same virus (HPV-6f in patient 01-101, Fig. 2 and 01-110, Fig. 3). There are also differences for one patient when he or she is followed for a long period of time. For example, Fig. 1 shows the variations in the quantity of viral DNA in 5 biopsy specimens from patient 01-202 for a 14 month period (lanes a-f) and illustrates that it is necessary to evaluate the response of the virus at the molecular level for a long period of time to distinguish natural variation from therapy induced differences. The analysis of patient 01-202 at the clinical level or the molecular level demonstrated improved disease control, but not elimination, while on interferon.

In contrast, patient 01-110 (Fig. 3) showed elimination of disease for 2 consecutive examinations at 4 months after 6 months of interferon therapy despite the presence of relatively high levels of viral DNA at the preceding examination. These results and the results of others who have demonstrated viral DNA in histologically normal tissue from patients in clinical remission (3) or in 1 patient who did not show evidence of clinical response to alpha interferon (14) suggest that assessment of interferon or other potential anti-viral agents in eliminating disease should be evaluated at the molecular as well as clinical levels. Therefore, we are continuing our molecular analyses of papillomavirus in patients receiving interferon therapy to attempt to determine if interferon is effective in reducing papillomavirus replication.

## ACKNOWLEDGMENTS

We would like to acknowledge the support of collaborating institutions at the Univ. of Nebraska, Oklahoma Univ., Univ. of Washington, Washington Univ., Univ. of

Southern California, Yale Univ., Baylor College of Medicine, Univ. of Iowa Hospitals, and The Hospital for Sick Children, Toronto. We also acknowledge Keith Peden for helpful discussions and Joy Marsh for assistance in the preparation of this manuscript.

## REFERENCES

1. Mounts P, Shah KV, Kashima HK (1982). Viral etiology of juvenile- and adult-onset squamous papilloma of the larynx. Proc Natl Acad Sci 79:5425.
2. Gissmann L, Wolnik L, Ikenberg H, Koldovsky U, Schnurch HG, zur Hausen H (1983). Human papillomavirus types 6 and 11 DNA sequences in genital and laryngeal papillomas and in some cervical cancers. Proc Natl Acad Sci 80:560.
3. Steinberg BM, Topp W, Schneider PS, Abramson A (1983). Laryngeal papillomavirus infection during clinical remission. New Engl J Med 308:1261.
4. Mounts P, Kashima HK (1984). Association of human papillomavirus subtype and clinical course in respiratory papillomatosis. Laryngoscope 94:28.
5. Finter NB, Fantes KH (1981). The purity and safety of interferons prepared for clinical use: The case for lymphoblastoid interferon. In Gresser I (ed): "Interferon," New York: Academic Press, p 65.
6. Kashima H, Leventhal B, Clark K, Dedo H, Donovan D, Lusk R, Muntz H, Singleton G, Weck P, Whisnant J (in preparation). Severity scoring and evaluation of clinical course in recurrent respiratory papillomatosis.
7. Mounts P, Shah KV (1984). Respiratory papillomatosis: Etiological relation to genital tract papillomaviruses. Prog Med Virol 29:90.
8. Braun L, Kashima H, Eggleston J, Shah KV (1982). Demonstration of papillomavirus antigen in paraffin sections of laryngeal papillomas. Laryngoscope 92:640.
9. Heilman CA, Law M-F, Israel MA, Howley PM (1980). Cloning of human papillomavirus genomic DNAs and analysis of homologous polynucleotide sequences. J Virol 36:395.
10. Haglund S, Lundquist P, Cantell K, Strander H (1981). Interferon therapy in juvenile laryngeal papillomatosis. Arch Otolaryngol 107:327.

11. Goepfert H, Sessions RB, Gutterman JU, Canair H, Dichtel WJ, Sulek M (1982). Leukocyte interferon in patients with juvenile laryngeal papillomatosis. Ann Otol Rhinol Largol 91:431.
12. McCabe BF, Clark KF (1983). Interferon and laryngeal papillomatosis: The Iowa experience. Ann Otol Rhinol Laryngol 92:2.
13. Bomholt A (1983). Interferon therapy for laryngeal papillomatosis in adults. Arch Otolaryngol 109:550.
14. Ikenberg H, Neumann-Haefelin D, Richthammer B, Wolfort W, Adler C-P, Bodo G, Gissmann L, zur Hausen H (1985). Interferon therapy for bronchial papillomatosis controlled by papillomavirus-DNA hybridization. Arch Otolaryngol 111:96.

**Papillomaviruses: Molecular and Clinical Aspects, pages 155–163**


# INFECTION OF THE ORAL CAVITY WITH GENITAL TRACT PAPILLOMAVIRUSES*

Zohreh Naghashfar,[1] Mark J. Kutcher,[2] Edward Sawada[3] and Keerti V. Shah[1]

[1]Department of Immunology and Infectious Diseases, School of Hygiene and Public Health, The Johns Hopkins University, Baltimore, Maryland, 21205
[2]School of Dentistry, University of Maryland, Baltimore, Maryland, 21201
[3]Maryland State Cancer Control Unit, Baltimore, Maryland, 21201

ABSTRACT Warts of the oral cavity are etiologically heterogeneous. In addition to HPV-13, a virus associated with focal epithelial hyperplasia in the oral cavity, genital papillomaviruses HPV-6 and HPV-16 are recovered from oral cavity lesions. The warts caused by genital papillomaviruses were asymptomatic, multiple or single, recurrent, and located in different parts of the oral cavity.

## INTRODUCTION

Papillomas are not uncommonly found in the oral cavity. The histologic entity "irritation fibroma" which is one of the most commonly accessioned lesions of the soft tissues of the oral cavity is sometimes the result of fibrosis in a previous papilloma. Clinically, papillary lesions of the oral cavity are exophytic and pedunculated, although they are occasionally sessile. The lesion is usually formed by numerous, small finger-like projections which give these benign tumors a verrucous or "cauliflower-like" surface. However, they are sometimes found as smooth, elongated single-stalked entities. Most are quite small, being only a few millimeters in diameter, although some have been reported to measure several centimeters.

*This work was supported by NIH grant #P01 AI-16959.

Many of the lesions retain normal mucosal coloration but those subjected to constant trauma become hyperkeratotic and take on a white coloration. Oral papillomas are found most commonly on the tongue, lips, buccal mucosa, gingiva, palate, and on or near the uvula. The lesions can occur at any age and have been reported in very young children and in those over 70 years of age.

Until recently warts at all sites were regarded as being caused by a single wart virus and warts were generally thought of as having no more than a nuisance value (1). However, investigations in the past ten years have completely changed this outlook. At least 31, individually distinct, human papillomaviruses (HPV) are recognized. The HPVs show considerable specificity with respect to site and morphology of the lesion. Almost all flat skin warts are caused by HPV-3 or HPV-10, common warts by HPV-2 or HPV-4 and plantar warts by HPV-1 or HPV-4. Five different HPVs, HPV-6, HPV-11, HPV-16, HPV-18 and HPV-31, predominantly infect the genital tract. HPV-6 and HPV-11 appear to be responsible for most of the condylomas in the genital tract as well as for most of the papillomas in the respiratory tract (2,3,4). A few of the HPVs have oncogenic potential. HPV-5 and HPV-8 are associated with squamous cell carcinomas which arise in macular lesions of the rare dermatological disorder, epidermodysplasia verruciformis (5). HPV-16 and HPV-18 are strongly associated with genital tract malignancies in the female and in the male (6,7). Identification of HPVs from a variety of genital lesions has shown that the clinical spectrum of wart virus infections is much broader than was previously recognized. In the genital tract, the viruses cause not only the exophytic, pedunculated growths readily identified as warts but they may also produce flat, barely raised lesions which may be difficult to detect without a colposcope. They also cause a variety of cellular atypias which have the potential for progression to malignancy.

The role of HPVs in the causation of skin warts is fully established, but the etiology of various types of oral papillomas is unclear. Viral papillomas of the oral cavity are probably the result of contact of the oral mucosa with one's own warts at other sites by autoinoculation or by contact with warts of another individual. Histologically oral warts are often classified as "verruca vulgaris" implying transmission from the common skin warts or as condylomas implying transmission of genital tract viruses.

However, the histologic criteria are ambiguous and not reliable with respect to the source of the virus.

## Investigations of Oral Cavity Lesions

Numerous previous studies have reported the presence of papillomavirus particles in oral cavity lesions (8,9,10). More recently, papillomavirus capsid antigen has been demonstrated in paraffin sections of oral lesions by immunoperoxidase tests with a genus-specific antiserum (11-15) (Table 1). The presence of capsid antigen is indicative of a productive infection and it correlates very well with the presence of viral particles in the tissue (16). The antigen was present in the nuclei of superficial cells of the epithelium. It was identified in 40%-100% of tissues diagnosed histologically as papilloma, condyloma, verruca vulgaris, leukoplakia, and focal epithelial hyperplasia but not in keratoacanthomas (Table 1). The antigen was reported to be present in areas adjacent to verrucous carcinoma (14) but was not detected in the carcinomas themselves. Because the serum reacts with capsids of all human and animal papillomaviruses, it is not useful in specifically identifying the infecting virus. Type-specific antisera to HPVs are not yet available.

TABLE 1

A SUMMARY OF INVESTIGATION FOR PAPILLOMAVIRUS CAPSID ANTIGEN IN ORAL LESIONS

| Investigator | Observation |
|---|---|
| Jenson et al. (11) | 18 of 29 verruca vulgaris |
| | 2 of 5 multiple papilomas |
| | 3 of 5 condylomata |
| | 0 of 28 keratoacanthomas |
| Lutzner et al. (20) | 2 of 2 FEH |
| Syrjanen et al. (14) | 8 of 12 in lesion adjacent to squamous cell carcinoma |
| Jin and Toto (12) | 8 of 11 verruca vulgaris |
| | 3 of 6 condyloma accuminatum |
| | 0 of 7 verrucous carcinoma |
| Loning et al. (13) | 5 of 6 oral papillomas |
| | 2 of 5 homogenous leukoplakia |
| | 2 of 2 nodular leukoplakia |
| Naghashfar et al. (15) | 6 of 15 papilloma or verruca vulgaris |

The specific diagnosis of an infecting genotype requires hybridization studies of tissue DNA with labeled viral DNA probes. These may be performed with DNA extracted from fresh or fresh-frozen tissues (2,3), or with cells spotted on filter and denatured *In situ* (17), or by *in situ* hybridization of paraffin sections or cell smears on glass slides (18,19) (Table 2). Most of the studies with oral tissues have been done with Southern transfer hybridization of DNA extracted from the lesions. This technique is very sensitive and can detect 0.1 genome copy/cell, but it requires fresh or fresh-frozen tissue. Diagnosis has also been made by *in situ* hybridization of paraffin sections of the tissue with radiolabeled probes. This technique is considerably less sensitive than the Southern transfer method for detection of the viral genome, but it can be performed on material that is collected, processed and stored in a routine manner.

TABLE 2

METHODS OF DIAGNOSIS OF PAPILLOMAVIRUS GENOTYPES

| Specimen | Method |
|---|---|
| DNA extracted from fresh tissues or cells | (i) Southern transfer hybridization, after transfer of electrophoretically separated cellular DNA fragments to filters (23) |
| | (ii) hybridization of denatured cellular DNA spotted on filter |
| Exfoliated cells | hybridization of cells spotted on filter and denatured *in situ* (17) |
| Cells or paraffin section of tissue on slide | *In situ* hybridization (18, 19) |

In contrast to the large amount of work done to characterize HPV genomes in skin and genital warts, investigations aimed at identifying the HPV genotypes in the oral cavity have been limited. They are summarized in Table 3. In the study of Lutzner et al. (20), the identity of the genotype was inferred from restriction enzyme digest pattern of the viral DNA but was not confirmed by hybridization studies. All of the other studies were based on hybridization of tissue DNAs with radiolabeled probes. In one instance, the genotype was identified by *in situ*

TABLE 3

PAPILLOMAVIRUS GENOTYPES IN THE ORAL CAVITY

| Investigator | Tissue | Genotype |
|---|---|---|
| Petzoldt and Pfister (24) | one case of FEH | HPV-1 |
| Lutzner et al. (20) | one case of verruca vulgaris | HPV-2* |
| Pfister et al. (21) | 3 of 6 cases of FEH | HPV-13 |
| Syrjanen et al. (23) | one case of FEH | HPV-13 |
| Loning et al. (13) | some leukoplakias | HPV-11 and 16 |
| Naghashfar et al. (15) | 3 of 8 cases of papilloma and in one paraffin section of an oral papilloma | HPV-6 and 16 |

*based on restriction enzyme digest pattern only

hybridization of a paraffin section. In all other cases, genotype identification was made by Southern transfer hybridization with extracted tissue DNA.

A unique virus, HPV-13, is associated with lesions of focal epithelial hyperplasia (FEH) (21), a condition described as limited exclusively to the oral cavity and having a predilection for certain ethnic groups (22). FEH has a high prevalence of 7% to 36% in Greenlandic Eskimos at different locations in Greenland. In the same areas, the prevalence in Caucasians was 0.3%. It is also found in up to 3.5% of American Indians in Central and South America. The disease is seen mainly in children of the American Indians but in all age groups of Greenlandic Eskimos (22). HPV-13 was recovered by Pfister et al. (21) in 3 of 6 cases of FEH and by Syrjanen et al. (23) in one case of FEH (Table 3). Petzoldt and Pfister (24) identified HPV-1 in one case of FEH.

HPVs characterized from oral cavity lesions other than FEH are papillomaviruses of the genital tract. Loning et al. (13) reported that HPV-11 and HPV-16 were recovered from some oral leukoplakias but the details of these studies are not yet published. We identified HPV-6 in three cases and HPV-16 in one case of oral cavity lesions (15). The lesions in our study were asymptomatic, multiple or single, recurrent, and located in different parts of the oral cavity. The HPV-16-associated lesion, and a previous lesion on the uvula of the same patient, are shown in Figure 1. In the study of genital warts, some of the HPV infections can be recognized only after colposcopic examination. Application of 5% acetic acid to the area makes the lesions more prominent. One of us (ES) has found that the same procedures are also useful in identification of HPV infections of the oral cavity.

FIGURE 1

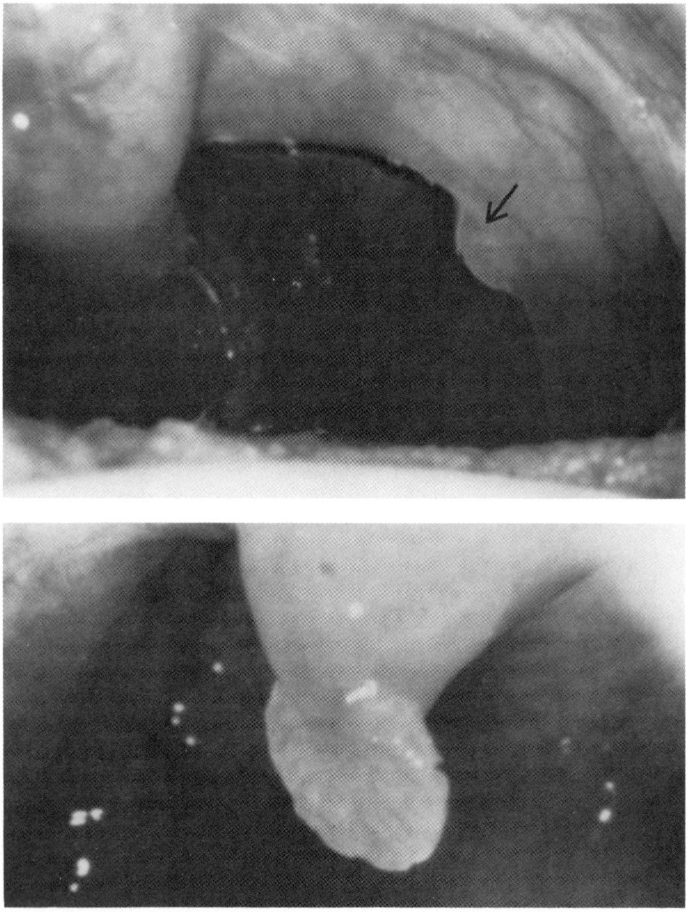

Fig. 1: A (top), lesion on posterior tonsillar pillar (arrow) from which HPV-16 was isolated; B (bottom), lesion on uvula of the same patient 8 months earlier. This lesion was not screened for viral genome.

## DISCUSSION

The results presented here show that warts in the oral cavity are etiologically heterogeneous and that genital tract viruses account for some of the warts in the oral cavity. Many sexually transmitted pathogens such as gonorrhea, syphilis and herpes simplex viruses are infections of both the genital and respiratory tracts. Papillomaviruses exhibit specificity with respect to the site of infection, so it is not surprising that viruses that infect the genital mucosa can also grow successfully in the oral mucosa. The contribution of HPVs that cause skin warts to oral cavities is not yet clear. The infection of the oral cavity with genital viruses may occur as a result of auto-inoculation, by oral contact with infected genitalia, or by contact with contaminated fomites. It is also possible that, as with laryngeal papilloma of juvenile onset, infection of the oral cavity may occur during fetal passage through an infected birth canal. The etiology, prevalence, pathogenicity, and epidemiology of HPVs in the oral cavity remain to be determined.

With respect to the pathogenic potential of oral HPVs, their possible role in oral cavity cancers deserves investigation. At least two of the genital tract viruses, HPV-16 and HPV-18, are strongly associated with cancers of the cervix, vulva and penis. Syrjanen et al. (14) have demonstrated productive papillomavirus infection in proximity to squamous cell carcinomas of the oral cavity and Eisenberg et al. (25) have found that verrucous carcinomas of the oral cavity display cytologic features of papillomavirus infections. Papillomaviruses have been implicated in the etiology of verrucous carcinomas of the genital tract. Investigation of oral cavity warts and malignancies with techniques which identify specific papillomavirus genotypes is likely to increase our understanding of these diseases.

## REFERENCES

1. Rowson KEK, Mahy BWJ (1967). Human papova (wart) virus. Bacteriol Rev 31:110-131.
2. Gissmann L, Diehl V, Schultz-Coulon JH, zur Hausen H (1982). Molecular cloning and characterization of human papilloma virus DNA derived from a laryngeal papilloma. J Virol 44:393-400.

3. Gissmann L, de Villiers EM, zur Hausen H (1982). Analysis of human genital warts (condylomata acuminata) and other genital tumors for human papilloma virus type 6 DNA. Intl J Cancer 29:143-146.
4. Mounts P, Shah KV (1984). Respiratory papillomatosis: Etiological relation to genital tract papillomaviruses. Prog Med Virol 29:90-114.
5. Orth G, Favre M, Breitburd F, Croissant O, Jablonska S, Obalek S, Jarzabek-Chorzelska M, Rzesa G (1980). Epidermodysplasia verruciformis: A model for the role of papilloma viruses in human cancer. In Essex M, Todaro G, zur Hausen H (eds): "Viruses in Naturally Occurring Cancers," Cold Spring Harbor Conferences on Cell Proliferation, Vol 7. New York: Cold Spring Harbor Laboratory, pp 259-282.
6. Durst M, Gissmann L, Ikenberg H, zur Hausen H (1983). A papillomavirus DNA from a cervical carcinoma and its prevalence in cancer biopsy samples from different geographic regions. Proc Natl Acad Sci USA 80:3812-3815.
7. Boshart M, Gissmann L, Ikenberg H, Kleinheinz A, Scheurlen W, zur Hausen H (1984). A new type of papillomavirus DNA, its presence in genital cancer biopsies and in cell lines derived from cervical cancer. EMBO J 3:1151-1157.
8. Frithiof L, Wersall J (1967). Virus-like particles in human oral papilloma. Acta Oto-laryngol 64:263-266.
9. Wysocki GP, Hardi J (1979). Ultrastructural studies of intraoral verruca vulgaris. Oral Surg, Oral Med, Oral Pathol 47:58-62.
10. Gross GE, Pfister H, Mittermayer C (1980). Papilloma virus particles in a fibroma of the tongue. Acta Dermatovener (Stockholm) 60:315-318.
11. Jenson AB, Lancaster WD, Hartmann DP, Shaffer EL Jr (1982). Frequency and distribution of papillomavirus structural antigens in verrucae, multiple papillomas, and condylomata of the oral cavity. Am J Pathol 107: 212-218.
12. Jin YT, Toto PD (1984). Detection of human papovavirus antigen in oral papillary lesions. Oral Surg, Oral Med, Oral Pathol 58:702-705.
13. Loning T, Reichart R, Staquet MJ, Bercher J, Thivolet J (1984). Occurrence of papillomavirus structural antigen in oral papillomas and leukoplakias. J Oral Pathol 13:155-165.
14. Syrjanen KJ, Pyrhonen S, Syrjanen SM, Lamberg M (1983). Immunohistochemical demonstration of human

papilloma virus (HPV) antigens in oral squamous cell lesions. Brit J Oral Surg 21:147-153.

15. Naghashfar Z, Sawada E, Kutcher MJ, Swancar J, Gupta J, Daniel R, Kashima H, Woodruff JD, Shah K (1985). Identification of genital tract papillomaviruses HPV-6 and HPV-16 in warts of the oral cavity. J Med Virol (submitted).
16. Ferenczy A, Braun L, Shah KV (1981). Human papillomavirus (HPV) in condylomatous lesions of the cervix. Am J Surg Pathol 5:661-670.
17. Wagner D, Ikenberg H, Boehm N, Gissmann L (1984). Identification of human papillomavirus in cervical smears by deoxyribonucleic acid _in situ_ hybridization. Obst Gynecol 64:767-772.
18. Beckmann AM, Myerson D, Daling JR, Kiviat NB, Fenoglio CM, McDougall JK (1985). Detection of human papillomavirus DNA in carcinomas by _in situ_ hybridization with biotinylated probes. J Med Virol (in press).
19. Gupta JW, Gendelman HE, Naghashfar Z, Gupta P, Rosenshein N, Sawada E, Woodruff JD, Shah KV (1985). Specific identification of human papillomavirus type in cervical smears and paraffin sections by _in situ_ hybridization with radioactive probes. Intl J Gyn Pathol (in press).
20. Lutzner M, Kuffer R, Blanchet-Bardon C, Croissant O (1982). Different papillomaviruses as the causes of oral warts. Arch Dermatol 118:393-399.
21. Pfister H, Hettich I, Runne U, Gissmann L, Chilf GN (1983). Characterization of human papillomavirus type 13 from focal epithelial hyperplasia Heck lesions. J Virol 47:363-366.
22. Praetorius-Clausen F (1972). Rare oral viral disorders (molluscum contagiosum, localized keratoacanthoma, verrucae, condyloma acuminatum, and focal epithelial hyperplasia). Oral Surg, Oral Med, Oral Pathol 34:604-618.
23. Syrjanen S, Syrjanen K, Ikenberg H, Gissmann L, Lamberg M (1984). A human papillomavirus closely related to HPV-13 found in a focal epithelial hyperplasia lesion (Heck disease). Arch Dermatol Res 276:199-200.
24. Petzoldt D, Pfister H (1980). HPV-1 DNA in lesions of focal epithelial hyperplasia Heck. Arch Dermatol Res 268:313-314.
25. Eisenberg E, Rosenberg B, Krutchkoff DJ, Conn F (1985). Verrucous carcinoma: A possible viral pathogenesis. Oral Surg, Oral Med, Oral Pathol 59:52-57.

Papillomaviruses: Molecular and Clinical Aspects, pages 165–180


# FURTHER STUDIES ON INTERFERON THERAPY IN JUVENILE LARYNGEAL PAPILLOMATOSIS[1]

Hans Strander, Stig Haglund, and P.-G. Lundquist[2]

Radiumhemmet and Department of Oto-Rhino-Laryngology, Karolinska Hospital, 104 01 Stockholm, Sweden

ABSTRACT The experience with interferon (IFN) therapy on patients with juvenile laryngeal papillomatosis (JLP) at the Karolinska Hospital is updated. Twelve cases have been treated and followed up after treatment. An antitumor effect has been documented for all cases. Various doses and schedules used have revealed that the success of leukocyte IFN treatment of JLP to a large extent depends on the dose. It is suggested that the dose optimum should be worked out in detail and that larger series of patients should be treated with this purpose in mind. Further studies on mechanisms involved in treatment effects are also necessary to optimize this type of therapy.

## INTRODUCTION

Human laryngeal papillomatosis of the juvenile type (JLP) (1, 2) is a benign tumor disease with viral association (3, 4, 5, 6). In some cases it can recur causing a chronic disease requiring extensive periodic surgical intervention in order to maintain an adequate airway (7).

[1]This work was supported by the Cancer Society in Stockholm and the Albert and Mary Lasker Foundation.
[2]Present address: Department of Oto-Rhino-Laryngology, University of Linköping, Linköping, Sweden

It has to be considered as an important disease dispite the fact that it is a rather uncommon disease as it usually affects young children and can cause severe symptoms.

The suspected viral etiology of JLP has lead to the development of various forms of adjuvant therapy to prevent recurrencies after surgery and has received general interest since similar diseases also can be found in the dermatological and gynecological areas (8). Up to the mid-seventies there were, however, no such treatments which lead to consistent effects. Meanwhile, the surgical techniques were improved and the use of $CO_2$ laser treatments have been of great benefit in the local control of the disease in the patients (9, 10).

In 1976 we undertook a pilot study at the Karolinska Hospital in order to see if treatment of this particular disease with systemic administration of human leukocyte interferon (IFN) therapy (11, 12) would be feasible. The initial results were reported from 1977 and on (13). Over the years we have updated the results and a few papers presenting more detailed information have been published (14, 15, 16).

At the time of writing we have treated and followed for extended periods of time 12 patients with this particular disease at the Karolinska Hospital. The present paper will give data on these 12 patients and provide some clinical impact for the future use of IFN therapy against this distressing disease.

## METHODS

The patients have all been followed for various periods of time at the Department of Oto-Rhino-Laryngology of the Karolinska Hospital in Stockholm. Whenever feasible the patients have gone home to their home districts where they also have been seen by local doctors on occasion. Surgical interventions were initially made by conventional means but over the last year laser excisions have been employed.

The human leukocyte IFN preparations have been obtained through professor K. Cantell of the Central Public Health Service, Helsinki, Finland, or dr H.-L. Kauppinen at the Red Cross Transfusion Service, Helsinki, Finland. Some patients have also been treated with IFN obtained through a joint project between the Karolinska Hospital and the University Hospital of Uppsala, Sweden. All the human leukocyte IFN preparations have been semi-purified, containing IFN at a purity of 1-6 x $10^6$ IU per mg protein, and prepared by methods employing Sendai virus as the IFN inducer (17, 18). The number of units has been determined through comparison to the international standard preparation 69/19.

IFN treatment was always given on an ambulatory basis and older patients were instructed to administer their own IFN. Younger patients received their IFN, which was always given i.m. at a dose of 3 x $10^6$ IU, by their parents or by district nurses.

## RESULTS

Case reports. Below follows a description of the 12 cases treated to date.

Case 1. (J.M.)-JLP was discovered in this 2 1/2-year-old girl in 1974. Thirteen endoscopic removals were followed by tracheostomy in December 1975 because of respiratory pathway obstruction. Complete occlusion of the larynx occured in January 1976 and therapy was initiated with human leukocyte IFN by giving injections 3 times weekly. In May 1976 only a thin mass of papillomatous tissue remained. In January 1977 a few papillomas were present. The vocal cords were free. Unfortunately a glottic web was present so the tracheostoma could not be removed. In March 1977 there was further diminuition. After 1 1/2 years of treatment it was decided to remove as much as possible of tumor tissue. In December 1977 active growth of papillomas still occured. They were removed. In January 1978 no further regression was observed and therapy with leukocyte IFN was discontinued. In March 1978 extensive increase in tumor activity occured. From June 1978 and on,tumor removal had to be done every month. In September 1978 IFN therapy was again initiated due to uncontrolled growth. Three injections were given per week. In October 1978 almost all papillomas had disappeared and in December 1978 the larynx was remarkably clean and the IFN was then only given twice weekly. In March 1979 there were no signs of tumor growth and it was then decided to give IFN once weekly only. In August 1979 no tumor was visible. In December 1979 IFN therapy was discontinued. In August 1980 there were no visible tumors. In March 1981 there were a couple of small papillomas which were removed. There were no signs of papillomatous growth in September 1981. An operation was performed in order to correct stenosis. In April 1984 decanylation could be performed. In December 1984 a split operation was performed and in February 1985 a laryngeal fissure. The patient has been free of papillomatosis for the last 4 years.

Case 2. (U.B.G.)-JLP was discovered in this 4-year-old girl in 1968. More than 25 endoscopic removals had been made up to 1975 when tracheostomy had to be performed due to tumor growth. In June 1976 the papillomatosis completely occluded the larynx and extended up to the base of the tongue. IFN therapy was initiated that month giving IFN 3 times weekly by i.m. injections. In January 1977 gradual diminuition of the tumors took place so the vocal cords became visible. The tracheostomy was closed. In June 1977 a thin layer of papillomatous tissue was present. IFN therapy was discontinued.

In August 1977 a considerable increase in the size of the papillomas occured. The tumors were removed and IFN therapy was started on a 3 times weekly basis. In November 1977 tumor growth had come to a halt. In January 1978 no active tumor growth was observed. IFN therapy was then reduced to injections given twice weekly. In February 1978 there was still no visible tumor growth. IFN was further reduced to one injection per week. In June 1978 some papillomas were observed. IFN was discontinued. In August 1978 exploding growth required tracheostomy. IFN was reinstituted in September on the 3 times weekly schedule. Five weeks later, in September 1978, a good air-way was present and the papillomatous growth had decreased. IFN therapy was then reduced to the twice weekly schedule. In June 1979 a sharp increase in tumor growth was noticed. IFN therapy was then again given 3 times weekly. In August 1979 a decrease in tumor activity was documented. IFN was continued 3 times weekly and in December 1979 there was an unchanged status. In January 1980 IFN therapy was halted. In June 1980 there was papillomatous tissue through the supraglottic space up to the arytenoid region and in August 1980 further endoscopic removals had to be done. Up to May 1981 the patient had to be operated almost every month since there was very active papillomatous growth.

In May 1981 it was decided to give the patient daily IFN treatment. At the next control endoscopy, after not even a month of treatment, there was no papillomatous tissue to remove and there were only a few small superficial papillomas present. It was then decided to reduce the treatment to the 3 times weekly schedule. In August there was no papillomatous growth to be seen. In November 1981 the patient was worse and there was massive growth in the whole larynx and it was again decided to give IFN daily. This was followed later with signs of papilloma regression. It was then again decided to give the patient IFN 3 times weekly. Control check ups in March and June 1982 showed abundant papillomatous growth. In September growth had continued and the whole larynx was covered by papillomatous tissue. Removals had to be undertaken in December 1982 and in February 1983. It was then decided to give IFN treatment only twice weekly after February 1983. Due to the presence of air obstruction it was again decided in April 1983 to give IFN 3 times weekly. In August 1983 there was abundant papillomatous growth and it was decided to go on giving IFN 3 times weekly. In October 1983 and January 1984 some papillomatous tissue was removed by laser treatment. IFN treatment was continued and in May 1984 there was almost no papillomatous tissue to be seen. In July 1984 it was decided to stop IFN treatment but after 2 months there was again abundant papillomatous growth. The patient has come for control check ups in October 1984, February 1985 and in March 1985 again with abundant papillomatous growth. It has now been decided to try to treat the patient with daily IFN therapy.

Case 3. (T.L.)-JLP was discovered in this 2 1/2-year-old boy in 1962. Fifty endoscopies had been performed before admission to our hospital. Before the initiation of IFN therapy in September 1977 removals had had to be done every second week for the previous 6 months. At endoscopy papillomatous tissue covered a large part of the larynx and IFN therapy was initiated 3 times weekly. In October 1977 there was a halt of the tumor growth and in December 1977 there was no further change in the extension of the papillomatous tissue. It was decided to remove as much as possible of the tumor and continue IFN therapy. In January 1978 there was no tumor activity and IFN was reduced to the twice weekly schedule. In October 1978 only few papillomas were present and IFN therapy was discontinued. In December 1978 there was accelerated growth and abundant papillomas. As much of the tumor mass as possible was removed and IFN therapy was again given 3 times weekly. In February 1979 there was no appearant increase in tumor size but there was still papillomatous tissue present. In April 1979 no change could be seen and IFN therapy was discontinued. In September 1979 there were a few solitary papillomas present and after removal the larynx was completely clean. There were still a few papillomas present in December 1979. Papillomatous growth then continued and removals had to be done in connection with a visit in August 1979, and after that on 18 occasions, the last one in January 1985. It has now been decided again to try to reinstitute IFN on this case to see whether it is possible to affect the distressing disease in this patient.

Case 4. (H.K.)-JLP was diagnosed in this 9-year-old boy in 1965. A large number of endoscopies had been performed up to 1977 when an endoscopy in September 1977 showed abundant papillomatous growth. A check up was made in October 1977. A few papillomas were present and IFN therapy was instituted 3 times weekly. During one year up to October 1978 no signs of tumor growth were present and IFN therapy was discontinued. Seven months later there was an inspection in May 1979 showing no visible tumor and the same negative result was obtained in October 1979. In January 1980 the patient complained of respiratory distress and an endoscopy showed almost complete tracheal obstruction caused by papillomatous growth. Tumor was removed and check ups were instituted more frequently and in June 1980 papillomas had to be removed again. There was almost complete tracheal obstruction and IFN therapy was reinstituted 3 times weekly. The situation improved and in August 1980 there were only solitary papillomas present. IFN therapy was continued up to October 1980. There was just a small papilloma present which was removed. There were also small papillomas present in March 1981 and in October 1981. In January 1982 there were signs of subglottic growth of papilloma tissue. It was removed and IFN therapy was instituted 3 times weekly up to May 1982. A control check up in June 1982 showed no signs of papillomatous growth. In November 1982 and also in September 1983 there were signs of small papillomas. There was a very small papilloma present in August 1984. This patient is free of symptoms and has presently no signs of papillomatous growth.

Case 5. (R.E.)-JLP was discovered in this 3 1/2-year-old boy in 1977. Due to very active papillomatous growth leading to 5 endoscopic removals during the 2 previous months it was decided in August 1978 to initiate IFN therapy and give it 3 times weekly. Initially in August 1978 there were abundant papillomas present bilaterally on the vocal cords and on the ventricular folds. In November 1978 there was a decrease in tumor activity leading to only few papillomas. In March 1979 the patient had developed a good voice. In June 1979 there was no apparent increase of tumor and there was an unchanged situation up to December 1979 when the status of the patient's condition was excellent with very slight papillomatous growth. It was then decided to stop IFN treatment. In February 1980 there was a tremendous recurrence with tumor growing all through the larynx. As much as possible of the tumor was removed and IFN therapy was reinitiated 3 times weekly. In August 1980 there were only a few solitary papillomas present.

This patient has all the time since been given IFN therapy at the same dose. Due to a difficult social situation it has been difficult to control his injections. He has had to be reoperated every third to every sixth month and still he has some signs of papillomatous activity. We have now decided to try to give him daily IFN injections and control the injections strictly.

Case 6. (C.S.)-In 1977 JLP was found in this 1 1/2-year-old boy. During 1977 4 endoscopies had to be done due to fulminant tumor growth. In February 1978 as much as possible of the tumor was removed and IFN therapy initiated 3 times weekly. In March 1978 there was still abundant papillomatous growth and again as much of the tumor was removed as possible. In April 1978 there was a sharp improvement in the status and only very few papillomas in the arytenoid region remained in the patient. In September 1978 there was still diminished tumor activity and it was then decided to give IFN twice weekly. In December 1978 there was no apparent tumor growth and IFN therapy was reduced to a once weekly schedule. In April 1979 there were no signs of tumor and it was then decided to discontinue IFN therapy. In August 1979 there was abundant papillomatous growth and the papillomas were surgically removed. In November 1979 there were moderate amounts of papillomas present and this situation prevailed through February 1980 and June 1980. It was then decided to reinitiate the IFN therapy and treatment was again given 3 times weekly. In August 1980 there were only few solitary papillomas present. In November 1980 one could see some papillomas which were removed and the patient was continued on IFN therapy. Small signs of papillomatosis were present in March 1981. In June 1981 there was very little left. In September 1981 there was moderate presence of papillomatosis and the papillomas were removed. In January 1982 there were more signs of papilloma growth. The papillomas were removed and the IFN therapy was continued at the same dose. In August 1982 there were signs of less activity and in November 1982 there was only one small papilloma remaining. Through check ups made in March, July and October, 1983, and February, May and September, 1984, and also March, 1985, there have been moderate papillomas present regularly. The patient has continued on the 3 times weekly schedule. We have now decided to give IFN as daily treatment to this patient.

Case 7. (C.C.)-JLP was seen in this 2-year-old boy in 1956. He had had tracheostomies twice and more than 40 endoscopies had been performed up to April 1976. Abundant tumor growth was present, the patient had almost no rima glottidis and the situation was considered severe. In 1977 the patient had to be operated several times and papillomas were abundant in large parts of the larynx. IFN therapy was initiated March 1978 3 times weekly. In April 1978, 1 month later, there was almost no recurrence of papillomas.

In August 1978 some papillomas were seen and extirpated. In September 1978 the same status was documented and in October 1978 nothing had to be removed. In February 1979 there were only few papillomas present. IFN therapy was then reduced to twice weekly injections. There was no appearance of tumor growth in March 1979 and it was then decided to give IFN only once a week. In August 1979 there was an increase in tumor size with reappearance of papillomas all through the larynx. IFN therapy was then given twice weekly. In September 1979 there were still abundant papillomas present and IFN therapy was initiated 3 times weekly. In October 1979 there was again diminished tumor activity and only superficial papillomas were present. In December 1979 there were only very few superficial papillomas present and IFN therapy was discontinued.

In January 1980 there was abundant papillomatous growth all through the vocal cords, the ventricular folds and the epiglottis. In March 1980 there were also abundant papillomas present and IFN therapy was reinitiated and the IFN was given 3 times weekly. In June 1980 there were papillomas present on the left side of the larynx. In July 1980 only a few superficial papillomas remained. The patient continued with 3 weekly injections. In December 1980 there was only very little papillomatous tissue to observe. The patient continued on IFN and through March, July and October there was very little papillomatous growth. The same was apparent at check ups in April, August and November in 1982 and the situation remained the same in March, July and October 1983. IFN therapy was then stopped.

In January 1984 there was again abundant growth of papillomas. They were growing everywhere in the larynx and they had to be removed by extensive surgery. This situation has prevailed during 1984 and the patient has had to be operated 6 times, the last time in March 1985. We are now trying to institute IFN therapy again and perhaps give the IFN at a daily dose.

Case 8. (J.L.)-JLP was discovered in this 3-year-old boy in 1979. He was operated 4 times during 1979 and 4 times during 1980 and abundant papillomatous growth was removed on each occasion. In December 1980 he had developed subglottic growth and it was then decided to institute IFN therapy 3 times weekly. In March 1981 he had a very small remnant of papilloma tissue present and in July 1981 he had no signs whatever of any papillomatous growth. Further control check ups after 1981, 2-3 times per year, have revealed no evidence for papilloma growth. IFN therapy was discontinued in March 1982. He is presently free of papillomas.

Case 9. (M.G.)-Papillomas were discovered in this 4 1/2-year-old boy in March 1973. Thirteen endoscopies with removal had to be done up to September 1978. In April 1981 the patient had been operated upon 19 times, the last time being in January 1981. It was then decided to give IFN 3 times weekly. Already in July 1981 the boy had improved and an inspection showed no signs at all of any papillomas. In January 1982 he had small papillomas and a few small papillomas were seen also in April and July 1982. A very small papilloma was found in October 1982 and a small one was also seen in June 1983. It was decided to stop IFN therapy. He had during a check up in November 1983 some more signs of papillomatosis but not much was present in February, May and September, 1984. He also had a small papilloma in February 1985. It has not yet been decided whether he should continue IFN therapy on a more long term basis as a prophylactic measure.

Case 10. (B.A.S.)-JLP was found in this 21-year-old boy in 1978. During the first year he had to be operated several times and when he come to the Karolinska Hospital in 1979 he had abundant papillomatosis in his larynx. From September 1979 IFN was given 3 times weekly. In November 1979 all his signs of papillomatosis were removed. At that time the picture was stationary. He had a couple of small papillomas in January and in March 1980 but there was a clear impression that the disease was less active. In May 1980 he only had very small signs of papillomatous growth and this was removed. IFN was then given according to the twice weekly schedule and from June and on on the once weekly schedule.. In October 1980 there was no papillomatosis seen and all the following check ups, the latest being made in February 1985, have shown a completely free larynx and no signs of papillomatosis.

Case 11. (J.F.)-JLP was discovered in this 5-year-old boy in 1960. He had very active disease requiring 50 endoscopies and removals up to 1979. At the time of initiation of IFN therapy there was abundant papilloma growth. The IFN was given 3 times weekly from October 1979 and on. There was still papillomatosis left after the last endoscopic removal. In November 1979 there was a complete remission.In December 1979 there was some papillomatosis seen which was removed but on the following endoscopy in January 1980 and February 1980 there were no signs of papillomatosis. A small papillomatosis growth was removed in August 1980. In November 1982 he was completely free of papillomatosis and the IFN therapy was then withdrawn. After that he has been completely free of his disease.

Case 12. (U.O.)-JLP was discovered in this 5 1/2-year-old boy in 1979. He had complained of horseness for 2 years and it was seen that he had papillomatous growth bilaterally. IFN therapy was initiated in September 1979 3 times weekly. He received the IFN for 1 year and there were then no signs of papillomas upon discontinuation. He has been free of his disease up to March 1985 when a solitary papilloma was removed. He has not received any IFN after 1980 and he has presently no signs of papillomatosis.

Infections. As already reported the frequency of infections in treated patients were reduced during IFN therapy (19).

Side effects. As mentioned earlier fever is the most common symptom in the patients but the reaction tends to subside upon repeated injections. The frequency of various side-effects occuring occasionally have been discussed previously (20).

Morphology. A degenerative pattern was found microscopically in the tumors of the treated patients and the tumor nuclei started to appear pyknotic and the cytoplasm became watery or shrunken. There was also loss of cellular contact and disapperance of desmosome bridges and loosening of filament. The intercellular space was vastly increased (16). Detailed ultrastructural observations in the treated patients have not yet been reported but will be so in due course.

## DISCUSSION

Our previous impression that human leukocyte IFN therapy can cause regression of papillomatous growth remains true. Similar observations have been made by others (21, 22, 23, 24, 25, 26, 27, 28, 29, 30, 31, 32, 33, 34, 35, 36). In the material to date at the Karolinska Hospital there are 7 complete remissions, 4 partial remissions and 1 minimal response (on the border line to partial remission). It is evident that IFN therapy at the present dose, which usually has been $3 \times 10^6$ IU given 3 times weekly, irrespective of body weight, seems to cause significant effects on papillomatous growth in these patients. Several problems remain to be solved in using this particular therapy.

First of all it has to be decided what type of IFN should be used in the treatment of these patients. We are continuing to use human natural leukocyte IFN, but we shall hear about results employing other types of preparations during this meeting. High purity of preparations should be aimed at especially since it seems that an almost pure IFN preparation has antitumor effects in another papilloma virus-associated disease, condylomata accuminata (37).

One problem which has to be solved when employing this type of therapy is a very important one. We can see from the case histories above that whenever IFN therapy is reduced by decreasing the dose or giving the therapy less frequently the results tends to become worse. Instead I think we should perhaps give daily treatment. It also seems difficult in many instances to stop IFN treatment. I think we have to follow the patients individually and use as much IFN as is required to cause complete regressions. After achieving complete regressions we have to decide how to continue. It is important that doctors involved in the treatment of this disease with various IFN preparations meet and discuss how to proceed since it is difficult to collect very large groups of patients. Also I think it is very important that every case is described in detail. Otherwise it will be difficult to compare different results.

It should now be possible, by using the more newly developed IFN preparations, to invidualize the treatment and give IFN on a $m^2$- or body weight-basis. It is obvious that older patients weighing more than the children ought to require higher doses to achieve complete remissions. Some trials can hopefully be made in a randomized manner comparing different schedules. In addition, it is important that we try to obtain all possible information from every patient treated with IFN therapy.

The most exiciting problem to solve will be to determine what is achieving the antitumor effect (38). It is not known in any tumor disease whether IFN exerts its main action directly on virus growth, on various viral functions, if it has other direct effects on growing tumor cells or if the most important effects are mediated through the host.

IFN therapy seems to be rather safe at the doses used in this report. Thousands of patients have received such treatments and there have been few incidences of severe short-term or long-term complications. It should be emphasized, though, that a patient treated for papillomatosis with IFN, developed a squamous cell carcinoma (39) and we have also a similar experience at the Karolinska Hospital, where a patient receiving IFN therapy for extensive wart formation, who had been kidney transplanted, receiving immunosuppressive therapy, later developed squamous cell carcinoma of the tongue (40).

In order to solve the problems brought up in this discussion research efforts have to take place in the areas of clinical research and theoretical biology and experimental work has to be pursued in tissue culture and in animals (41,42).

## ACKNOWLEDGEMENTS

We acknowledge a gift from Professor Kari Cantell, Central Public Health Laboratory, Helsinki, Finland, for the human leukocyte interferon preparations used in the early part of this study and also for collaboration over the years. The staff of the Department of Oto-Rhino-Laryngology of the Karolinska Hospital is greatfully acknowledged.

## REFERENCES


1. Szpunar J (1977). Juvenile laryngeal papillomatosis. Otolaryngol Clin North Am 10, 67.
2. Cohen SR, Seltzer S, Geller KA, Thompson JW (1980). Papilloma of the larynx and tracheobronchial tree in children. A retrospective study. Am Otol 89, 497.
3. Quick CA, Faras A, Crzyzele R (1978). The etiology of laryngeal papillomatosis. Laryngoscope 88, 1789.
4. Mounts P, Shah KV, Kashima H (1982). Viral etiology of juvenile-and adult-onset squamous papilloma of the larynx. Proc Natl Acad Sci USA 79, 5425.
5. Gissman L, Diehl V, Schulz-Coulon HJ, zur Hausen H (1982). Molecular cloning and characterization of human papilloma virus DNA derived from a laryngeal papilloma. J Virol 44, 393.
6. Gissman L, Wolnik L, Ikenberg H, Koldovsky U, Schnürch HG, zur Hausen H (1983). Human papillomavirus types 6 and 11 DNA sequences in genital and laryngeal papillomas and in some cervical cancers. Proc Natl Acad Sci USA 80, 560.
7. Cacura W (1977). Langzeitbeobactung bei juvenilen Kihlkopf-papillomen nach chirurgischer abtragung und ultraschollbehandlung. Laryngol Rhinol Otol 56, 133.
8. Overall Jr JC (1984). Dermatologic viral diseases. In Galasso GJ et al (eds):"Antiviral Agents and Viral Diseases in Man", New York: Raven Press,p 247.
9. Strong M, Vaughan C, Cooperband S, Healy G, Clemente M (1976). Recurrent respiratory papillomatosis: management with the $CO_2$ laser. Ann Otol Rhinol Laryngol 85, 508.
10. Dedo HH (1978). Epitomes:use of carbon dioxide laser technology in laryngeal and pharyngeal surgery. West J Med 129, 330.
11. Strander H (1983). The role of interferon in disease. In Burke DC, Morris AG (eds):"Interferons:From Molecular Biology to Clinical Application", Cambridge: Cambridge Univ Press, p 7.
12. Strander H (1985). Interferon treatment of human neoplasia. Adv Cancer Res, in press.
13. Cantell K, Strander H, (1977). Human leukocyte interferon for clinical use. In Högman CF, Lindahl-Kiessling K, Wigzell H (eds):"Blood leukocytes. Functions and use in therapy", Stockholm: Almqvist and Wicksell, p 73.

14. Haglund S, Lundquist PG, Cantell K, Strander H (1981). Interferon therapy in juvenile laryngeal papillomatosis. Arch Otolaryngol 107: 327.
15. Haglund S, Lundquist PG, Ingimarsson S, Cantell K, Strander H (1982). Interferon therapy in juvenile laryngeal papillomatosis. In Terry WH, Rosenberg S (eds): "Immunotherapy of Human Cancer", New York: Year Book Publ, p 407.
16. Lundquist PG, Haglund S, Carlsöö B, Strander H, Lundgren E (1984). Interferon therapy in juvenile laryngeal papillomatosis. Otolaryngol Head Neck Surg 92:386
17. Cantell K, Hirvonen S, Kauppinen HL, Myllylä G (1981). Production of interferon in human leukocytes from normal donors with the use of Sendai virus. Methods Enzymol 78:29.
18. Cantell K, Hirvonen S, Koistinen V (1984). Partial purification of human leukocyte interferon on a large scale. Methods Enzymol 78: 499.
19. Ingimarsson S, Cantell K, Carlström G, Strander H (1980). Virus infections and recurrence of osteosarcoma in patients receiving human leukocyte interferon. Int J Cancer 26: 395.
20. Ingimarsson S, Cantell K, Strander H (1979). Side effects of long-term treatment with human leukocyte interferon. J Infect Dis 140: 560.
21. Leventhal B, Kashima H, Levine A, Levy H (1981). Treatment of recurrent laryngeal papillomatosis with an artificial interferon inducer (poly IC-LC). J Pediatr 99: 614.
22. Göbel U, Arnold W, Wahn V, Treuner J, Jürgens H, Cantell K (1981). Comparison of human fibroblast and leukocyte interferon in the treatment of severe laryngeal papillomatosis in children. Eur J Pediatr 137: 175.
23. Leventhal B, Kashima H, Whisnant JK, Tuttle RL (1982). Human lymphoblastoid IFN (HLBJ) in juvenile laryngeal papillomatosis: Initial experience in a multicenter phase III trial. Third Ann Intern Congr Interferon Res, Miami. Abstract.
24. Bomholt A (1982). Interferon therapy of laryngeal papillomatosis in adults. Third Ann Intern Congr Interferon Res, Miami. Abstract.
25. Goepfert H, Sessions RB, Gutterman JU, Cangir A, Dichtel WJ, Sulek M (1982). Leukocyte interferon in patients with juvenile laryngeal papillomatosis. Ann Otol Rhinol Laryngol 91: 431.

26. Schouten TJ, Weimar W, Bos JH, Bos CE, Cremers CWRJ, Schellekens H (1982). Treatment of juvenile laryngeal papillomatosis with two types of interferon. Laryngoscope 92: 686.
27. McCabe B, Clark KF (1983). Interferon and laryngeal papillomatosis. The Iowa experience. Ann Otol Rhinol Laryngol 92: 2.
28. Sessions R, Goepfert H, Donovan D, Dichtel W, Gutterman J (1983). Further observations on the treatment of recurrent respiratory papillomatosis with interferon: a comparison of sources. Ann Otol Rhinol Laryngol 92: 456.
29. Bomholt A (1983). Interferon therapy for laryngeal papillomatosis in adults. Arch Otolaryngol 109: 550.
30. Weck PK, Kashima H, Leventhal B, Tuttle RL, Whisnant JK (1983). Evaluation of human lymphoblastoid interferon (HLBJ) in juvenile laryngeal papillomatosis: initial results in a phase II study. Antiviral Res, Abstract 1: 2.
31. Sessions RB, Dichtel WJ, Goepfert H (1984). Treatment of recurrent respiratory papillomatosis with interferon. Ear Nose Throat J 63: 488.
32. Lusk RP, McCabe BF, Clark KF (1984). Interferon and laryngeal papillomatosis. A follow-up of the Iowa experience. In Zoon KC, Noguchi PD, Liu TY (eds): "Interferon: Research, Clinical Application; and Regulatory Consideration", New York: Elsevier Sci Publ, p 169.
33. Shouten TJ, van den Broek P, Cremers CWRJ, Bos JH, Bos CF (1984). Personal communication.
34. Lodemann E, Kornhuber B, Gerein V, v Ilberg CH (1984). Personal communication.
35. Whisnant JK, Kashima H, Leventhal B, and the participating Wellferon JLP Centers (1984). Interferon treatment of juvenile laryngeal papillomatosis: the design of a cooperative trial with Wellferon. Presented at the third TNO/ISIR Congress on the biology of the interferon system. Heidelberg Oct 21-25. In press.
36. Healy G, Myers MW, Galasso GJ (1984). Personal communication.
37. Ling P, Einhorn N, Einhorn S, Secher D, Strander H (1985). Unpublished results.
38. Gresser I (1982). How does interferon inhibit tumor growth? Phil Trans R Soc London B 299: 69.
39. Shouten TJ, van den Broek P, Cremers CWRJ, Jongerius CM, Meyers JWR, Vooys P (1983). Interferons and bronchogenic carcinoma in juvenile laryngeal papillomatosis. Arch Otolaryngol 109: 289.

40. Strander H, Borglund E (1985). Unpublished results.
41. Turek LP, Byrne JC, Lowy DR, Dvoretzky I, Friedman RM (1982). In Merigan TC, Friedman RM, Knox CF (eds): "Interferons", UCLA Symp Molec Cell Biol, vol XXV, New York: Academic Press, p 181.
42. Lodemann E, Kornhuber B, Gerein V, v Ilberg CH (1984). (2'-5') Oligo (A) synthetase as a monitor of interferon action in juvenile laryngeal papillomatosis. J Interferon Res 4: 283.

**Papillomaviruses: Molecular and Clinical Aspects, pages 181–182**


# INTERFERON IN RECURRENT RESPIRATORY PAPILLOMATOSIS- A MULTICENTER CONTROLLED CLINICAL TRIAL.

G.B. Healy, M.D., A.L. Trowbridge, R.N.
Department of Otolaryngology,
The Children's Hospital, Boston, MA 02115

ABSTRACT The objective of this national randomized controlled clinical trial is to evaluate the effectiveness of Human Leukocyte Interferon in combination with laser surgery versus laser surgery alone in the treatment of Pediatric Recurrent Respiratory Papillomatosis. Patient enrollment began in January of 1983 and ended in February of 1985. A total of 123 patients from 31 participating centers were enrolled with 62 randomized to receive Interferon therapy.

Human Leukocyte Interferon was administered intramuscularly at a dosage of $2mu/m^2$ daily for the first week then 3 times a week for 1 year to 50% of the patients randomized into the trial. Patients in both arms were evaluated endoscopically at entry, 1 month, 3 months, and then every 3 months for 2 years. At each endoscopy the extent of gross papilloma in the larynx and tracheobronchial tree was mapped pre-operatively and post-operatively according to 42 specific anatomical locations on detailed topgraphic data forms. The degree of pre-op and post-op obstruction in the larynx and/or tracheobronchial tree was documented in terms of percent airway obstruction.

Interferon's potential effect on the growth and development of children was also evaluated. Physical growth parameters were obtained on all patients at each visit and plotted by one individual on NCHS growth charts and computerized by percentiles. The developmental parameters were tabulated on special age appropriate developmental forms at 6 month intervals and reviewed by the Children's Hospital Developmental Team.

In the first 25 months of the trial, 13 patients (10%) experienced some form of Interferon toxicity. Of the 123 patients evaluated, 7 (5%) experienced LFT elevations, 5(4%) experienced transient neutropenia, and 1 experienced general malaise, persistent fever, muscle aches and cramps, post injection. Of the 7 with elevated LFT's, 2 remained stable on full dose after 1 alteration while 5 required frequent alterations, maintaining normal LFT's on half dose only. All patients with transient neutropenia remained stable on full dose after 1 alteration. Two of the 5 neutropenias were most likely due to concurrent acute illnesses and not to the Interferon. No further toxcities have been reported in the last 6 months.

The degree of disease involvement, as reported on these data forms, will be serially evaluated to test if the extent of involvement at fixed points in time is different for the two treatment groups. The total number of sites involved, the location of new sites in relation to the original, contralateral disease and spread to adjacent anatomic areas will be considered. The primary analysis will enter on time to relapse in relation to treatment and baseline data.

To date, two interim statistical analyses have been completed by an outside contracted group of statisticians. All participating investigators, including the Boston group, remain blinded to any salient results. In order to maintain objectivity in the collection of data, the statistical results will not be available until the study has terminated.

# IV. THERAPEUTIC APPROACHES TO PAPILLOMAVIRUS INFECTIONS

Papillomaviruses: Molecular and Clinical Aspects, pages 185–200


# CLINICAL APPROACHES TO HUMAN PAPILLOMA VIRUS DISEASES: THE USE OF INTERFERONS

Phillip K. Weck and John K. Whisnant

Department of Immunology & Oncology
Burroughs Wellcome Co.
Research Triangle Park, NC 27709

ABSTRACT Therapeutic approaches for the human papilloma virus (HPV) associated diseases have been multiple. Physical removal of these usually benign epithelial proliferative lesions has been accomplished by surgical and chemical methods. Elimination of visible disease provides immediate therapy, and perhaps emotional relief for the patient, but it often fails to eradicate the underlying virus infection. Antiviral drug use for these diseases has been limited due to the lack of appropriate in vitro systems and animal models for testing new chemotherapeutics against HPV replication. The human interferons have proven clinically active in several of the papilloma virus diseases. These biological agents are good choices for treatment of HPV infections because they exhibit antiviral, antiproliferative, and immunomodulating activities. This manuscript will review the use of interferons in the treatment of two HPV-associated diseases: recurrent respiratory papillomatosis, and condyloma acuminata or genital warts.

## INTERFERON

### The System

It is recognized now that the interferon system consists of multiple proteins with diverse biological activities (1). The existence of three major types of interferons based on cell source has been recognized for some time. In recent years, a standardized nomenclature has been adopted for the interferons: alpha for leukocyte, beta for fibroblast, and gamma for immune interferon

(2). Advances in biochemical characterization of these polypeptides and isolation of the genes coding for them has expanded our understanding of this system. At least eighteen alpha interferon genes (3), as many as five beta interferon genes (4), and a unique gamma interferon gene (5) have been identified in a few years. However, understanding the biological properties, interactions, and *in vivo* functions of these genes' products remains far from complete. The ability to produce large quantities of interferons by sophisticated large-scale cell culture (6) and recombinant DNA methodology (7) has provided ample material to answer many questions. The expanded use of these biological agents in human clinical trials will add to the knowledge of the interferon system, its role in immune surveillance, inhibition of viral replication, and regulation of cell proliferation. Clinical experience to date has revealed that these multi-faceted proteins are potent and effective against a few, certainly not all, malignancies and viral infections.

Mechanism

The general role of interferons in the host's defense mechanisms has been associated historically primarily with acute viral infections. Circulating levels of biologically active interferon can be detected within the first few days of natural infection, experimental challenge, or virus vaccination. Consequently, interferons were thought to be produced only during cycles of active viral replication. Recent work in murine models suggests interferons may be involved at undetectable levels to sustain an antiviral status in immune cells that normally respond to virus infections (8). This study demonstrated that low levels of alpha and beta interferon in normal mice induce basal levels of 2'-5' oligoadenylate synthetase in macrophages and that neutralization of these interferons *in vivo* led to a decline in synthetase levels and increased sensitivity of macrophages to virus infections. If such systems are active in man, then a breakdown in this antiviral status could lead to an increased incidence of viral infection. Variability in basal endogenous interferon levels from one individual to another would explain why some patients suffer from multiple viral infections while others have relatively few. Thus, the interferon system may be a continuously functioning component of immune surveillance for combatting both acute and chronic virus infections.

## Initial Clinical Use

Exogenous interferons have been used to treat many viral infections in humans because of their potent effects on virus replication. Following discovery of these antiviral properties (9), it was logical that the first clinical trials in man involved local interferon application prior to virus challenge. An early controlled trial demonstrated that interferon derived from monkey cell cultures applied at the site of inoculation prevented vaccination against smallpox (10). In a separate study, this same interferon was shown effective in the treatment of vaccinial keratitis (11). These two initial reports demonstrated the activity of a primate interferon in man and led to additional trials in viral infections, primarily those classified as chronic or latent. The development of techniques to produce human interferon from peripheral blood leukocytes by Cantell and co-workers (12) was a major breakthrough and provided the material for many of the early trials. It is not within the scope of this review to address the many antiviral clinical studies performed with interferons. Rather, the following section will review primarily the use of interferons against two epithelioproliferative disorders associated with HPV infection: recurrent respiratory papillomatosis, and condyloma acuminata or genital warts.

# PAPILLOMA VIRUS DISEASES

## Clinical Virology

Diseases associated with the human papilloma viruses include a long list of clinical manifestations ranging from common skin warts to rare conditions such as recurrent respiratory papillomatosis and epidermodysplasia verruciformis (Table 1). Many of these will be considered in greater detail in other sections of these proceedings.

TABLE 1
HUMAN PAPILLOMA VIRUS TYPES
ASSOCIATED CLINICAL MANIFESTATIONS

| HPV Type | Associated Clinical Condition |
|---|---|
| 1 | Plantar warts, deep myrmecia |
| 2 | Common skin warts |
| 3 | Flat, mild EV |
| 4 | Keratotic skin and plantar warts |
| 5 | Macular EV |
| 6 | Laryngeal papillomas & genital warts |
| 7 | Butchers' warts |
| 8 & 9 | Macular, flat EV |
| 10 | Flat skin warts |
| 11 | Respiratory papillomas & cervical warts |
| 12 | Macular, flat EV |
| 13 | Focal hyperplasia |
| 14 & 15 | Macular, flat EV |
| 16 | Squamous cell carcinoma, Bowen's papulosis |
| 17 | Macular, flat EV |
| 18 | Squamous cell carcinoma, Bowen's papulosis |
| 19 - 25 | Macular, flat EV |

These warty conditions in man are linked to virus infection of the subepithelial layers of the skin. The first evidence for viral involvement was obtained by transfer of warts by a cell-free supernatant from papilloma tissue in self-inoculation experiments (13,14). The presence of viral particles in human tissue was proven by light and electron microscopy of genital wart biopsies (15,16). Such studies resulted in identification of the DNA-containing human papilloma viruses and their classification in the Papovaviridae family. Although these viruses cannot be propagated by standard in vitro methodology, thus preventing fulfillment of Koch's postulates for an infectious agent, organ culture experiments (17) and direct DNA hybridization in biopsy specimens (18,19) have established a likely viral etiology. Viral replication appears dependent on cellular differentiation because viral genome copy number increases as cells rise through the dermal and epidermal layers to the surface. This results in a "transformed" cell which multiplies rapidly giving rise to a benign skin growth, or wart, with overproduction of keratin. HPV replication is highly site-specific. For example, the HPV-6 found in genital warts (20) does not infect or readily multiply in skin epidermal cells and conversely, HPV-2 found in common warts (21) cannot be detected in cells of genito-urinary mucosal surfaces. Removal of these verrucous growths by various methods often results in regrowth which probably is due to incomplete eradication of the underlying viral infection. Recurrence of HPV-associated lesions and development of severe or extensive disease may be associated with altered immunity, especially localized immune response at the site of infection. The very nature of these HPV infections, therefore, makes interferon therapy a logical approach. The antiviral effects, even at low doses, should limit viral replication in new or regenerating epithelium. Cell cycle inhibitory or antiproliferative effects of interferon should slow the rapid growth of transformed epidermal cells. The immunomodulatory effects, such as stimulation of cytotoxic T-lymphocytes to kill virus-infected cells, should shift the immune balance in favor of the host. A combination of these three interferon actions may ultimately result in clearance of visible lesions and elimination of the viral DNA responsible for the transformation events.

## Interferon in Respiratory HPV

Recurrent respiratory papillomatosis (RRP) is an uncommon disease clearly associated with HPV infection (22,23). It afflicts the larynx and airway both of children and adults requiring multiple surgical excisions of papillomatous tissue to relieve airway compromise and poor voice quality. In the very young, it can become life-threatening when the airway is completely occluded. Table 2 summarizes published results of interferon studies in RRP in Europe and the U.S.A. Based on an anecdotal observation of plantar wart regression in a cancer patient receiving leukocyte interferon, the Swedish group began interferon therapy in a patient with juvenile onset RRP in January 1976 (24). The authors of this publication concluded that: 1) papilloma growth could be controlled, 2) regrowth occurred when interferon was reduced or discontinued, 3) papillomas regressed when interferon was re-initiated, 4) papillomas showed degeneration on interferon exposure and 5) virologic, pathologic, mechanistic, and dose-dependent questions remained to be answered in order to optimize interferon therapy of this disease. Two studies performed in the U.S. at M.D. Anderson Hospital/ Baylor College of Medicine (25) and the University of Iowa (26) corroborated the Swedish findings; however, the number of patients experiencing complete clearance of disease was somewhat lower (32-37% versus 53%). A follow-up study by the Houston group demonstrated that re-treatment of nine patients with leukocyte interferon from a different source resulted in responses similar to the initial trial (27). As a result of the early positive results in children, a study was conducted in Denmark to treat adults (28). Eight patients were treated for three weeks prior to surgery resulting in reduced tumor size in 5 individuals. Following surgery, interferon therapy was re-instituted for 5 months resulting in recurrence of small papillomas in only one patient. Follow-up evaluations off therapy for 7-11 months showed recurrence in 4 patients. Limited comparisons of alpha and beta interferons for severe juvenile onset RRP have been reported from the Netherlands (29) and Germany (30). Although only two patients were treated at each center, both groups observed better disease control with leukocyte interferon.

These reported high response rates have resulted in implementation of two large controlled trials in the U.S. One employs a highly purified human lymphoblastoid interferon (interferon alfa-N1, WELLFERON®) and the second, a partially purified leukocyte interferon derived by the Cantell method. The multi-center randomized cross-over trial with human lymphoblastoid interferon is designed to provide six months of therapy and six months of observation off drug (31,32). Patients must have severe disease requiring tracheostomy or surgical excisions three times in the six months prior to entering the trial. Randomization to observation or intramuscular administration of WELLFERON is followed by cross-over to the appropriate option. Disease evaluations are made at two month intervals and include disease diagrams, estimates of lesion sizes, anatomic level of disease, and estimates of cross-sectional airway compromise. Sixty patients randomized to interferon versus observation will be compared. Intra-patient comparison for each individual treated and observed will be important in substantiating reported clinical impressions. A comparison will be made also between the two groups after the six month cross-over. Clinical impressions from investigators and nurses are that the majority of patients benefit from interferon therapy. Parents have reported that children miss fewer days of school and participate more in peer group activities.

Interferon in Genital HPV

Condyloma acuminata, or genital warts, are benign fibro-epithelial tumors associated with HPV-6 infection. DNA hybridization and restriction enzyme analyses have shown close homology with HPV-11 and both viruses can be found in biopsies of genital warts or laryngeal papillomas (33,34). Studies using cloned HPV-6 genomic sequences have shown that 93% of all genital warts contain DNA sequences homologous to HPV-6 (34). Condyloma acuminata has a preference for moist environments especially mucosal surfaces. These epithelial proliferations have a predilection for the genital area and are found frequently in sexually active males and females. The disease presents in females as verrucous lesions on the perineum, vaginal or vulvar mucosa, or as flat leukoplakic lesions on the cervix. Males have penile lesions or warty growths on the perianal and/or rectal surfaces. The usual treatment of condyloma acuminata is topical application of caustic or keratolytic agents such as podophyllin (35). Topical treatments of trichloroacetic acid, 5-fluorouracil or colchicine have been tested experimentally with limited success. Recurrences are common and resistant/recurrent disease usually requires cryotherapy, surgical excision, or laser therapy.

The results of seven published reports on interferon therapy for genital warts are summarized in Table 3. Early trials by Ikic and colleagues (36,37) with a crude preparation of leukocyte interferon first demonstrated response to interferon. The Yugoslavian investigators employed interferon in a Vaseline-lanolin ointment with a 90% response rate in the preliminary trial (36). A second placebo-controlled trial reported clearing of disease in 4 of 10 interferon-treated patients and 2 spontaneous regressions in 11 placebo-treated patients (37). A pilot study by Scott and Csonka (38) demonstrated the effect of single intralesional injections of beta interferon in male patients. These results were encouraging in light of the small amounts of interferon injected into individual warts (38). A series of studies by two Israeli groups extended these observations by showing that topical application of a beta interferon ointment (39) or intralesional and intramuscular injections of a beta interferon solution caused significant regression of genital warts (40). In the latter studies, the authors concluded that intramuscular injection was the most suitable mode of administration of beta interferon. Intralesional administration of leukocyte derived interferon was tested in an open study in 8 patients with condyloma acuminata and 2 patients with giant condylomata of Bushke-Lowenstein (41). Five of the eight patients with condyloma acuminata experienced complete clearance of disease; the dose and schedule were not standardized but based on lesion surface area. Geffen and colleagues (41) suggested that efficacy of intralesional therapy may be related to duration of disease rather than size of individual lesions. In addition, they noted that local intralesional injections did not influence regression of adjacent or nearby lesions. In a separate study, systemic leukocyte derived interferon was reported successful in a patient with persistent and severe condyloma acuminata when given daily for 4 weeks (42). In all studies, three to six month follow-up periods showed that recurrence was rare in patients who experienced complete clearance. A pilot study with human lymphoblastoid interferon (interferon alfa-Nl, WELLFERON®) has supported the findings for systemic therapy in severe recurrent genital warts (43). In this study, doses of 5 $MU/m^2$ caused significant decreases in total white counts necessitating dose reductions in all patients. An on-going study is designed to compare 1 and 3 $MU/m^2$ doses of WELLFERON in patients with persistent disease (44). Preliminary analysis indicates that the patients respond at both doses and that interferon-related side effects are dose-dependent.

Additional Use of Interferon

Other HPV-associated diseases have been treated with interferons but in very limited studies. Intramuscular injections of large doses of leukocyte derived interferon over 3-4 months produced softening and reduced

TABLE 2

CLINICAL EXPERIENCE WITH INTERFERONS
IN RECURRENT RESPIRATORY PAPILLOMATOSIS

| | Sweden (24) | Houston (25) | Iowa (26) | Denmark (28) | Netherlands (29) | Germany (30) | USA/Multicenter (31,32) |
|---|---|---|---|---|---|---|---|
| Interferon | Leuk. | Leuk. | Leuk. | Leuk. | Beta, Leuk. | Beta, Leuk. | Alfa-N1 (WELLFERON®) |
| Dose | 3 MU | 2 MU/m$^2$ | 3 MU | 1,4 MU | 3 MU | 2 MU, 1 MU | 5 MU/m$^2$ |
| Schedule | tiw | qd, tiw | tiw | qd x 20<br>qod x 50 | tiw | qd x 28<br>qod 6-12 mos | qd x 28<br>tiw x 20 |
| No. Patients | 17 | 16 | 19 | 8 | 2 | 2 | 66 |
| Age Range (yrs.) | 2-29 | 2-35 | 2-42 | 30-65 | 6,8 | 5,4 | 1-44 |
| No. Excisions | 2-50 | <300 | -- | N.A. | N.A. | N.A. | 4-34/yr. |
| Disease Duration (yrs.) | 0.5-19 | 1-25 | 1-30 | 2-31 | 6,17 | 2.5-4 | 0.2-39 |
| Cleared | 53% | 37% | 32% | 87% | 50% | 50% | N.A. |
| Improved | 41% | 63% | 58% | 13% | 50% | 50% | N.A. |

( ) Indicates reference number of published report summarized.

THZZ/85/0183
amc/17/9/15

TABLE 3

CLINICAL EXPERIENCES WITH INTERFERONS
IN THE TREATMENT OF CONDYLOMA ACUMINATA

| | Yugoslavia (36) | Yugoslavia (36) | Israel (39) | England (38) | Israel (40) | USA (41) | USA (43) |
|---|---|---|---|---|---|---|---|
| Interferon | Leuk. | Leuk. | Beta | Beta | Beta | Leuk. | Alfa-N1 (WELLFERON®) |
| Route | Topical | Topical | Topical | I.L. | I.M. | I.L. | I.M. |
| Dose | 0.04 MU | 0.04 MU | N.A. | 300U | 2 MU | 3, 8.5 MU | 5 MU/m$^2$ |
| Schedule | 5-6 x/d | 5-6 x/d | qd | 1x | qd | 2x/wk | qdx28, tiw x 2wks |
| Duration | 2-8 wks | 2-8 wks | 4 wks | 1 wk | 10 d | 5 wks | 6 wks |
| No. Patients | 40 | 10 | 18 | 12 | 11 | 10 | 17 |
| Dis. Severity | Unknown | Unknown | Mild, Primary | Recurrent Primary | Mild, Primary | Severe | Severe, Recurrent |
| Complete Clearance | 36 | 4 | 14 | 1 | 9 | 5 | 8 |
| Partial Clearance | N.A. | 6 | 4 | 4 | 0 | 3 | 7 |

( ) Indicates reference number of report summarized.

THZZ/85/0183
amc/17/9/16

scaling of lesions in two patients with extensive body warts (45). Double-blind, placebo-controlled intralesional injections in one of these patients resulted in progressive regression of interferon treated warts. Vaginal flat condylomas have been treated successfully in a double-blind, placebo-controlled trial with a leukocyte interferon cream (46). Five of eight treated patients showed remissions as judged by colposcopy, however, all had cells typical of condyloma upon cytological testing. Treatment of flat condylomas has become important because of their frequent association with cervical dysplasia and possible transition from benign growths to malignant cervical carcinoma. Common or plantar warts also respond to interferon therapy. Intralesional injections of human lymphoblastoid interferon (WELLFERON®) to seven patients resulted in complete clearance in four and partial clearance in two individuals (47). Changes in the wart such as softening or reduction in size were noted often after only a few injections.

## REFERENCES

1. Stewart WE (1981). "The Interferon System." New York: Springer-Verlag.

2. Wiranowska-Stewart M (1981). Interferons: types alpha, beta and gamma. In Hadden JW, Stewart WE (eds): "Lymphokines," Clifton Press, p 133.

3. Weissmann C (1981). The cloning of interferon and other mistakes. In Gresser I (ed): "Interferon" vol. 3, London: Academic Press, p 101.

4. Sehgal PB, May LT, Sagan AD (1983). Isolation of novel human genomic DNA clones related to human interferon - beta 1 cDNA. Proc Natl Acad Sci USA 80:3632.

5. Gray PW, Goeddel DV (1982). Structure of the human immune interferon gene. Nature (London) 298:859.

6. Finter NB, Fantes KH (1980). The purity and safety of interferons prepared for clinical use: the case for lymphoblastoid interferon. In Gresser I (ed): "Interferon" vol. 2, London: Academic Press, p 65.

7. Nagata S, Taira H, Hall A, Johnrud L, Streuli M, Escodi J, Boll W, Cantell K and Weissmann C (1980). Synthesis in E coli of a polypeptide with human leukocyte interferon activity. Nature (London) 284:316.

8. Gresser I, Vignaux F, Belardelli F, Tovey MG, Maunory MT (1985). Injection of mice with antibody to mouse interferon alpha/beta decreases the level of 2'-5' oligoadenylate synthetase in peritoneal macrophages. J Virol 53:221.

9. Isaacs A, Lindenmann J (1957). Virus interference. I The interferon. Proc Royal Soc B147:258.

10. Scientific Committee on Interferon (1962). Effect of interferon on vaccination in volunteers. The Lancet i:873.

11. Jones BR, Galbraith JEK, Al-Hussaini MK (1962). Vaccinial keratitis treated with interferon. The Lancet i:875.

12. Cantell K (1977). Prospects for the clinical use of interferons. Med Biol 55:69.

13. Ullman EV (1923). On the etiology of the laryngeal papilloma. Acta Otolar 5:317.

14. Ishikawa K (1936). Fukuoka Otol 8:68.

15. Dunn AEG, Ogilule MM (1968). Intranuclear virus particles in human genital wart tissue: observation of ultrastructure of the epidermal layer. J Ultrastructure Res 22:282.

16. Oriel JD, Almeida JD (1970). Demonstration of virus particles in human genital warts. Br J Venereal Dis 46:37.

17. Steinberg BM, Abramson AL, Meade RP (1982). Culture of human laryngeal papilloma cells in vitro. Otolaryngol Head Neck Surg 90:728.

18. Gissman L, Diehl V, Schultz-Coulon HJ, zur Hausen H (1981). Molecular cloning and characterization of human papilloma virus DNA derived from a laryngeal papilloma. J Virol 44:393.

19. Steinberg BM, Topp WC, Schneider PS, Abramson AL (1983). Laryngeal papillomavirus infection during clinical remission. N Engl J Med 308:1261.

20. deVilliers E-M, Gissman L, zur Hausen H (1981). Molecular cloning of viral DNA from human genital warts. J Virol 40:932.

21. Orth, G, Favre M, Croissant O (1977). Characterization of a new type of human papillomavirus that causes skin warts. J Virol 24:108.

22. Mounts P, Shah KV, Kashima H (1982). Viral etiology of juvenile and adult onset squamous papilloma of the larynx. Proc Natl Acad Sci USA 79:5425.

23. Mounts P, Kashima H (1984). Association of human papillomavirus subtype and clinical course in respiratory papillomatosis. Laryngoscope 94:28.

24. Haglund S, Lundquist PG, Cantell K, Strander H (1981). Interferon therapy in juvenile laryngeal papillomatosis. Arch Otolaryngol 107:327.

25. Goepfert H, Sessions RB, Gutterman JU, Cangir A, Dichtel WJ, Sulek M (1982). Leukocyte interferon in patients with juvenile laryngeal papillomatosis. Ann Otol Rhinol Laryngol 91:431.

26. McCabe BF, Clark KF (1983). Interferon and laryngeal papillomatosis: the Iowa experience. Ann Otol Rhinol Laryngol 92:2.

27. Sessions RB, Goepfert H, Donovan DT, Dichtel WJ, Gutterman JU (1983). Further observations on the treatment of recurrent respiratory papillomatosis. Ann Otol Rhinol Otolaryngol 92:456.

28. Bomholt A (1983). Interferon therapy for laryngeal papillomatosis in adults. Arch Otolaryngol 109:550.

29. Schouten TJ, Weimar W, Bos JH, Bos CE, Cremers CWRJ, Schellekens H (1982). Treatment of juvenile laryngeal papillomatosis with two types of interferon. Laryngoscope 92:686.

30. Göbel U, Arnold W, Wahn V, Treuner J, Jurgens H, Cantell K (1981). Comparison of human fibroblast and leukocyte interferon in the treatment of severe laryngeal papillomatosis in children. Eur J Pediatr 137:175.

31. Weck PK, Kashima H, Leventhal B, Tuttle RL, Whisnant JK (1983). Evaluation of human lymphoblastoid interferon in juvenile laryngeal papillomatosis. Antiviral Res Abstr 1(2) P-117.

32. Whisnant JK, Kashima H, Leventhal B et al (1984). Interferon treatment of juvenile laryngeal papillomatosis: the design of a cooperative trial with Wellferon. In Kirchner H, Schellekens H (eds): "Biology of the Interferon System," Amsterdam: Elsevier, p 601.

33. Gissmann L, zur Hausen H (1980). Partial characterization of viral DNA from human genital warts (condyloma acuminata). Int J Cancer 25:605.

34. Gissmann L, deVilliers E-M, zur Hausen H (1982). Analysis of human genital warts (condyloma acuminata) and other genital tumors for human papillomavirus type 6 DNA. Int J Cancer 29:143.

35. von Krogh G (1978). Topical treatment of penile condyloma acuminata with podophyllin, podophyllotoxin and colchicine. Acta Derm Venereol (Stockholm) 58:163.

36. Ikic D, Orescanin M, Krusic J, Cestar Z, Alac Z, Soos E, Jusic D, Smerdel D (1975). Preliminary study of the effect of human leukocyte interferon on condylomata acuminata in women. In "Proc Symposium on Clinical Use of Interferon," Zagreb, Yugoslav Academy, p 223.

37. Ikic D, Bosnic N, Smerdel S, Jusic D, Soos E, Delmar N (1975). Double blind clinical study with human leukocyte interferon in the therapy of condylomata acuminata. In "Proc Symposium on Clinical Use of Interferon," Zagreb, Yugoslav Academy, p 229.

38. Scott GM, Csonka GW (1979). Effect of injections of small doses of human fibroblast interferon into genital warts. Br J Venereal Dis 55:442.

39. Marcovici R, Peretz BA, Paldi E (1983). Human fibroblast interferon therapy in patients with condyloma acuminata. Isr J Med Sci 19:104.

40. Schonfeld A, Nitke S, Schattner A, Wallach D, Crespi M, Hahn T, Levavi H, Yarden O, Shoham J, Doerner T, Revel M (1984). Intramuscular human interferon-beta injections in treatment of condylomata acuminata. Lancet i:1038.

41. Geffen JR, Klein RJ, Friedman-Kien AE (1984). Intralesional administration of large doses of human leukocyte interferon for the treatment of condyloma acuminata. J Inf Dis 150:612.

42. Einhorn N, Ling P, Strander H (1983). Systemic interferon alpha treatment of human condylomata acuminata. Acta Obstet Gynecol Scand 62:285.

43. Gall SA, Hughes CE, Weck P, Whisnant J (1984). Interferon for the treatment of resistant condyloma acuminata. Gynecol Oncol 17:264.

44. Weck PK, Gall SA, Micha JP, Reichman RC (1984). Wellferon (human lymphoblastoid interferon) in the treatment of resistant and recurrent condyloma acuminata. Antiviral Res Abstr 1(3):97.

45. Pazin GJ, Ho M, Haverkos HW, Armstrong JA, Breinig MC, Wechsler HL, Arvin A, Merigan TC, Cantell K (1982). Effects of interferon-alpha on human warts. J Interferon Res 2:235.

46. Vesterinen E, Meyer B, Cantell K. Purola E (1984). Topical treatment of flat vaginal condyloma with human leukocyte interferon. Obstet Gynecol 64:535.

47. Gibson JR, Harvey SG (1984). Interferon in the treatment of persistent viral warts. Dermatologica 169:47.

Papillomaviruses: Molecular and Clinical Aspects, pages 201–215


# LYMPHOBLASTOID INTERFERON FOR THE THERAPY OF CONDYLOMATA ACUMINATA:

## AN INTER-STUDY COMPARISON OF TWO DOSE REGIMENS

Stanley A. Gall, M.D.[1], Connie E. Hughes, R.N.[2], Kenneth Trofatter, Jr., M.D.[2], John Whisnant, M.D.[3], Phillip K. Weck, Ph.D.[3]

Department of Obstetrics and Gynecology
Duke University Medical Center
Durham, NC 27710

ABSTRACT Condylomata acuminata or genital warts, are verrucous growths frequently found in sexually active females and males. Modes of therapy include keratolytic agents such as podophyllin, trichloroacetic acid or 5 fluoro-uracil with recurrent disease treated with cryotherapy, surgical excision or laser. Approximately 5% of patients will have persistent condyloma despite current therapy. Our trials were designed to treat patients who failed conventional therapy and to evaluate the efficacy, toxicity and tolerance of intramuscular and intralesional administration of Wellferon® (human lymphoblastoid interferon). Patients were required to have condyloma present for at least 6 months and received at least ten podophyllin treatments. Warts were evaluated with bidimensional measurements on a divided grid drawing, by photographs, and by biopsies for histological

[1]Present Address: Department of Obstetrics and Gynecology, University of Illinois - Chicago, 840 S. Wood Street, Chicago, IL 60612.

[2]Present Address: Department of Obstetrics and Gynecology, Duke University Medical Center.

[3]Present Address: Burroughs Wellcome Co., Research Triangle Park, NC 27709

evaluation and viral DNA typing. Blood was obtained for hematological and immunological testing. Interferon was administered I.M. at 5 MU/$m^2$ daily for 28 days then three times a week for two additional weeks. Evaluations were done weekly for four weeks then every other week. Patients with total disappearance of condylomata were considered complete responders (CR) while a partial response was a 50% or greater decrease in lesion area and no response was no change or less than 50% decrease in size. Patients experiencing CR were observed 6 months; those who were PR continued to receive interferon three times per week for 6 weeks and if the patient was NR, intralesional therapy was offered. Complete blood count, liver and renal tests were obtained. Additional patients were treated with doses of 3 MU/$m^2$ administered daily for 14 days following by three times per week dosing for an additional four weeks. Analysis of response showed an overall approximate CR of 67% and PR of 20%. Additional therapy of PR patients with excision or cryotherapy improved the cure rate to greater than 90%.

Condylomata acuminata are fibro-epithelial tumors of viral etiology. The papillomatous lesions exhibit a predilection for the genital area where they may be found with increased frequency in sexually active females and males. Condylomata have been recognized as a disease entity since antiquity being located on the external genitalia and as a vaginal lesion. More recently, the importance and recognition of the flat cervical lesion has occurred. Successful innoculation of human volunteers with unfiltered material from a penile condyloma were produced after a period varying from 3-9 months. The agent of condylomata acuminata was identified with electron microscopy by Dunn and Ogilvie in 1968 (1) and Ariel and Almeida in 1970 (2). The usual locations of condylomata acuminata are the labia, perineum, anus, cervix and vaginal mucosa (3).

Virus particles observed in condyloma are members of the papovaviridae family (4) and share the morphology and size (55 NM) of papillomaviruses. These particles have an icosahedral capsid with capsomeres (5). Their genome is composed of a supercoiled covalently closed circular double stranded DNA molecule with a molecular weight of approximately 5 x $10^3$ daltons (6).

The usual clinical sign of condylomata acuminata is the appearance of rough warty papillomas on the perineum, labia major, labia minor, clitoris, perineum, anus and vaginal mucosa. Warty lesions can also be present on the cervix but flat condyloma on the cervix usually referred to as leukoplakia, are more common. The virus is thought to be sexually transmitted in most cases and it has been estimated that more than 900,000 new infections occur in the United States annually. The detailed epidemiology has not been done because the disease is not reportable to health authorities and because the agent has not been convincingly grown in tissue culture. The incubation period in humans is 2-6 months. Viral spread is from cell to cell with a proliferation of epithelial cells causing the resultant lesion. The spontaneous regression rate for untreated patients with first episode condylomata acuminata of the vulva is 33% within a six month period.

Papillomaviruses are found in a variety of human warty lesions: skin warts, plantar warts, oral and laryngeal papillomas and lesions of epidermodysplasia verruciformis. The prevailing scientific thought until recently suggested that these lesions had the same etiologic agent. However, completion of DNA hybridization studies has revealed a number of serotypes of human papilloma virus (HPV). Initially five serotypes were described (7) but more than thirty-one are now known. The HPV type identified in condylomatous tissue has been designated HPV-6 (8) and shares DNA homology with papillomaviruses found in laryngeal papillomas HPV-11 (9). Hybridization studies using cloned HPV-6 genomic sequences have shown that 93% of all genital warts contain DNA sequences homologous to this virus, however, tissue from cervical, vulva or penile carcinomas contain no detectable HPV-6 DNA (8).

Evidence for viral involvement in cervical carcinoma has come from cloning experiments that identified another HPV-type, HPV-16, in cervical cancer biopsies (10). Therefore, HPV types 6, 11, 16 and 18 infect the genital tract with type 6 and 11 found in genital warts but seldom found in invasive squamous cell carcinoma (8,10). However, HPV types 16 and 18 were found almost exclusively in high grade cervical intraepithelial neoplasia and invasive cancer (9).

In the last several years it has been recognized that HPV commonly infects the cervix and produces acuminata warts as well as flat warts which appear as leukoplakia when stained with acetic acid. These lesions contain mild cytologic atypia and cells with densely staining irregular nuclei and perinuclear halos (koilocytotic atypia) (11). This information has been extremely helpful in clarifying some of the confusion related to early abnormal lesions of the cervix. It is clear that many lesions classified as cervical epithelial neoplasia grade I (CIN I) are in fact HPV-induced flat condylomata with a high spontaneous regression rate. This information helps explain the high rate of reversion to normal cytology of patients with CIN I and implies and strengthens the concept of a viral precursor for malignant cervical disease.

Meisels and Morin reported HPV of the cervix was found in 1.69% of 234,715 women during a mass screening program in Canada during the years 1975 to 1979. Condyloma of the cervix represented the most prevalent squamous lesion diagnosed during this 5-year period (12). Condylomata acuminata co-existed with dysplasia and neoplasia in 25.6% of the lesions.

The concept that the majority of invasive squamous carcinomas of the genital tract are preceded by a precursor stage of development has been widely accepted. Morphologically, precursor conditions are recognized by comparing the nuclear and cytoplasmic alterations at comparable levels in normal and abnormal squamous mucosa. These include nuclear enlargement, hyperchromasia, increased number of mitosis (normal and abnormal) and alterations of the cellular arrangement (polarity). The differentiation of the cytoplasm is abnormal, incomplete or lacking. The current terms used to designate these changes are dysplasia-CIS or CIN I, II, III.

Because the concept of HPV acting as a carcinogen, co-carcinogen or a promotor of CIN is exciting and probable, the therapy of patients with HPV becomes of paramount interest. Many modes of treatment have been employed for the removal or eradication of genital warts. Some of the methods of therapy have utilized the finding of HPV typing in designing therapy protocols. Most therapy plans for HPV have utilized the application of caustic or keratolytic agents (13). Application of 25% podophyllin in benzoin, trichloroacetic acid or 5-fluoro-uracil for mild or primary lesions is often successful. Recurrent or persistent disease usually requires cryotherapy, surgical excision or laser therapy. Recurrences are common (14). Surgical techniques are painful and leave scars while laser techniques leave raw surfaces which may heal poorly, especially with extensive intravaginal application. In addition, systemic reactions to topical podophyllin have been reported and it is contraindicated in pregnancy because of mutagenicity (15).

Experimental therapies such as autologous vaccines (16), colchicine (13) and dinitrochlorobenzene sensitization (DNCB) (17) have had sporadic use and limited success. Studies with topically applied leukocyte interferon have demonstrated the responsiveness of genital warts to this type of therapy (18,19,20).

The research studies published to date have not defined the experimental subjects in detail. This becomes of critical importance in judging the outcome of therapy because greater than 33% of patients with initial HPV infection will undergo spontaneous regression within 6 months without therapy. The previously cited therapy studies whether using interferon or other agents have not defined the patients as to length of disease, severity of disease or previous treatment.

Persistent condylomata acuminata can cause considerable discomfort, personal trauma, hygiene problems and an increased threat of CIN. Since most individuals who develop condylomata acuminata are cured with simple therapies, i.e., podophyllin, it is appropriate to consider patients who do not respond to conventional treatment as being abnormal and in need of more intensive evaluation and therapy.

The present studies were designed to treat patients with condylomata acuminata who failed conventional therapies and were considered to have resistant and persistent condylomata acuminata. The studies were also designed to evaluate the efficacy, toxicity, and tolerance of intramuscular and intralesional administration of human lymphoblastoid interferon (Wellferon®).

## METHODS

A pilot study and treatment of an additional group of patients were conducted at Duke University Medical Center from December 1982 to December 1984. All patients had resistant and persistent condylomata acuminata as evidenced by the presence of warts for at least six months and had received ten or more podophyllin applications or equivalent treatments. Histological confirmation of condylomata acuminata was required. An informed consent approved by the institutional review board was signed by each patient.

Patients were excluded if any of the following were present: 1) concomitant corticosteroids, cytotoxic immunosuppression or radiotherapy; 2) immunological therapy within the previous three months or known major immunodeficiencies; 3) hepatic dysfunction; 4) nursing women; 5) pregnancy or inadequate contraceptive practice 6) malignant degeneration in biopsied tissue; 7) anemia (hemoglobin less than 10 gm/dl), thrombocytopenia (less than 1,000,000/$mm^3$), leukopenia (less than 4,000/$mm^3$); 8) renal dysfunction manifested by a serum creatinine greater than 1.4 mg/dl.

## STUDY DESIGN

Patients were evaluated by a routine medical history and physical examination and were admitted to the clinical research unit for two days for observation while the interferon was started. Documentation of the genital warts was done by recording the bidimensional measurements of each wart on a divided grid of the external genitalia. Photographs were made initially and at each follow-up examination. Biopsies were obtained for routine histology and for DNA typing. Blood was obtained for routine hematological evaluation including platelet count and for relevant chemistries: BUN, creatinine, SGOT, SGPT and bilirubin. A urinalysis was obtained. Hematological, hepatic and renal blood tests were repeated weekly when the patient was receiving daily interferon and every two weeks when the patient was receiving interferon three times per week.

In our initial series of patients, blood was obtained at the initial visit and every two weeks for the following two tests: T-cell subsets (T-helper, T-suppressor), phytohemagglutinin (PHA), concanavalin A (con A), and pokeweed mitogen (PWM) stimulation of lymphocytes, IgG, IgA, IgM determinations and interferon levels. Patients were sensitized for delayed hypersensitivity reactions to dinitrochlorobenzene.

Wellferon® (human lymphoblastoid interferon) was initiated by two different dosing and administrative protocols. The first protocol was studied on seventeen patients who received interferon by intramuscular (I.M.) injections at a dose of 5 $MU/m^2$ daily for 28 days followed by the same dose three times per week for two additional weeks. A second regimen employed interferon I.M. at 3 $MU/m^2$ daily for two weeks, followed by the same dose for an additional four weeks. In both protocols an initial assessment of response was made after six weeks of therapy and additional therapy depended on this clinical assessment.

Wellferon is a highly purified preparation of alpha interferons derived from viral induction of the human lymphoblastoid cell line Namalwa (16). Dose modifications were made if patients encountered severe side effects or clinical laboratory toxicities following interferon administration.

Measurements of condylomatous lesions were made upon entry and every two weeks. Protocol evaluations were made after six weeks of therapy and at the end of the study based on the following disease assessment: Complete Response (CR) total disappearance of the condylomata, Partial Response (PR) 50% or greater decrease in the condyloma size, No Response (NR) any change less than a 50% decrease in the products of the bidimensional measurements.

Patients who entered the initial trial received interferon at the dose of 5 $MU/m^2$, and judged to be CR were observed for six months while those who were PR after six weeks of therapy continued to receive interferon three times per week for an additional six weeks. If no response occurred the patient was offered intralesional therapy (I.L.) at a dose of 1 $MU/m^2$ twice weekly for four weeks or until the condyloma disappeared. All NR patients were offered intralesional therapy.

Twenty-three patients were treated with interferon at 3 MU/$m^2$. Patients received daily I.M. injections for two weeks followed by three times a week for four weeks. Patients judged to have a complete response were observed for six months while patients with PR were continued on the same dose for an additional four weeks. Those patients who were NR had their interferon dose escalated (those receiving 1 MU/$m^2$ were increased to 3 MU/$m^2$ and those at 3 MU/$m^2$ were increased to 5 MU/$m^2$).

Symptomatic side effects including fever, chills, fatigue, malaise, nausea/vomiting and headache were recorded daily by the patients. Clinical laboratory values and side effects were evaluated weekly while the patient was receiving daily interferon and every two weeks while the patient was receiving three times/week (T.I.W.) injections. Dose modification was made on the basis of a standardized severity grading system.

## RESULTS

Seventeen patients were entered on the initial protocol at the dose of 5 MU/$m^2$. Twenty-three patients received 3 MU/$m^2$ on the second protocol. Various characteristics of patients in each treatment group are listed in Table 1.

TABLE 1

TRIAL BY INITIAL DOSING SCHEDULE

| | 5 MU/$m^2$ | 3 MU/$m^2$ |
|---|---|---|
| N | 17 | 23 |
| Mean Age (Yr.) | 31.2 | 30.5 |
| Range, Age, (Yr.) | 18-48 | 8-59 |
| Female | 17 | 23 |
| White | 14 | 19 |
| Black | 3 | 4 |

Sixteen of the seventeen patients who were initially treated with 5 MU/$m^2$ were evaluable (Table 2). The first patient treated withdrew after eight injections because of nausea and vomiting. After six weeks of therapy, 4/16 (25%) were judged to be complete responders while 11/16 (69%) were PR and 1/16 (6%) demonstrated no response.

Eleven patients received an additional six weeks of T.I.W. therapy with four patients showing a CR. Four patients received intralesional therapy with a complete response in three. Three patients refused intralesional therapy. At the conclusion of the protocol 11/16 (69%) were completely cured of their condylomata. Additional detailed measurements and laboratory evaluations of patients on this pilot study have been summarized elsewhere (21,22).

TABLE 2

PATIENT RESPONSES TO INTERFERON 5 $MU/m^2$

| | 6 Weeks | % | End | % |
|---|---|---|---|---|
| CR | 4 | 25 | 11 | 69 |
| PR | 11 | 69 | 4 | 25 |
| NR | 1 | 6 | 1 | 6 |
| Evaluable | 16 | 94 | 16 | 94 |
| Not Evaluable | 1 | 6 | 1 | 6 |

Twenty-three patients were treated with an initial interferon dose of 3 $MU/m^2$ and twenty-one were evaluable, (Table 3). Two patients withdrew from the study because of difficulty in coming to the clinic or a loss of interest in the self-administered I.M. injections. After six weeks of therapy 6/21 (28%) demonstrated CR, 10/21 (48%) were PR and 5/21 (24%) were NR. The 10 patients who were PR were given four additional weeks of interferon at 3 $MU/m^2$ T.I.W. and 2 patients became complete responders. The 5 patients who were NR were given an additional four weeks of interferon at 5 $MU/m^2$ T.I.W. and one showed a complete response. At the conclusion of 10 weeks of the protocol 9/21 (43%) were judged to be CR, 8/21 (38%) PR and 4/21 (19%) NR. Following the conclusion of the protocol, six patients who were PR or NR were given the options of surgical excision or cryotherapy for remaining disease.

TABLE 3

PATIENT RESPONSE TO INTERFERON 3 $MU/m^2$

| | 6 Weeks | % | 10 Weeks | % |
|---|---|---|---|---|
| CR | 6 | 28 | 9 | 43 |
| PR | 10 | 48 | 8 | 38 |
| NR | 5 | 24 | 4 | 19 |
| Evaluable | 21 | 91 | 21 | 91 |
| Not Evaluable | 2 | 9 | 2 | 9 |

The kinetics of lesion regression is of great interest. The lesion size at patient entry varied from 0.6 to 160 sq cm. Measurements after two weeks show marked reductions in those patients destined to be CR or PR with responses continuing at a slower rate over the next four weeks. If wart regression had not started by the fourth week it was unlikely to occur.

The biologic side effects including fever, chills, fatigue, nausea/vomiting, malaise and headache were recorded by the patient on each dosing day. All patients in each group demonstrated fever of greater than 38°C to temperatures as high as 40.3°C accompanied by chills with the initial I.M. injection of interferon. The fever was usually of less than 12 hours in duration and did not occur unless a dosing lapse of greater than three days was present. The most prevalent chronic side effects were those of fatigue and malaise being greatest during the times interferon was administered daily. All side effects were greatly reduced with T.I.W. dosing and were milder in patients receiving doses of 3 $MU/m^2$ as compared to symptoms in patients at 5 $MU/m^2$.

In patients receiving 5 $MU/m^2$, significant decreases in mean white counts, lymphocytes, neutrophils, eosinophils and platelets were noted between days 0 and days 8, 15, 22, 29 and 43. Significant changes in mean hemoglobin levels occurred from day 22 onward. All patients had some reduction in neutrophils. Seven patients had a single absolute granulocyte count $<1,000/mm^3$ but none experienced infectious sequelae. No patient experienced a bleeding diathesis as a result of platelet count reductions of at least $50,000/mm^3$ in 14/16 patients. Hematological abnormalities were markedly diminished in the 3 $MU/m^2$ group with only 2/23 (9%) requiring dosage reduction for a white count of $<3,000/mm^3$.

All patients in the 5 $MU/m^2$ group manifested increases of SGPT and SGOT with minimal elevations over baseline. All hepatic abnormalities returned to normal values with dose reduction. Only one patient receiving interferon at the dose of 3 $MU/m^2$ required dose reduction.

Immunological evaluation showed T-cell helper/suppressor ratios and mitogenic stimulation of lymphocytes to be normal. The average OKT4/OKT8 ratio for 12 patients was 2.23 (range 1.2 to 3.7) whereas 31 laboratory controls had an average of 2.04 (range 0.5/03.6). In addition, all patients tested had an adequate and normal response to PHA, Con A and PWM as compared to a group of control patients.

Determinations of immunoglobulins A and G in the serum showed no change in level throughout the study period. In contrast, IgM levels were elevated.

Dosing alterations were used as a measure of toxicity and efficacy (Table 4). When no response was present the dose was escalated and when moderate to severe toxicity was present, the dose was reduced.

TABLE 4

DOSING CHANGES IN PATIENTS TREATED WITH WELLFERON

| Initial Dose | N | Dose Decreased | % | Dose Increased | % |
|---|---|---|---|---|---|
| 5 $Mu/m^2$ | 17 | 17 | 100 | 0 | 0 |
| 3 $Mu/m^2$ | 23 | 1 | 4 | 5 | 22 |

All dose reductions were due to biologic side effects or laboratory abnormalities of hematologic or hepatic function. All occurred between 1 to 2 weeks of therapy and dosage escalations occurred after ten weeks of therapy.

## DISCUSSION

Condylomata acuminata recognized for centuries as an external disease entity has been linked recently to development of neoplasia of the cervix, vagina and vulva. In addition, it is estimated that more than 900,000 new cases are present in the U.S. yearly. While the vast majority of patients with condylomata acuminata can be treated by simple procedures, a small percentage of patients are resistant to conventional therapy. Some of these patients show evidence of modified immune status as evidenced by the presence of measurable endogenous interferon levels, elevated IgM levels, or an increased number of patients not responding to DNCB sensitization. In contrast, serum IgA and IgG levels, OKT4/OKT8 ratios and mitogen stimulation indices are normal. Therefore, the exact defect in the immune system remains ill-defined.

Exogenous topical interferon was first reported by Ikic et al. (18,19) in 1975 with the application of a vaseline-lanolin ointment of a crude leukocyte interferon. This resulted in the complete response of 36/40 women treated for a period of 4-12 weeks. Schonfeld et al. (20) used I.M. injection of fibroblast interferon (IFN-β) and claimed an 80% complete response rate. The patients treated by Ikic and Schonfeld were largely untreated patients rather than patients with resistant and persistent disease.

The objectives of our studies were to evaluate the efficacy, biologic side effects and tolerance of varying doses of interferon. Statistical analysis of the efficacy of these and two other dosing schedules are in progress. The manifestation of biologic side effects appear to be dose dependent. Although all patients manifest fevers with the first I.M. injection, all other symptoms are markedly diminished with lower doses. Patients receiving 5 $MU/m^2$ daily will manifest some unpleasant side effects but these were never life threatening. The side effects diminish substantially when T.I.W. dosing is used and particularly at the 3 $MU/m^2$ dose.

Hematological aberrations were the most prominent laboratory abnormalities in response to interferon, however, no serious clinical effects were noted. The hematological aberrations occurred mainly in patients receiving 5 $MU/m^2$ on a daily basis.

The clinical trials with Wellferon® at various dosing schedules have demonstrated that this interferon is active in the treatment of resistant and persistent condylomata acuminata. Patients who manifest this variety of warts seem to have an immunodeficiency syndrome which is not well defined. Further therapy trials are indicated in association with surgical excision and/or laser therapy.

REFERENCES

1. Dunn AEG, Ogilvie MM (1968). Intranuclear virus particles in human genital wart tissues: Observations on the ultrastructure of the epidermal layer. J Ultrastruct Res 22:282.

2. Ariel JD, Almeida JD (1970). Demonstration of virus particles in human genital warts. Br J Vener Dis 46:37.

3. Woodruff JD, Peterson WF (1958). Condyloma acuminata of the cervix. Am J Obstet Gynecol 75:1354.

4. Feuner F (1976). Classification and nomenclature of viruses. Intervirology 7:54.

5. Klug A, Finch AT (1965). Structure of viruses of the papilloma-polyoma Type I human wart virus. J Mat Biol 11:403.

6. Gissman L, ZurHausen H (1976). Human papilloma viruses: physical mapping and genetic heterogenecity. Proc Nat Acad Sci USA 73:1310.

7. Coggin JR, ZurHausen H (1979). Workshop in Papilloma viruses and Cancer. Can Res 39:545.

8. Gissman L, Devilliers EM, ZurHausen H (1982). Analysis of human warts (condyloma acuminata) and other genital tumors for human papilloma virus type 6 DNA. Int J Cancer 29:143.

9. Gissman L, Diehl V, Schulte-Colon HJ, ZurHausen H (1982). Molecular cloning and characterization of human papilloma virus DNA derived from a laryngeal papilloma. J Virol 44:493.

10. Gissman L, Wolnik L, Ikenburg H, Koldousky U, Schnurch HG, ZurHausen H (1983). Human papilloma virus types 6 and 11 DNA sequences in genital and laryngeal papillomas and in some cervical cancers. Proc Natl Acad Sci USA 80:560.

11. Richart RM (1975). Cervical intraepithelial neoplasia. In Somers SC (ed): "Genital and Mammary Pathology Decennial" 1966-1975. New York, Appleton-Century-Crofts p 1-28.

12. Meisels A, Morin C (1981). Human papilloma virus and cancer of the uterine cervix. Gynec Oncol 12: 5-111.

13. Von Krogh G (1978). Topical treatment of penile condyloma acuminata with podophyllin, podophyllotoxin and colchicine. Acta Dermatol (Stockholm) 58:163.

14. Rasmussen JE (1981). Warts and what to do about them. Drug Therapy 11:65.

15. Fisher AA (1981). Severe systemic and local reactions to topical podophyllin resin. Cutis 28:233.

16. Finter NB, Fantes KH (1981). The purity and safety of interferons prepared for clinical use. The case of lymphoblastoid interferon. In Gresser I, (ed): "Interferon" Academic Press 3:65.

17. Foster DC, Woodruff JD (1981). The use of dinitrochlorobenzene in the treatment of vulvar carcinoma in situ. Gynecol Oncol 11:330.

18. Ikic D, Bosnic N, Smerdel S (1975). Double blind clinical study with human leukocyte interferon in the therapy of condyloma acuminata. Proc Symp Clinical Use of Interferon, Zagreb pp 229-233.

19. Ikic D, Orescanin J, Krusic Z (1975). Preliminary study of the effect of human leukocyte interferon on condyloma acuminata in women. Proc Symp Clinical Use of Interferon. Zagreb pp 233-228.

20. Schonfeld A, Nitke S, Schattner A (1984). Intramuscular human interferon-β injections in treatment of condyloma acuminata. Lancet 1:1038.

21. Gall SA, Hughes CE, Weck P, Whisnant J (1984). Interferon for the treatment of resistant condyloma acuminata. Gynecol Oncol 17:264.

22. Gall SA, Hughes CE, Mounts P, Madden DL, Segreti A, Weck PK, Whisnant J (1985). The efficacy of human lymphoblastoid interferon (Wellferon®) in the therapy of resistant condyloma acuminata. N Engl J Med (manuscript submitted).

**Papillomaviruses: Molecular and Clinical Aspects, pages 217–233**


# NATURAL LEUKOCYTE INTERFERON FOR TREATMENT OF CONDYLOMATA ACUMINATA A RANDOMIZED, DOUBLE-BLIND, PLACEBO CONTROLLED STUDY[1]

Alvin E. Friedman-Kien, M.D., Terry F. Plasse, M.D., Patricia Cremin, R.N., Brenda Castro, R.N., Helen Badiak, B.S., Jeremy R. Geffen, B.S., David Fedorczyk, M.S., and J. Richard Trout, Ph.D.

Department of Dermatology, New York University School of Medicine, New York, New York, Interferon Sciences, Inc. New Brunswick, New Jersey, and Department of Statistics, Rutgers University, New Brunswick, New Jersey

ABSTRACT Thirty-four patients with genital warts, 33 of whom had received prior therapy, were treated intralesionally with either natural leukocyte (alpha) interferon (IFN) or placebo. Patients were treated twice weekly for eight weeks; patients randomized to interferon received a median dose of 600,000 IU per treatment, with the dose dependent on the amount needed to saturate the warts. Eighteen patients were allocated to IFN, of whom 12 are evaluable for efficacy. Thirteen of 16 placebo patients are evaluable for efficacy. Toxicity consisted primarily of fever (10 IFN, 1 placebo patient) and an influenza-like syndrome (7 IFN, 0 placebo patients). These effects were self-limited and occurred no later than after the seventh injection. Ten of the twelve (83%) IFN but only 1/13 (8%) placebo patients had complete

[1]This work was supported by Interferon Sciences, Inc., the Howard Gilman Foundation, the Sara Chait Foundation and the Rita and Stanley H. Kaplan Cancer Center.

disappearance of all treated warts by the end of therapy or the first follow-up visit three weeks later (P=0.0002). One additional IFN and 1 placebo patient had at least 90% decrease in the volume of treated warts by the end of therapy or first follow-up visit. In this heavily pretreated group of patients, natural leukocyte IFN was highly effective as compared to placebo in inducing complete regression of all treated warts.

## INTRODUCTION

Condylomata acuminata (genital warts) are benign epithelial tumors caused by the human papilloma virus (HPV). The lesions tend to occur in the genital and perianal areas, and they can assume various morphological configurations (1). Condyloma lesions can be highly contagious: it has been reported that up to 70% of exposed partners of patients with condylomata either have or develop these lesions (2). Condyloma acuminatum is now recognized to be one of the most common sexually transmissible diseases in the United States. It is estimated that in 1981 there were 946,000 physician consultations for condylomata acuminata as compared to 295,000 consultations for genital herpes infections (3).

Treatment methods currently in use include topical application of varying concentrations of caustic agents such as podophyllum and trichloroacetic acid 5-flourouracil, surgical excision, electrodessication and/or curettage under local anesthesia, cryotherapy with liquid nitrogen, carbon dioxide laser irradiation, and intralesional injections of bleomycin (4). Following each of these treatments, patients commonly experience pain and considerable discomfort for several days. Immunotherapy with autologous vaccine has also been used with variable results (5,6). These treatment methods are often ineffective. Repeated therapy is usually required due to persistence or recurrence of the previously treated lesions and the frequent development of new lesions in the same regions (8,9,10).

Despite the fact that HPV has not yet been successfully grown in tissue culture, during the past few years up to twenty-five different subtypes of HPV have been identified by electron microscopy, immunohistochemistry, agarose gel electrophoresis, and DNA hybridization techniques (11,12). The demonstration of specific subtypes of the virus has occurred in benign skin warts, anogenital condylomata acuminata and warts of the uterine cervix (13,14). Correlations have also recently been established between HPV-induced condylomata and malignant carcinoma of the penis, vulva, and uterine cervix (15-21). The HPV has also been identified in normal laryngeal epithelial cells, as well as in overt papilloma tissues of patients with juvenile laryngeal papillomatosis (22). This disease, which is thought to be transmitted to the infant through contact with maternal condyloma lesions during vaginal delivery (23-25), often requires frequent surgical removal of the lesions due to multiple recurrences in patients aged 3 months to 70 years (22).

Human interferons (IFN) are known to have a spectrum of biological activities, including the in vitro and in vivo inhibition of viral replication in infected cells and the suppression of cell proliferation (26,27). Other properties attributed to IFN include enhancement of monocyte phagocytosis, antibody-dependent cell-mediated cytotoxicity, and natural killer cell activity (26,27). The combination of these effects as well as the relatively low toxicity of IFN reported in previous human trials has led to their clinical testing in different viral infections and tumors, including various types of warts such as condylomata (28-32).

In recent years, several studies have specifically tested the therapeutic efficacy of topical human leukocyte (alpha) IFN in patients with condylomata acuminata, with some success (33-35). Temporary as well as long term remissions have also been reported in patients with juvenile laryngeal papillomatosis treated with parenteral human leukocyte (alpha) IFN (36,37). Further clinical investigations on the long term treatment of laryngeal papillomatosis with systemic IFN are currently in progress (38). Finally, results of a pilot study which tested the effects of intralesional injections of human fibroblast (beta) IFN in patients with genital warts suggested that the "small dose" injections of IFN given may have inhibited the growth of the injected warts as compared with that of uninjected lesions (39). A randomized trial of intramuscular human fibroblast interferon has demonstrated efficacy (40).

In our preliminary open study (41), eight patients with classical condylomata acuminata were treated with biweekly intralesional injections of natural human leukocyte (alpha) IFN for 5 to 14 weeks. Five of the eight had complete resolution of all treated warts. We have now conducted a randomized, double blind, placebo-controlled trial to confirm our initial findings.

## PATIENTS AND METHODS

Forty patients have been enrolled to date, of whom 34 have either completed treatment or withdrawn from the study. All patients gave informed consent. All females were instructed to use an effective means of contraception and none was known to be pregnant or lactating during treatment. All but one interferon patient and all placebo patients had received prior treatment with standard modalities, including one or more of the following: chemocautery with podophyllum or trichloroacetic acid, cryotherapy with liquid nitrogen, surgical treatment including $CO_2$ laser, electrodessication and curettage. No patient with severe concommitant disease, e.g., immunodeficiency states, was entered into the study, and no patient had any immunostimulation, e.g. BCG, within one month prior to entry. None of the patients received other specific therapy for warts while on the study. Analysis by treatment allocation of the 34 patients evaluated thus far revealed no significant differences in patient characteristics (Table 1) or prior therapy (Table 2).

Patients were treated with either interferon or a placebo, which consisted of the same vehicle as was used for the interferon preparation. The interferon used was monoclonal antibody purified natural leukocyte (alpha) interferon produced by Interferon Sciences, Inc., New Brunswick, NJ. Interferon production was induced by Sendai virus in pooled buffy coat human leukocytes. The base of each lesion was injected with approximately 0.05 ml of medication (about 250,000 IU for IFN-treated patients) for each 25 $mm^2$ area. In our preliminary study (41), this was found to be sufficient to saturate the condyloma lesions. Patients were treated twice weekly for eight weeks or until complete disappearance of all treated warts, whichever came first. Patients who missed injections were treated for up to nine weeks. After therapy, patients were examined

TABLE 1
PATIENT CHARACTERISTICS

| | Interferon | Placebo |
|---|---|---|
| Number | 18 | 16 |
| Male/Female | 14/4 | 12/4 |
| Age, median (years) | 29.9 | 25.7 |
| Race: White | 13 | 14 |
| Black | 3 | 2 |
| Other | 2 | 0 |
| Median time since initial episode, years | 1.3 | 1.8 |
| Location of treated warts | | |
| Penis | 12 | 12 |
| Vulva | 3 | 4 |
| Scrotum | 3 | 1 |
| Perineum | 4 | 2 |
| Number of warts | | |
| Median | 6.5 | 6 |
| Range | 3 to 10 | 2 to 10 |
| Area of warts ($mm^2$) | | |
| Median | 55 | 42 |
| Range | 12 to 382 | 12 to 185 |
| Volume of warts ($mm^3$) | | |
| Median | 50 | 38 |
| Range | 6 to 382 | 12 to 237 |

periodically for three months.

A patient was considered to have been adequately treated if he or she:

a) completed a total of 16 treatments or was treated for nine weeks, whichever came first, or
b) had complete disappearance of all treated warts before the end point noted in (a), or
c) had progressive disease, defined as at least a 25% increase in the volume of one or more of the patient's treated warts, while on treatment.

A complete response was defined as complete disappearance of all treated lesions within the treatment period or by the time of the first follow-up visit after completion of therapy.

In order to determine if any dissimilarities exist

TABLE 2
PRIOR THERAPY

| | Interferon | Placebo |
|---|---|---|
| Number | 18 | 16 |
| Number of patients who received prior therapy | 17 | 16 |
| Number of patients who received prior therapy for lesions treated in this study | 6 | 10 |
| Median number of prior courses of therapy | 3 | 3 |
| Range | 0 to 8 | 1 to 8 |
| Median time since start of last treatment (weeks) | 13.6 | 16.9 |
| Range | 1.4 to 376.9 | 1.4 to 83.1 |
| Number of patients who had received previous treatment with: | | |
| Podophyllum | 14 | 14 |
| Trichloroacetic acid | 2 | 5 |
| Cryosurgery | 3 | 6 |
| Surgical excision | 5 | 3 |
| Electrodessication | 5 | 5 |
| $CO_2$ Laser | 3 | 0 |
| Autologous Vaccine | 1 | 0 |

between the interferon and placebo groups regarding patient characteristics, prior therapy, treatment compliance, adverse effects, laboratory findings, or response to therapy, Fisher's Exact Chi-Square Tests and Wilcoxon Two Sample Tests were used. The curves in Figure 3 were determined by the Kaplan and Meier product-limit method and depict probabilities for complete disappearance of warts as a function of time. The logrank test was used to analyze differences between the curves. Tick marks along the curves represent censored patients. Progressive-disease patients who withdrew from the study are assumed to have censored times equivalent to the longest recorded time within the appropriate treatment group.

## RESULTS

### Tolerance and Toxicity

A total of 34 patients have been either adequately treated (12 IFN, 13 placebo) or withdrawn from the study (6 IFN, 3 placebo). All 34 patients are evaluable for toxicity. Reasons for withdrawal are indicated in Table 3. The median volumes given to interferon- and placebo-treated patients for initial treatment sessions were 0.19 ml and 0.18 ml respectively (ranges 0.06 ml to 0.34 ml for interferon and 0.06 ml to 1.31 ml for placebo).

TABLE 3
TREATMENT COMPLIANCE

| | Interferon | Placebo |
|---|---|---|
| Number | 18 | 16 |
| Adequately treated | 12 | 13 |
| Completed three months' follow-up | 6 | 5 |
| Withdrawals | 6 | 3 |
| Lost to follow-up | 0 | 1 |
| Relocated | 3 | 2 |
| Fever or flu-like syndrome | 3 | 0 |

As the volume of medication injected decreased with decreasing size of warts present, over the course of therapy, the interferon group received a smaller volume of medication than the placebo group. The dose of interferon administered per treatment and the total dose given during the entire course of therapy are shown in Table 4.

Side effects were self-limited and usually mild (See Table 5). While some patients had slight transient discomfort from the injections, the majority noted that these treatments were preferable to standard forms of therapy. The most common side effect of intralesional IFN was fever, usually accompanied by an influenza-like syndrome, including malaise, myalagias and headache. Fever was noted by 10 of the 18 interferon-treated

TABLE 4
INTERFERON ADMINISTERED (N = 18)

| | Median | Range |
|---|---|---|
| For all patients (n=18) | | |
| Total dose, IU | $7.0x10^6$ | 0.6 to $16.4x10^6$ |
| Initial dose, IU | $1.0x10^6$ | 0.3 to $1.8x10^6$ |
| Average dose per treatment session, IU | $0.6x10^6$ | 0.3 to $1.3x10^6$ |
| Number of treatment sessions | 13 | 1 to 16 |
| For complete responders (n=10) | | |
| Total dose, IU | $9.9x10^6$ | 2.5 to $16.4x10^6$ |
| Initial dose, IU | $1.1x10^6$ | 0.3 to $1.8x10^6$ |
| Average dose per treatment session, IU | $0.6x10^6$ | 0.3 to $1.3x10^6$ |
| Number of treatment sessions | 15.5 | 7 to 16 |

patients but by only one of the placebo-treated patients. Side effects usually disappeared within several hours and in no case did they last longer than a

TABLE 5
ADVERSE EFFECTS

| | Patients Reporting Adverse Effect | |
|---|---|---|
| | Interferon | Placebo |
| N= | 18 | 16 |
| Number of patients with side effects | 14 | 5 |
| Fever | 10 | 1 |
| Myalgias | 7 | 0 |
| Headache | 7 | 0 |
| Malaise | 4 | 0 |
| Backache | 2 | 0 |
| Significant pain at injection site | 2 | 3 |
| GI discomfort | 1 | 1 |
| Light-headedness | 1 | 1 |
| Inguinal adenopathy | 1 | 0 |
| Local Pruritus | 1 | 2 |
| Tongue hyperaesthesia | 1 | 0 |

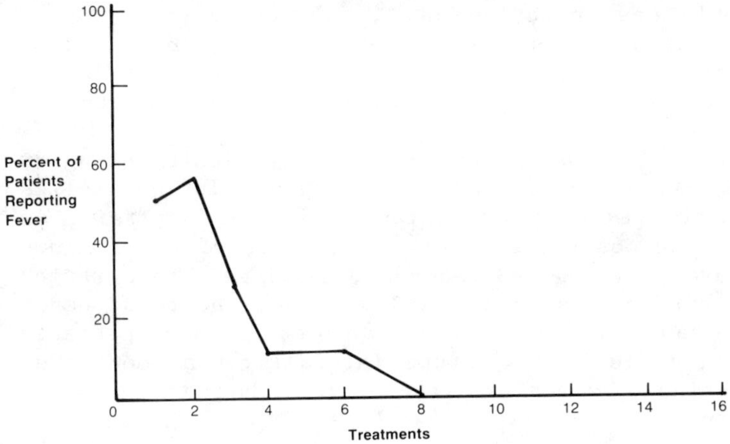


FIGURE 1. Percentage of interferon patients reporting fever after injection

day. There was no relationship between initial IFN dose and occurrence of fever. Symptoms were severe enough to induce 3 patients to discontinue treatment, 2 subjects

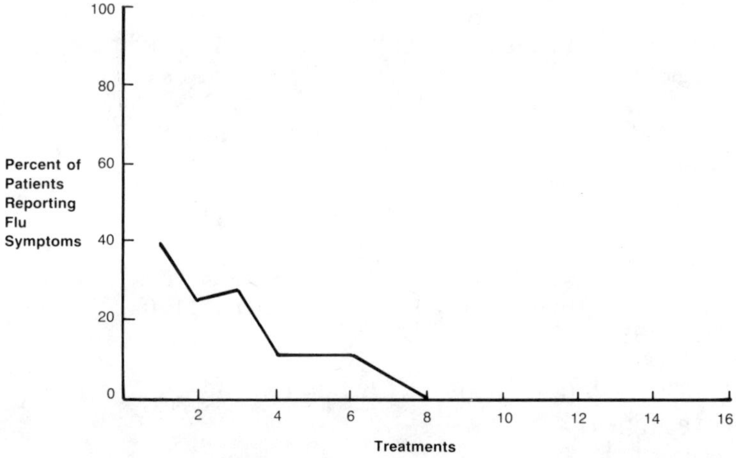


FIGURE 2. Percentage of interferon patients reporting influenza-like syndrome after injections

after only one injection and 1 subject after 2 injections. The symptoms disappeared with continued therapy in the other patients, as shown in Figures 1 and 2. No interferon patient experienced fever after more than 7 injections.

Figure 2 shows the percentage of patients noting an influenza-like syndrome after treatment. Influenza-like syndrome is defined, for purposes of this analysis, as the simultaneous presence of two or more of the following: fever, myalagias, headache, malaise. The duration of this syndrome was usually less than 1 hour and never longer than one day. While 7 of the IFN patients developed a flu-like syndrome initially, none continued to experience symptoms after more than the seventh injection.

TABLE 6
LABORATORY FINDINGS
PRE-THERAPY TO WEEK 4

| Change In | Interferon | Placebo |
|---|---|---|
| Leukocyte count ($1^{-1}$) | | |
| Median | $0.4x10^9$ | $0.7x10^9$ |
| Range | -0.6 to $3.7x10^9$ | -3.4 to $5.2x10^9$ |
| Granulocyte count ($1^{-1}$) | | |
| Median | $2.3x10^9$ | $0.6x10^9$ |
| Range | -0.2 to $3.5x10^9$ | -3.4 to $5.9x10^9$ |
| Hemoglobin (gm/dl) | | |
| Median | 0 | -0.3 |
| Range | -0.7 to 0.2 | -1.2 to 1.5 |
| Platelet count ($1^{-1}$) | | |
| Median | $-20.0x10^9$ | $18.0x10^9$ |
| Range | -60.0 to $2.0x10^9$ | -19.0 to $37.0x10^9$ |
| SGOT (U/ml) | | |
| Median | -8.0 | -2.5 |
| Range | -10.0 to 18.0 | -12.0 to 11.0 |
| Creatinine (mg/dl) | | |
| Median | 0 | 0 |
| Range | -0.1 to 0.3 | -0.1 to 0.3 |
| Total protein (gm/dl) | | |
| Median | -0.2 | -0.1 |
| Range | -0.6 to 0.6 | -0.4 to 1.1 |
| Albumin (gm/dl) | | |
| Median | -0.1 | 0.25 |
| Range | -0.3 to 0.6 | -0.4 to 0.7 |

A summary of significant laboratory data is shown in Table 6. No clinically significant changes in blood counts or chemistries occurred in any patient studied. The decrease in platelet count in IFN patients was statistically significant relative to the mild increase in placebo patients (P=0.009). However, no IFN patient had a platelet count less than 172 x $10^9$. The median platelet count went from 318 x $10^9$/l to 272 x $10^9$/l for IFN patients, as compared to a change from 238 x $10^9$/l to 250 x $10^9$/l for placebo patients.

Response To Therapy

As shown in Table 7, response to IFN therapy, as compared to placebo, was dramatic. Eighty-three percent (10/12) of interferon- vs. only 8% (1/13) of placebo-treated patients had complete disappearance of all treated warts by the end of therapy or by the first follow-up visit (p=0.0002). Furthermore, although the number of patients in each group was small, the effect of treatments was seen in patients with refractory as

TABLE 7
RESPONSE TO THERAPY

| | Interferon | Placebo | P-Value |
|---|---|---|---|
| Number adequately treated | 12 | 13 | |
| Complete responders by end of therapy (%) | 6 (50) | 0 (0) | 0.005 |
| Complete responders by first follow-up visit (%) | 10 (83) | 1 (8) | 0.0002 |
| At least 90% decrease in volume (%) | 11 (92) | 2 (15) | 0.0002 |
| Patients developing additional warts while on therapy (%) | 5 (42) | 9 (69) | 0.163 |
| Patients who had complete response of all additional warts (%) | 3 (60) | 1 (11) | 0.095 |
| Patients with refractory warts who had complete response (%) | 4 (100) | 1 (11) | 0.007 |
| Patients with recurring warts who had complete response (%) | 6 (75) | 0 (0) | 0.030 |

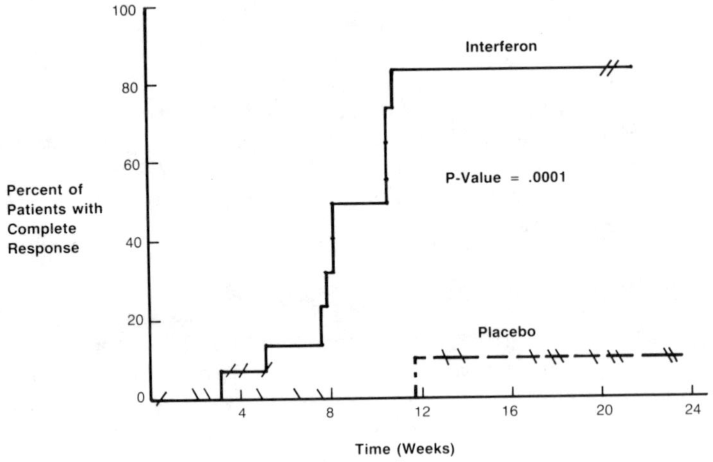


FIGURE 3. Time to complete disappearance of warts

well as recurrent warts. Four out of 4 IFN vs. 1/9 placebo patients with refractory warts had a complete response (p=0.007). Those who had recurrent warts also responded with 6/8 complete responders in the IFN group as compared to 0/4 on the placebo group (p=0.03).

Eleven of 12 IFN-treated vs. 2 of 13 placebo-treated patients had at least a 90% reduction in total volume of warts (p=0.0002).

Figure 3 shows the time to complete disappearance of all treated warts. The median time to complete response was 73 days for interferon patients, but was not reached for placebo patients (P=0.0001).

Of the 5 IFN patients who developed new lesions while on study, 3 had complete response of all new lesions. One of 9 placebo patients with new lesions appearing during the study had complete response (P=0.095, see Table 7). The median number of treatments to the new warts was 5 (3-13) for IFN patients, as compared to 11 (0-14) for placebo patients.

Patients have now been followed for a median of 11.5 weeks from the end of treatment (range 0 to 22 weeks). Two IFN patients who had complete responses had relapses 5 and 7 weeks after the end of treatment. Those patients each received a total of $9.9 \times 10^6$IU over

15 and 16 treatments, respectively. The placebo patient with a complete response had not relapsed after 14 weeks of follow-up.

## DISCUSSION

In this group of heavily pretreated patients, intralesional injections of alpha interferon were very effective in resolving genital warts. Six IFN but no placebo patients achieved complete responses during the treatment period. Four more IFN and 1 placebo patient had complete disappearance of their lesions by the time of their first follow-up visit. Two of the 10 IFN patients had relapses within a short time after therapy. They have not been retreated. We do not know whether they are truly refractory to IFN therapy or just need a longer period of treatment to achieve a sustained response. Although we have not yet developed long term follow-up data on this group, we have continued to see the patients from our open study (41). With a minimum follow-up of one year, none of the five complete responders has had a relapse of their treated warts.

Compared to other modalities, the intralesional form of therapy had a high degree of patient acceptance. Standard therapies are routinely quite painful for a prolonged period, whereas only 11% (2/18) of interferon-treated patients and 19% (3/16) of placebo-treated patients reported significant pain. Of these, only one placebo patient reported severe pain. The treatment is not difficult to administer. Unlike destructive therapies, interferon did not produce ulcerations similar to those experienced by many patients with standard therapy. Rather, in most cases, the lesions resorbed, first flattening and then disappearing. Thus there was no incidence of secondary infections, which are common in patients treated with standard therapies.

While fever, often accompanied by influenza-like symptoms, was present initially in many patients, it subsided rapidly. Several patients became quite anxious about this initially. In only one case, however, was therapy discontinued at the investigator's suggestion. With antipyretics and reassurance that the symptoms would not persist, most patients were able to tolerate the fevers, which were usually mild.

Recent work has implicated HPV in causation of several types of cancers (16,42,43). Podophyllum itself may also be carcinogenic (44). Elimination of the virus, which may occur with interferon treatment, may eliminate the potential for development of cancers due to HPV infection.

The optimal dose and schedule for intralesional IFN administration has not yet been determined. Despite the transient systemic side effects initially seen in most patients, the dose of IFN administered was not enough to prevent development of new warts in several of the patients treated. However, 3/5 patients did have complete regression of the new warts when the new lesions were treated directly. Response of the new warts was much more rapid than that of the pre-existing lesions. This observation suggests that warts may respond more rapidly if treated early. On the other hand, those IFN patients who had only partial responses might have benefited from a longer course of therapy.

Further studies involving different doses and varied schedules of administration are underway. Since it is possible that different strains of HPV may respond differently to treatment, virus typing may also aid in helping to determine the optimum therapeutic regimen. It is clear, however, in this group of patients with genital warts resistant in many cases to standard therapy, that natural leukocyte interferon was safe and effective in causing regression of the disease.

## REFERENCES

1. Oriel JD (1971). Natural history of genital warts. Br J Vener Dis 47:1-13.
2. Morton RS (1979). The other STD's. A synopsis. Publication no. 40-45. Department of Health and Human Services, Washington, D.C.
3. Centers for Disease Control (1983). Condyloma acuminatum-United States, 1966-1981, MMWR 32:306-8.
4. Margolis S (1982). Therapy for condylomata acuminata. Rev Inf Dis 4: S829-36.
5. Biberstein H (1944). Immunization therapy of warts. Archives of Dermatology and Syphilology 50:12.

6. Malison MD, Morris R, Jones LW (1982). Autogenous Vaccine therapy for condylomata acuminatum. Br J Vener Dis 58:62-5.
7. Abcarian H, Sharon N (1982). Long-term effectiveness of the immunotherapy of anal condyloma acuminatum. Dis Colon Rectum 25:678.
8. Friedman-Kien AE (1977). Minor viral diseases of the skin and mucosal surfaces, in Harrison's Principals of Internal Medicine. Eds.: G Thorn, R Adams, E Braunwald, K Isselbacher, R Petersdorf, New York, McGraw Hill, pp. 1027-30.
9. Simmons PD (1981). Podophyllum 10% and 25% in the treatment of ano-genital warts. Comparative double-blind study. Br J Vener Dis 57:208-9.
10. Simons PD, Langlet F, Thin RNT (1981). Cryotherapy versus electrocautery in the treatment of genital warts. Br J Vener Dis 57:232-4.
11. Syrjanen KJ (1984). Current concepts of human papillomavirus infections in the genital tract and their relationship to intraepithelial neoplasia and squamous cell carcinoma. Ob Gyn Survey 39:252-65.
12. Lutzner MA (1983). The human papilloma viruses. A review. Arch Dermat 119:631-5,
13. Kryzyzek RA, Watts SL, Anderson DL, et al (1980). Anogenital warts contain several distinct species of human papillomavirus. J Virology 36:236-44.
14. Gissman L, de Villiers E-M, zur Hausen H (1982). Analysis of human genital warts (condylomata acuminata) and other genital tumors for human papillomavirus type 6 DNA. Int J Cancer 29:143-6.
15. zur Hausen H (1976). Condylomata acuminata and human genital cancer. Cancer Research 36:794.
16. Crum CP, Ikenberg H, Richart RM, Gissman L (1984). Human papilloma virus type 16 and early cervical neoplasia. N Engl J Med 310:880-4.
17. Crum CP, Braun LA, Shah BKV, et al. (1982). Vulvar intraepithelial neoplasia: Correlation of nuclear DNA content and the presence of a human papilloma virus (HPV) structural antigen. Cancer 49:468-71.
18. Reid R, Stanhope CR, Herschman BR, et al. (1982). Genital warts and cervical cancer. 1. Evidence of an association between subclinical papilloma virus infection and cervical malignancy. Cancer 50:377-87.

19. Lynch PJ (1982). Warts and cancer. The oncogenic potential of human papilloma virus. Amer J Dermatopathology 4:55-60.

20. Friedman-Kien AE (1976). Giant condyloma of Buschke-Lowenstein, in Cancer of the Skin. Eds.: R Andrade, S Gumport, G Popkin, T Rees, Philadelphia, WB Saunders.

21. Steffen C (1982). Concurrence of condylomata acuminata and bowenoid papulosis. Confirmation of the hypothesis that they are related conditions. Amer J Dermatopathology 4: 5-8.

22. Steinberg BM, Topp WC, Schneider PS, Abramson AL (1983). Laryngeal papilloma virus infection during clinical remission. N Engl J Med 308:1261-4.

23. Cook TA, Cohn AM, Brunschwig JP, et al. (1973). Wart viruses and laryngeal papillomas. Lancet 1:782.

24. Quick CA, Watts SL, Kryzyzek RA, Faras AJ (1980). Relationship between condylomata and laryngeal papillomata. Clinical and molecular virological evidence. Ann Otol Rhinol Laryngol 89: 467-71.

25. Quick CA, Faras A, Kryzyzek R (1978). The etiology of laryngealpapillomatosis. Laryngoscope 88:1789-95.

26. Berman B, Frankfort HM (1982). The human interferon system. Int J Dermatology 21:12-8.

27. Ho M (1982). Recent advances in the study of interferon. Pharmacological Reviews 34:119-29.

28. Vesterinien E, Meyer B, Purola E, Cantell K (1984). Treatment of vaginal flat condyloma with interferon cream. Lancet 1:157.

29. Ikic D, Trajer D, Cupak K, et al (1981). The clinical use of human leukocyte interferon in viral infections. Int J Clin Pharmacology, Therapy, and Toxicology 19:498-505.

30. Uyeno K, Ohtsu A (1980). Interferon treatment of viral warts and some skin diseases, in The Clinical Potential of Interferons, Proceedings of the International Conference on Clinical Potentials of Interferons in Viral Diseases and Malignant Tumors. Eds.: R Kono, J Vilcek, Tokyo, University of Tokyo Press.

31. Pazin GJ, Ho M, Haverkos HW, et al (1982). Effects of interferon-alpha on human warts. J Interferon Research 2: 235-243.

32. Scott JM (1983). Papillomas, in Interferon and Cancer. Ed: K Sikora, New York, Plenum Press.
33. Ikic D, Orescanin M, Krusic J, et al(1975a). Preliminary study of the effect of human leukocyte interferon on condyloma acuminata in women. Proc Symposium Clin Use Interferon, Zagreb, Yugoslav Acad Sci Arts.
34. Ikic D, Bosnic N, Smerdel S, et al (1975b). Double blind clinical study with human leukocyte interferon in the therapy of condylomata acuminata. Proc Symposium Clin Use Interferon, Zagreb, Yugoslav Acad Sci Arts.
35. Ikic D, Brnobic A, Jurkovic-Vukelic V, et al (1975c). Therapeutical effect of human leukocyte interferon incorporated into ointment and cream on condylomata acuminata. Proceedings: Symposium on Clinical use of Interferon, Zagreb, Yugoslav Acad. Sci Arts.
36. Haglung S, Lundquist P, Cantell K, Strander H (1981). Interferon therapy in juvenile laryngeal papillomatosis. Arch Otolaryngol 107:327.
37. McCabe BF, Clark KF (1983). Interferon and laryngeal papillomatosis. The Iowa experience. Ann Otol Rhinol Laryngol 92:2-7.
38. McCabe BF. Personal communication, 1984
39. Scott GM, Csonka GW (1979). Effect of injections of small doses of human fibroblast interferon into genital warts. A pilot study. Br J Vener Dis 55:442-5.
40 Schonfeld A, Schattner A, Crespi M, et al (1984). Intramuscular Human Interferon-β Injections in Treatment of Condylomata Acuminata. Lancet pp. 1038.
41. Geffen JR, Klein RJ, Friedman-Kein AE(1984). Intralesional Administration of Large Doses of Human Leukocyte Interferon for the Treatment of Condylomata Acuminata. J Infect Dis 150:612-625.
42. Rhatigan RM, Jimenez S, Chopskie EJ (1972). Condyloma acuminata and carcinoma of the penis. South Med J 65: 423.
43. Charlewood GP, Shippel S (1953). Vulval condyloma acuminata as a premalignant lesion in the Bantu. S Afr Med J 27: 149-151.
44. Svindland, HB (1984).
Eur J Sexually Transmitted Diseases 1:165-7.

Papillomaviruses: Molecular and Clinical Aspects, pages 235–247


# CHEMOTHERAPY OF PAPILLOMAVIRUS INFECTIONS

Brigid G. Leventhal, and Haskins K.Kashima

Johns Hopkins Hospital,Baltimore, Maryland, 21205

ABSTRACT Antimitotic agents (podophyllin, colchicine) can cause regression of papillomas with topical application. Antimetabolites or DNA intercalators (5FU, Bleomycin) can cause regression given locally or systemically. Potential combinations with alpha interferon include:antiproliferative agents (DFMO); immune active agents (cymetidine); antiviral agents (acyclovir, AraA); and multiple interferons or interferon inducers.

The papillomaviruses are small DNA viruses that are widespread in nature and induce benign squamous epithelial tumors in many higher vertebrates, including man. None of the papillomaviruses has yet been successfully propagated in long term tissue culture in the laboratory. This means that any study of the efficacy of a particular therapeutic agent will have to be in vivo, either in a whole animal model or in man. There are specific difficulties in assessing clinical response in this group of diseases. First, for many patients this is a multicentric disease which is difficult to quantitate, even with direct visualization. One is usually trying to make a three dimensional measurement on a two dimensional scale. Second, a number of these benign tumors undergo spontaneous regression, and so all therapeutic studies should be controlled, and patient numbers are small in some categories. Finally, these tumors, although initially benign, have a distinct propensity to undergo malignant degeneration, particularly in the presence of a cocarcinogen such as ionizing radiation (1) or cigarette smoke, so that agents such as alkylators probably should not be tried.

Historically antimitotic agents such as podophyllin and colchicine have been most widely employed in the local control of this disorder. In a large trial in patients with penile condylomata acuminata (2) von Krogh compared concentrated ethanolic preparations of podophyllin, podophyllotoxin and colchicine in a total group of 227 previously untreated patients. The overall response rate was 99 or 44%. All preparations appeared to be equally effective but there was more severe adverse irritative effects with the colchicine (17%) than with the podophyllin derivatives (2-4%). This investigator makes the point that measurable levels of podophyllin in the serum will appear if the area treated is large enough, and systemic side effects including hypotension and myelosuppression can be seen with this local therapy. Dedo (4) has used local application of podophyllin to lesions of laryngeal papillomatosis and feels that in this site as well, disease control is better than with surgery alone.

The antimetabolite, 5 fluoruracil has also been widely studied particularly in patients with penile condylomata. Von Krogh (2) felt that a 5% cream when topically applied was more effective, than a 1% ethanol solution. With the prolonged treatment for an average of 4 weeks that was required in the patients with recalcitrant disease, there was a 40% incidence of adverse effects, again principally irritative. These results and some of others are summarized below:

## Table 1

Chemotherapy of Papillomas

5 FU

| Site | Concentration | Vehicle | % Response | % Adverse Effects | | | References |
|---|---|---|---|---|---|---|---|
| | | | | None | Slight | Severe | |
| Penis | 5% (2 weeks) | cream | 40 | 60 | 40 | 0 | 2,4 |
| | 5% (4 weeks) | cream | 60 | 20 | 40 | 40 | 2,6 |
| | 1% | 70% ethanol | 35 | 42 | 58 | 0 | 2 |
| Larynx | 0.5-5% | aerosol | 75 | 10 | 50 | 40 | 7 |

Weimar et al. (5) have developed a suppository of 5% 5FU for insertion into the male or female urethra with responses in 12/12 treated patients. Wallin (6) compared 5 fluorouracil with podophyllin and found that 10/27 treated with 5 FU and 14/31 treated with podophyllin remained disease free for 4-9 months There was no significant difference between these two results and some of the patients who failed to respond to the initial therapy responded to the other after they were crossed over. Only one patient receiving podophyllin reported side effects, while more than half the patients receiving 5 FU reported side effects, some serious enough to make them stop using the cream.

Smith and coworkers (7) administered repeated instillations of 5 FU at concentrations from 0.5 to 5% into the larynx and tracheobronchial tree. They saw inhibition of papilloma regrowth in 6/8 patients. The major limitation to drug effectiveness was the requirement for its frequent administration, i.e. more than once daily. Toxicities included tracheal bleeding, peristomal inflammation, bronchospasm and coughing.

Hasumi and coworkers (8) applied idoxuridine ointment on condyloma acuminatum of the female genital tract in a randomized double blind study. Six of six treated patients had regression of disease lasting for at least three months. In the 5 placebo treated patients there was progression in one patient and no change in the other four. Their rationale for selecting this agent was that it was antiviral as well as a DNA synthesis inhibitor in mammalian cells. Kerstein (9) treated rectal papillomas by the instillation of a gauze pack soaked in thio TEPA. This was effective in 2 of 2 patients, however thio TEPA in view of its alkylating activity, does not seem an ideal agent for treatment of this disease. An intriguing example of topical therapy is a single case report of a patient with extensive anal and perianal condylomata treated by Holcombe (10) with methylene blue dye and phototherapy. Dr. Holcombe postulated that the dye acted as a photosensitizer in his patient. In view of the current interest and effectiveness of the use of porphyrins as photosensitizers for argon laser therapy in the treatment of endobronchial cancer, this lead may deserve follow up in respiratory papillomatosis.

Bleomycin has been administered via several different routes to patients with papillomas. Figueroa (11) injected Bleomycin intralesionally at doses between 0.5 and 5 mg at intervals of two to three weeks in patients with rectal condylomata. Seven of ten patients responded, however this seems like an uncomfortable and inefficient way of treating disease. Hagedorn (12) treated one patient with oral florid papillomatosis with intra carotid artery Bleomycin. This seems unnecessarily invasive, since it is probable that the agents would have been just as effective if administered intravenously. Mehta and Herold (13) administered intravenous bleomycin at doses of 7 units/m2 twice weekly to a total dose of 240 U/m2 to a patient with severe endotracheal disease. There was a complete response. Unfortunately bleomycin is a drug for which the total lifetime dose is limited since above a cumulative dose of 400U pulmonary fibrosis regularly occurs.

Systemic anticancer agents have not often been used in this disease, although Doll et al.(14) report a case of one patient with coexistent embryonal carcinoma of the testis whose penile and perianal papillomata regressed when he was treated with bleomycin, platinum and velban and another woman with ovarian carcinoma whose papillomas regressed on systemic 5 Fluorouracil. There are also case reports of methotrexate having an effect when given systemically.

Immune stimulants and antiviral agents are obviously logical choices for therapy of this viral disease. The most widely used has been interferon which has been discussed at length earlier in this symposium. The majority of patients show a response to interferon but it is often incomplete and disease tends to recur once the drug is stopped. For this reason a search has been made for compounds that it would be logical to combine with interferon in this disease. Interferon has a number of effects as part of or in addition to its antiviral effects which might account for response in this disease. This topic has recently been reviewed (15) and categories of activity are shown below.

TABLE 1

| Biologic response modification by interferons |
|---|
| Interferon induced proteins |
| Cell surface changes |
| Immune effector cell function |
| Antiproliferative effects |

There are a number of changes at the cell surface. Cell membrane lipids are altered and this process may require the catalytic function of prostaglandin synthetase and superoxide dismutase (16). Inhibitors of the former such as aspirin, or of the latter such as diethyldithiocarbamate (DDC) may inhibit the antiviral action of interferon. Tovey et al. (17) have shown however that concentrations of indomethacin and aspirin which inhibit the formation of prostaglandins and prevent the interferon induced increase in the intracellular concentration of cyclic GMP, have no effect on the development of the interferon induced antiviral state. This leads to the interesting speculation that these activities could be tested separately in a clinical setting to see which is responsible for the effect in papillomatosis. Short of such a controlled experiment, however, it seems prudent, to give acetoaminophen for control of symptoms to patients receiving interferon. Interferon causes other changes in the cell surface. Histocompatibility antigens increase as do glucocorticoid receptors. Beta 2 microglobulins also increase. It is quite conceivable that one day antibodies or immune cells specifically reactive against an antigen which is much increased by the action of interferon may represent the ideal combintation therapy. Interferon also alters immune effector cell function. It increases target specific T cell cytotoxicity. NK and K cell activity increase as does phagocytosis by macrophages. Interferon has also been shown to enhance lymphotoxin induced target cell killing in the absence of a cytotoxic cell (18).

Suppressor T cells may be produced as a late phase of the proliferative immune responses. Cimetidine has been shown to inhibit the formation of suppressor T cells which arise in response to the presence of animal tumors and to have an antitumor effect in these models. Cimetidine presumably inactivates the suppressor T cells by blocking an H2 type histamine receptor on their surface, and might be expected to be synergistic with interferon. Cimetidine alone had no effect when given to 12 patients with condylomata (19). The combination of cimetidine and interferon has been felt to induce regression in patients with malignant melanoma who would not have been expected to respond to either drug alone (20) and therefore may be worthy of investigation in papillomatosis.

The effect of interferon which is felt most likely to account for the responses in papillomatosis and in tumors is the antiproliferative effect. This is at least in part because human tumors grown in nude mice will have their growth slowed in the presence of human interferon, which should not affect the immune system of the mouse (15). The antiproliferative effects of interferon might, of course, be increased by the concurrent administration of any one of a number of cancer chemotherapeutic agents as has been seen in a number of human tumor models (21), however the toxicity and potential carcinogenicity of most of these agents make them less than ideal candidates for therapy in papilloma virus disease.

In malignant cells the enzyme ornithine decarboxylase is often increased as polyamine synthesis accompanies cell division. One agent which has a definite antiproliferative effect and which is synergistic with interferon in some in vitro systems is the ornithine decarboxylase inhibitor, difluoromethylornithine (22,23). It appears in the studies by Sunkara that the effect in this cell line is not due to a synergistic effect on polyamine synthesis, however. These authors postulate that polyamines inhibit the phosphorylation of chain initiation factor EIF 2. Decrease of intracellular polyamines would enhance the phosphorylation of EIF 2 by interferon induced protein kinase resulting in inhibition of protein synthesis and cell death.

Another group of agents which are being discussed elsewhere in this symposium are retinoids. This group of compounds are known to show antiproliferative and differentiation effects on epithelial tissues in animals and humans; however it should be remembered that papillomavirus replicates most actively in the more differentiated layers of the epithelium, and there is logical reason to fear that these tumors might increase their viral load in the presence of retinoids.

In addition to trying to kill the cells which support virus growth and replication, it would be ideal to use agents which kill the virus directly. Although there is no known agent which can strictly be called anti papilloma virus, several agents which have antiviral effects in other systems have been tried or suggested for therapy in papillomatosis. Work with acyclovir has shown rather dramatically that acyclovir is more effective in the presence of interferon in a viral system where acyclovir itself is active, namely dendritic keratitis caused by the herpes simplex virus (24). There are conflicting reports as to whether the combination is effective in cytomegalovirus infections where acyclovir does not have independent activity (25) and, of course, there is no direct reason to feel that acyclovir would have antiviral effects in a papillomavirus system. An early report of another antiviral agent, adenine arabinoside, in six children with laryngeal papillomatosis was encouraging with positive responses seen in three (26). Combination of adenine arabinoside with interferon appears more effective than either drug alone in control of hepatitis B infection; however adenine arabinoside both alone and in combination with interferon shows rather alarming dose related gastrointestinal and central nervous system toxicity (27). The former include nausea, vomiting, diarrhea and hypokalemia. The latter include peripheral neuropathy with pain and dysesthesias, and central signs including tremor, ataxia, dysgraphia, myoclonic seizures and coma. This drug should not be given by investigators who can not monitor blood levels.

Most papilloma therapy has used alpha interferon. There is now increasing evidence that combinations of interferons may be more effective than one type alone. Borden and coworkers (15) suggest that with the cloned interferons it may be possible to select for a particular activity, even within alpha interferons as a group. Beta interferons have generally not been as effective as alpha in the treatment of papillomatosis (28,29). There is experimental evidence that gamma interferon may potentiate the effect of alpha interferon in certain tissue culture systems (30) and certain tumor cell lines may show independent sensitivity to interferon and to the double stranded RNA products such as Poly (I) Poly (C) which serve as interferon inducers (31). This might make combination therapy with interferon and double stranded RNA logical. When poly inosinic polycytidylic acid was given to patients with papillomatosis it was felt to be effective in 4/10 courses (32,33). This group of patients, perhaps because of their frequent exposure to hepatotoxic anesthetics, had to have therapy stopped in four courses because of hepatotoxicity and hepatotoxicity was noted in four other courses. Thus is was felt that this formulation of Poly ICLC was too toxic for long term use. It was of interest that in the three patients where data was available, interferon production in response to double stranded RNA was excellent, thus showing that the disease state itself was not due to a deficiency in their native ability to make interferon in response to other stimuli.

## REFERENCES

1. Majoros M, Parkhill EM, Devine KD (1964). Papilloma in the larynx in children. Am J. Surg. 108:470.
2. von Krogh G, (1981). Condyloma Acuminata. Acta Derm. Venereol. (Suppl.). Stockholm 191:1.
3. Dedo HH, and Jackler RH (1982). Ann. Otol. Rhinol. Laryngol. 91:425.
4. Bringel PJP, and Arruda RD (1982). 5 Fluorouracil cream 5% in the treatment of intraurethral condylomata acuminata. Brit. J. Urol. 54:295.
5. Weimar GW, Milleman LA, Reiland TL and Culp DA (1978) 5 Fluorouracil urethral suppositories for the eradication of condyloma acuminata. J. Urol. 120:174.
6. Wallin J (1977) 5 Fluorouracil in the treatment of penile and urethral condylomata acuminata. Brit. J. Vener. Dis. 53:240.
7. Smith HG, Healy GB, Vaughan CW and Strong MS (1980) Topical chemotherapy of recurrent respiratory papillomatosis. A preliminary report. Ann. Otol. 89:472.
8. Hasumi K, Kobayashi T, and Ata M (1984) Topical idoxuridine for genital condyloma acuminatum. Lancet 1:968.
9. Kerstein ID (1977). Thiotepa in the management of anorectal condylomata acuminata: Report of two cases. Dis. Col. & Rect. 20:625.
10. Holcombe RG (1981). Methylene blue dye in the management of condylomata acuminata. J. La State Med. Soc. 133:68.
11. Figueroa S, and Gennaro AR (1980). Intralesional bleomycin injection in treatment of condyloma acuminatum. Dis. Col.& Rectum 23:550.
12. Hagedorn M, Weigel K, and Petres J (1978). Treatment of oral florid papillomatosis with Bleomycin. Arch. Dermatol. 114:1083.

13. Mehta P, and Herold N (1980). Regression of juvenile laryngobronchial papillomatosis with systemic bleomycin therapy. J. Ped. 97:479.
14. Doll DC, Wasserman PI (1979). Anticancer agents in condyloma acuminatum. New Engl. J. Med. 301:1288.
15. Borden EC (1984). Progress toward therapeutic application of interferons -- 1979-1983. Cancer 54(Suppl):2770.
16. Chandrabose KA, Pottathil R, Borden EC, Fox R, and Cuatrecasas, P (1982). The possible roles of prostaglandin synthetase and cytoplasmic superoxide dismutase in interferon action in homologous cells. In "Prostaglandins and Cancer: First international conference," New York: Alan R. Liss, p.345.
17. Tovey MG, Gresser I, Rochette-Egly C, Begon-Lours-Guymarho J, Bandu MT, Maury C (1982). Indomethacin and aspririn do not inhibit the antiviral or anti-proliferative actions of interferon. J. Gen Virol. 63:505.
18. Williams TW and Bellanti JA (1983). In vitro synergism between interferons and human lymphotoxin induced target cell killing. J. Immunol. 130:518.
19. Rampen FHJ, van Everdingen JJE (1982). Inefficacy of cimetidine in condylomata acuminata. Br. J. Vener Dis. 58:275.
20. Flodgren P, Borgstrom S, Jonsson PE, Lindstrom C, Sjogren HO (1983). Metastatic malignant melanoma: Regression induced by combined treatment with interferon HuIFN alpha (Le) and cimetidine. Int. J. Cancer 32:657.
21. Borden EC, Balkwill FR (1984). Preclinical and clinical studies of interferons and interferon inducers in breast cancer. Cancer 53:783.

22. Sunkara PS, Prakash NJ, Mayer GD, Sjoerdsma A (1983). Tumor suppression with a combination of alpha difluoromethyl ornithine and interferon. Science 219:851.
23. Rosenblum MG, Gutterman JU (1984). Synergistic antiproliferative activity of leukocyte interferon in combination with alpha difluoromethylornithine against human cells in culture Cancer Res. 44:2339.
24. de Koning EWJ, van Bijsterveld P, Cantell K (1983). Combination therapy for dendritic keratitis with acyclovir and alpha-interferon Arch. Ophthalmol. 101:1866.
25. Spector SA, Tyndall M, and Kelley E, (1982). Effects of acyclovir combined with other antiviral agents on human cytomegalovirus. Am. J. Med. 73:36.
26. Pritchard J, Marshall WC, Eggerding C, Pracy R, Evans JNG, Tymm G, Innes A, and Singh A (1980). Treatment of Laryngeal papillomatosis. Lancet 11:1383.
27. Sacks SL, Scullard GH, Pollard RB, Gregory PB, Robinson WS, Merigan TC (1982). Antiviral treatment of chronic hepatitis B virus infection: pharmacokinetics and side effects of interferon and adenine arabinoside alone and in combination. Antimicrob. agents chemother. 21:93.
28. Gobel U, Arnold W, Wahn V, Treuner J, Jurgens H, and Cantell K (1981). Comparison of human fibroblast and leukocyte interferon in the treatment of severe laryngeal papillomatosis in children. Eur. J. Ped. 137:175.
29. Schouten T, Weimar W, Bos JH, Bos CE, Cremers CWRJ, Schellekens H (1982). Treatment of juvenile laryngeal papillomatosis with two types of interferon. Laryngoscope 92:686.
30. Schiller JH, Groveman DS, Schmid SM, Willson JKV, Cummings KB and Borden EC (in press). Synergistic antiproliferative effects of human recominant alpha 54, beta ser, and gamma interferons on human cell lines of various histogenesis.

31. Hubbell HR, Liu R, and Maxwell B (1984). Independendent sensitivity of human tumor cell lines to interferon and double stranded RNA. Cancer Res. 44:3252.
32. Leventhal BG, Kashima H, Levine AS and Levy HB (1981). Treatment of recurrent laryngeal papillomatosis with an aritificial interferon inducer (poly ICLC). J. Ped. 99:614.
33. Leventhal BG, Whisnant J, Kashima, HK, Levy HB (in press) Recurrent respiratory papillomatosis J. Biol. Resp. Modifiers.

Papillomaviruses: Molecular and Clinical Aspects, pages 249–255


# RESPONSE OF HUMAN PAPILLOMA-ASSOCIATED DISEASES TO RETINOIDS (VITAMIN A DERIVATIVES)[1]

S.A. Weiner[2], F.L. Meyskens, Jr.[3], E.A. Surwit[2]
D.S. Alberts[3], and N.S. Levine[3]

Departments of Medicine and OB/GYN
University of Arizona and Arizona Cancer
Center, Tucson, AZ 85724

We have investigated the effect of retinoids on HPV-associated diseases, including cervical dysplasia (CD), laryngeal papillomatosis (LP), and epidermodysplasia verruciformis (EDV). For patients with CD we have used a cervical cap with an inert collagen sponge insert to deliver B-trans retinoic acid (TRA, vitamin A acid); the cap is changed daily for a total of 4 days. We conducted a phase I trial in which 10/22 patients treated with hi dose TRA experienced a complete response. We determined that a concentration of 0.37% TRA was safe for phase II efficacy trials. Patients received the initial treatment and were retreated every 3 months for 2 days for 9 months. They were evaluated before each course by colposcopy, cytology, and if both were negative, by biopsy. Six months after therapy had been stopped, 20 patients were evaluable for response. Complete responses (CR) were shown in 10 and no responses in 10 patients. A phase III randomized trial against placebo is planned. We have also treated 5 patients with refractory LP using oral 13-cis-retinoic acid (13cRA). Two sustained CR's were obtained. Using an ethyl ester derivative of retinoic acid (Etretinate) Bichler has reported CR's in 28 of 42 patients with LP. We have also documented a PR in a patient with severe EDV using oral 13 cRA.

1. This work was supported by NCI Grant #CA 27502
2. 1501 N. Campbell, University of AZ, Dept. OB/GYN
3. 1501 N. Campbell, University of AZ, Dept. Internal Medicine

# INTRODUCTION

Vitamin A and its natural and synthetic derivatives (retinoids), have been shown to be capable of modulating the differentiation of normal and abnormal cells in vitro and in vivo.(1,2) Retinoids may also act as antipromoters, preventing the phenotypic expression of malignancy initiated by a variety of carcinogens. We have investigated their effect on a variety of human papilloma virus (HPV) associated diseases, including cervical dysplasia, laryngeal papillomatosis (LP) and epidermodysplasia verruciformis (EDV). This report will present the preliminary results of a number of clinical trials involving the use of retinoids in the treatment of HPV associated conditions.

## Background in Chemoprevention

Clearly, the most significant impact that can be made on cancer mortality is in the realm of prevention. Three major areas exist towards which intervention can be directed.(3) Primary prevention consists of preventing exposure to known carcinogens. Examples would include abstinence from tobacco or eliminating asbestos from the work place. Efforts in this area obviously need to be directed toward social and political change. Secondary prevention involves modulating the initiation or promotion phase of carcinogensis using various biologic response modifiers. This can involve the use of antioxidants (Vitamin E, butylated hydroxytoluene, etc.) to quench free radicals, thereby functioning as antiinitiators in preventing cell damage resulting from various carcinogens. Alternatively, antipromoters (retinoids, proteases, steroids) can be used to prevent the phenotypic expression of malignancy in the transformed cell. The cervical epithelial cell infected with human papilloma virus is an example of the latter. The use of retinoid compounds to prevent the development of cervical neoplasia is a natural extension of this concept. The biologic effects of retinoids that make them useful as chemoprevention agents can be divided into 2 main categories: 1) their modulation of immune response; 2) their effect on cellular differentiation.

Although the specific mechanisms remain unclear, numerous animal studies have confirmed the role of retinoid compounds as enhancers of both cellular and humoral immunity. (1) In murine systems, the cytoxicity of killer T cells and stimulated macrophages to tumor cells was augmented using retinoid acid.(1) Enhancement of graft rejection using either retinoic acid or retinyl palmitate has also been noted in mouse models.(1) Humoral response in mice has been shown to be enhanced when retinol, retinal or retinoic acid was administered prior to an immunologic challenge with bovine gamma globulin.(1) The exact role that immunomodulation plays in human systems remains to be determined. Retinoids have long been known to be modulators of cellular differentiation. As early as 1965 Chu and Malmgren demonstrated that 10% Vitamin A palmitate was able to prevent the induction of cervical carcinomas initiated by 10% DMBA in Syrian hamsters.(4) Numerous other animal models have confirmed the ability of retinoids to function as antipromoters. Not only are these compounds capable of preventing malignant transformation, but they have been shown capable of altering established malignant cell lines. This has been demonstrated in embryonal cell carcinoma, melanoma, promyelocytic leukemia, breast carcinoma and cervical carcinoma, to name a few.(2,5) Therefore, it is a logical extension of this concept to attempt to use retinoids clinically to prevent the phenotypic expression of neoplasia induced by papilloma virus as well as to reverse established preneoplsia.

## RESULTS

### Cervical Dysplasia

Phase I trial of trans retinoic acid (TRA). Patients with mild, moderate or severe cervical dysplasia were selected for a phase I trial of TRA administered topically using a cervical cap with a collagen sponge insert for topical drug delivery.(6) The retinoic acid and delivery device were changed daily for four days. A starting concentration of 0.05% was chosen and escalated until unacceptable vaginal toxicity was encountered at a concentration of 0.484%. Patients were assessed for signs of systemic and local toxicity. Systemic effects were mild and not dose related. Cervical inflammation was seen in a majority of patients, 22 of 35. Vaginal toxicity was minimal in 23 patients, and only 3 patients experienced severe toxicity requiring discontinuation of treatment, and this was seen at the highest concentration (.48%) of TRA. Clinical follow up of these patients revealed that 10/22 (45%) patients treated at a higher drug concentration had a CR vs only 2/14 (14%) patients treated with lower doses of TRA. Responses were seen in all histologic grades. (unpublished data)

Phase II trial of trans retinoic acid (TRA). A phase II trial, utilizing the optimal concentration of trans retinoic acid,as defined in the phase I trial, of .372%,was initiated and completed.(7) All patients underwent an induction regimen of 4 consecutive 24 hour applications using the cervical cap and collagen sponge as described in the phase I trial. In addition, at 3 month intervals thereafter, patients had maintenance treatments for 2 consecutive 24 hour applications for three additional treatments. Toxicity was evaluated for both the induction and maintenance regimens. A clear relationship existed between the duration of exposure to retinoids, that is, the 4 days of treatment in the induction regimen versus the 2 days of treatment in the maintenance regimen, for both local and systemic toxicity. Two+ vulvar/vaginal toxicity was more prevalent in the induction regimen. The systemic toxicity was essentially limited, with a few exceptions, to the induction regimen only. Twenty-five patients were entered into this trial and 20 were fully evaluable (mild dysplasia, 8; moderate dysplasia, 10; severe dysplasia, 2). Complete disappearance of disease was noted in 10/20 (50%) patients. No significant benefit from retinoids was obtained in 10/20 (50%) patients.

Phase I trial of retinyl acetate (RA). We have recently completed a phase I trial of retinyl acetate, and compared two delivery systems, the cervical cap vs the vaginal applicator.(unpublished data) Thirty-three patients were entered into the study. With dose escalation of retinyl acetate, vulvo-vaginal toxicity became significant in patients treated with the vaginal applicator. At a dose of 18 mg, 3/5 patients had moderate vulvar toxicity and 2/5 had moderate or severe vaginal toxicity. Dose limiting toxicity has not been reached with the cervical cap. Early clinical follow up has failed to reveal significant disease regression. CR's were seen in only 7/27 (26%) patients treated with the cervical cap and 0/10 patients treated with the vaginal applicator. This lends validity to the fact that the observed regression rates seen with TRA in our phase I and II studies probably represent true pharmacologic effect and not just spontaneous regression or placebo effect.

In summary, of 56 patients treated with TRA for cervical dysplasia, 20/42 (47.6%) had a CR when higher concentrations of TRA were used, vs only 2/14 (14%) patients treated with lower concentrations. Preliminary data from the phase I trial of RA does not reveal evidence for clinical activity in cervical dysplasia.

## Laryngeal Papillomatosis

Five patients with recurrent laryngeal papillomatosis were entered into a trial of 13-cis-retinoic acid (0.5--2.0 mg/kg/day PO) and evaluated for toxicity and regression of disease. All patients had at least 3 surgical excisions (median 6) during the preceding 12 months. Two patients experienced a complete response (6-24 months). One patient experienced a partial response for 5+ months. Toxicity was limited, with all patients experiencing mild to moderate cheilosis. Mild conjuctivitis, balanitis and triglyceridemia were seen in one patient each. It is recommended that future trials of 13-cis-retinoic acid for LP utilize 1/mg/kg/d and continue treatment for 4-6 months after attainment of a CR.

## Epidermodysplasia Verruciformis

Experience with this disease is limited; however, 1 patient experienced a 50% decrease in the total mass of lesions after therapy with isotretinoin at 2 mg/kg/d.(9) Therapy had to be discontinued due to skin toxicity and prompt relapse subsequently occurred. Other investigators have also had isolated case reports of similar responses, and these have been seen in patients with HPV-5 and HPV-3 lesions. (10,11)

## DISCUSSION

### Clinical Role of Retinoids

The preliminary results of our studies appear to indicate that certain retinoid compounds may be useful in treating disorders of cellular differentiation associated with human papilloma virus infection. However, the exact clinical role remains to be determined. Our studies in cervical dysplasia confirm the observation that different retinoids may have widely diverse effects and that efficacy may be dependent not only on the histology or pathogenesis of the lesion, but also on the choice of compound. Indeed, certain in vitro properties of retinoids have been demonstrated which suggest that these compounds could function as promoters of carcinogenesis in certain situations. So, although preliminary results are encouraging, further clinical trials are needed before the concept of utilizing biologic response modifiers (and retinoids in particular) for chemoprevention can be widely endorsed.

## REFERENCES

1. Lotan, R: Effects of vitamin A and its analogues (retinoids) in normal and neoplastic cells. Biochem Biophy Acta 605:33, (1980).
2. Peck, GL: Chemoprevention of cancer with retinoids. Gynecol Oncol 12:5331, (1981).
3. Meyskens, FL: Chemoprevention of Head and Neck Cancer. "Investigative Techniques in the staging of Head and Neck Cancer", Head and Neck Cancer RE Wittes, ed. John Wiley and Sons Ltd.
4. Chu, EW and Malmgren, RA: An inhibitory effect of vitamin A on the induction of tumors of forestomach and cervix in the Syrian hamster by carcinogenic polycyclic hydrocarbons. Cancer Res 25:884-885, (1965).
5. Meyskens, FL: Modulation of abnormal growth by retinoids: A clinical perspective of the biological phenomenon. Life Sci 28: 2323-2327, (1981).
6. Meyskens, FL, Graham, V, Chvapil, M, et al: A phase I trial of B-all-trans-retinoic acid delivered via a collagen sponge and cervical cap for mild or moderate intraephithelial neoplasia. JNC 71:921-925, (1983).

7. Surwit, EA, Alberts, D, Dorr, R, et al: A phase II trial of trans-retinoic acid (Vitamin A acid) in the treatment of cervical dysplasia (intraepithelial neoplasia). Proc Am Soc Clin Oncol C-678 (1984).
8. Alberts, DS, Coulthard, SW, Meyskens, FL: Regression of Aggressive Laryngeal Papillomatosis with 13-Cis-Retinoic Acid (Accutane ). Arch Otolaryn (in press)
9. Meyskens, FL, Gilmarkin, E, Alberts, DS et al: Activity of Isotretinoin Against Squamous Cell Cancers and Pre neoplastic Lesions, Cancer Treat Rep, 66: 1315-19, (1982).
10. Lutzner, MA; Blanchet-Bardon, C Oral Retinoid Treatment of Human Papillomavirus type 5 Induced Epidermodysplasia Verruciformis. NEJM 302:1091, (1980).
11. Jalbonska, S, Obalek,S, Wolska,H, Jarabek-Charzelska, M RO 10-9359 in Epidermodysplasia Verruciformis. Preliminary Report in Retinoids Advances in Basic Research and Therapy. Orfanos, CE et al, Eds. Springer-Verlog Berlin, (1981).

Papillomaviruses: Molecular and Clinical Aspects, pages 257–271


# DEVELOPMENT OF A RECOMBINANT DNA VACCINE AGAINST BOVINE PAPILLOMAVIRUS INFECTION IN CATTLE

William P. Pilacinski, Donald L. Glassman,[1] Kimberly F. Glassman, David E. Reed, Melissa A. Lum, Richard F. Marshall, Charles C. Muscoplat

Molecular Genetics, Inc.
Minnetonka, MN 55343

ABSTRACT L1 and L2, the two large open reading frames (ORF) in the nontransforming region of the bovine papillomavirus type 1 (BPV-1) genome have been cloned and expressed in *E. coli*. *E. coli* produced L1 and L2 proteins elicit rabbit α-sera which reacts with BPV-1 by ELISA and IP; however, the L1 protein gives a more consistent neutralizing response in the inhibition of transformation of mouse C127 cells by BPV-1 virions. Two *E. coli* bacterins expressing the L1 ORF protect vaccinated calves against BPV-1 challenge.

## INTRODUCTION

Bovine papillomavirus (BPV) produces benign proliferative lesions (warts) on the skin and other epithelial surfaces of cattle, its natural host. Typically the warts regress and disappear within a few months to a year; however, occasionally they become quite large and persist indefinitely. Warts on the teats of dairy cattle may interfere with lactation and penile warts may have an impact on breeding programs. The presence of warts also affects the value of an animal for show or sale.

[1]Present address: College of Veterinary Medicine, University of Minnesota, St. Paul, MN 55108

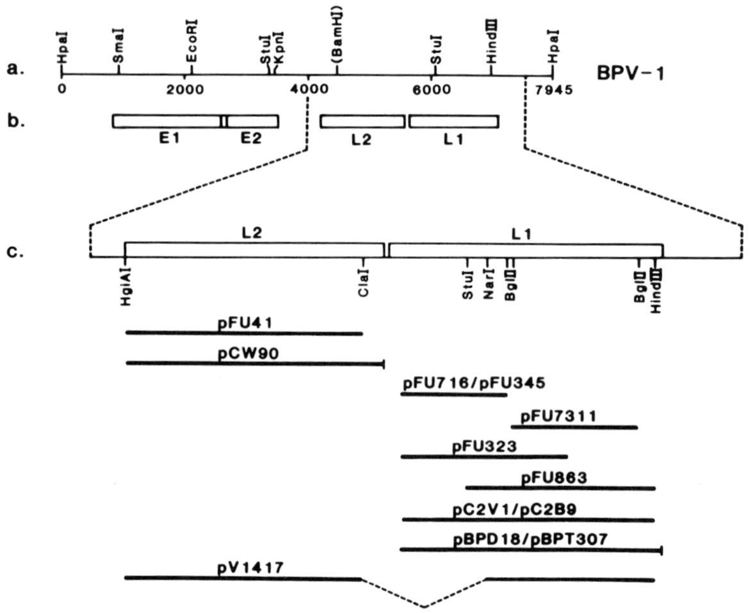


FIGURE 1 a. Linear restriction map of BPV-1. Positions of restriction sites are from sequence determined by Chen et al. (8). The BamHI site is in parenthesis because the BPV-1 isolate we cloned does not have this site. b. The four largest open reading frames in the BPV-1 genome; E1 and E2 overlap in different reading frames. Direction of transcription would be from left to right. c. Expansion of L1 and L2 open reading frames. The lines below each reading frame delineate the regions expressed in the designated plasmid. Plasmids pCW90, pBPD18 and BPT307 utilize the natural translation termination codon at the end of their respective reading frames. pC2B9 is fused out of phase with the E. coli β-gal gene. All remaining plasmids are fused in phase with β-gal.

The BPV virion has a naked, icosahedral capsid and a double stranded DNA genome of about 8000 base pairs (bp) and is closely related to viruses that infect humans, dogs, and rabbits (1,2,3). Of the six distinct types of BPV which have been isolated from wart tissue and described (4,5,6,7), BPV-1 and BPV-2 are the predominant types found in warts on dairy and beef cattle within the U.S.

BPV cannot be grown in cell tissue culture nor has it been successfully produced in laboratory animals; therefore, conventional methods of vaccine production cannot be used. However, recent studies have contributed greatly to understanding the molecular biology of BPV. Of greatest interest to us was the complete DNA sequence of the BPV-1 genome (8) and the assignment of RNA transcripts from transformed cells and from BPV-1 infected wart tissue to specific regions of the BPV-1 genome (9,10). These and other studies (11) suggested that most of the BPV-1 major coat protein was encoded within the L1 and possibly the L2 open reading frames (see figure 1). With this information we initiated a project to develop a vaccine against BPV-1 infection using recombinant DNA technology, the results of which are presented in this report.

## RESULTS

### Construction of Expression Plasmids Containing BPV-1 DNA

Figure 1C shows the regions of either the L2 or L1 ORF contained in the plasmids designated. pFU41 contains a fusion of a small β-gal leader peptide, the L2 ORF from the HgiAI to the ClaI sites, and the β-gal gene from the ClaI site through its terminus. pCW90 is an analogous construction containing the L2 terminus unfused to β-gal. Both gene fusions are expressed from the *E. coli* wild-type *lac* promoter.

pFU716, pFU345, pFU323, pC2V1, pC2B9, pBPD18 and pBPT307 contain a small λ *cro* leader peptide fused to the L1 ORF, 76 bp downstream from the ATG. This was done by BAL31 nuclease digestion from a PvuII site within the L2 ORF and subsequent ligation to the λ *cro* leader peptide DNA sequence. pFU7311 and pFU863 are fused to the λ *cro* peptide at the BglII and StuI sites within the L1 ORF, respectively. pFU716 is fused to β-gal at the first BglII site in L1; pFU7311, at the third BglII site; pFU863, pC2V1 and pC2B9, at the HindIII site; and pFU345 and pFU323 at the points indicated after BAL31 digestion from the carboxy termini. pBPD18 and pBPT307 contain the L1 ORF carboxy-terminus unfused to β-gal.

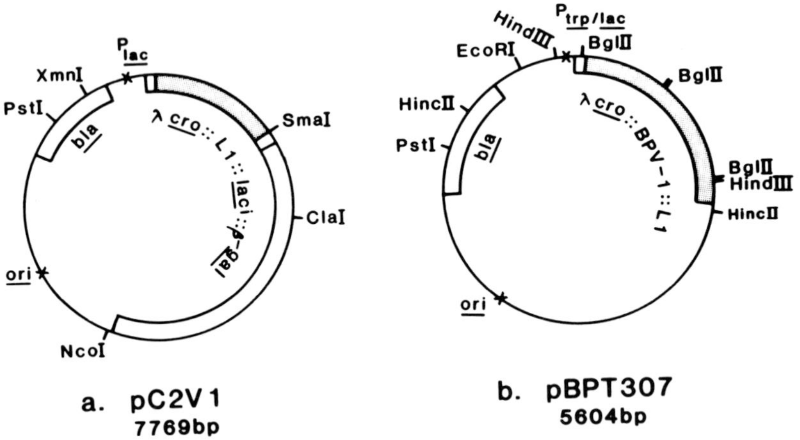


FIGURE 2. Diagrammatic representations of: a. pC2V1, a plasmid containing a λcro::BPV-1 L1::laci::β-gal fusion expressed by the lac promoter. This plasmid is representative of the BPV-1::β-gal constructions. The details of pC2V1's construction were described previously (12). b. pBPT307, a plasmid containing a λcro::BPV-1 L1 fusion expressed by a hybrid trp/lac promoter. It was constructed from pBPD18 which was described previously (12). pBPT307 is the only construction containing the "high level" hyrbid trp/lac promoter; all other constructions contain wild type or UV5 lac promoter. The stippled area indicates BPV-1 DNA.

The pBPT307 gene fusion is expressed from an *E. coli* trp/lac hybrid promoter, all other L1 constructions are expressed from the lac UV5 promoter. pV1417 contains a fusion of the L2 and L1 ORFs at the ClaI and NarI sites, respectively, with a β-gal leader peptide and terminus. It is expressed from a wild-type lac promoter.

Figure 2 shows a diagram of two plasmids, pC2V1 and pBPT307, which are representative, respectively, of the β-gal fused and naturally terminating BPV-1 constructions.

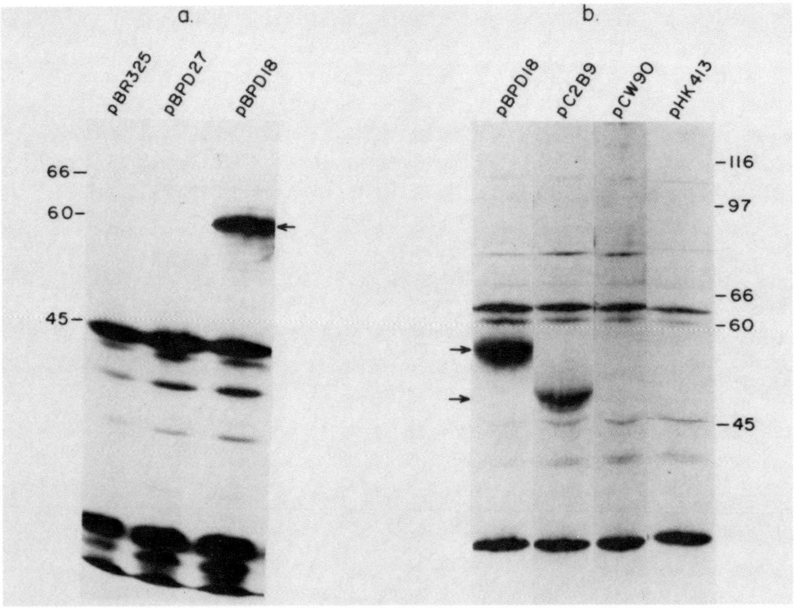


FIGURE 3. IP of $^{35}$S-methionine-labelled *E. coli* containing the indicated plasmid. The supernatants from cell lysates were precipitated with rabbit anti-BPV-1 sera and electrophoresed through SDS-polyacrylamide gel. pBR325 and pHK413 are non-BPV-1 DNA containing control plasmids. pBPD27 is a non-expressing co-isolate of pBPD18 [see (12) for details of construction]. pC2B9 was constructed from pBPD18 and resulted in the deletion of approximately 5000 daltons from the protein produced by pBPD18. Arrows show the positions of unique, BPV-1 specific proteins. The positions of standards and their molecular weights in kilodaltons are also shown.

## Expression of BPV-1 Proteins

All plasmids constructed were transformed into *E. coli* K12 strain NF1829. This strain contains an F'*lac*I$^{Q1}$ plasmid and over produces the *lac* repressor which allows efficient repression of transcription from the *lac* or hybrid *trp*/*lac* promoter when present on a multi-copy plasmid.

Rabbit α-sera generated against purified BPV-1 was used to immune precipitate (IP) $^{35}$S-methionine labelled E. coli cultures containing some of the plasmids described above. Protocols were described previously (12) and the results are presented in Figure 3. pBPD18 shows a BPV-1 specific band at the expected MW of about 51K. pC2B9, which contains a deletion of BPV-1 DNA present in pBPD18, shows a smaller MW BPV-1 specific band. pBPD27 is an out of translational reading frame co-isolate of pBPD18 and thus shows no BPV-1 specific protein band. pCW90 does not show a BPV-1 specific protein band although subsequent experiments suggest that it should be capable of producing the L2 ORF protein. No BPV-1 specific proteins are produced by either the pBR325 or pHK413 control plasmids.

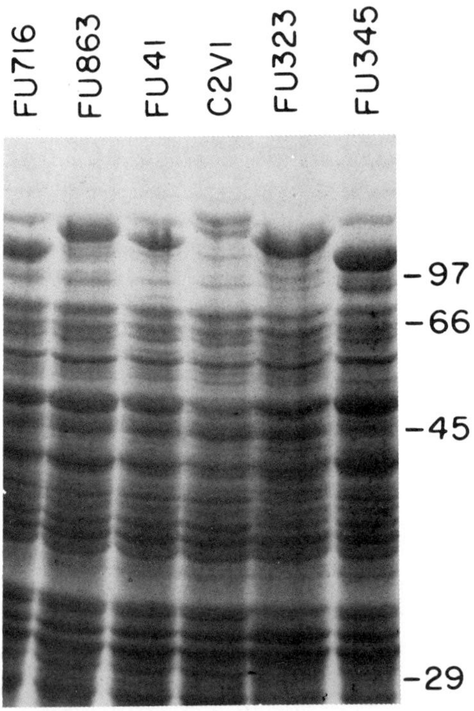


FIGURE 4. Coomassie-stained PAGE of lactose induced E. coli containing the indicated plasmids, all of which are BPV-1::β-gal fusions. The large (greater than 97K MW) bands which vary in size between the different plasmids are the BPV-1::β-gal fusion proteins.

To increase the stability and aid in the purification of the BPV-1 specific proteins, portions of L1 and L2 ORFs were fused to the β-gal gene as described above. Polyacrylamide gel electrophoresis (PAGE) of lactose induced E. coli cells containing some of these plasmid is shown in Figure 4. It shows large (greater than 97K) MW bands corresponding to proteins of the sizes expected of the various BPV-1::β-gal gene fusions.

In order to increase the expression level of the non-β-gal fused L1 ORF protein, the lac promoter was replaced by the hybrid trp/lac promoter, which has been shown to be a high-level promoter (13). Figure 5 shows the results of an induction experiment with E. coli containing pBPT307 and subsequent purification of the aggregated λcro::L1 fusion protein. The uninduced cells showed a small amount of read through. Both lactose and IPTG induced equally well when added at early mid-log growth in L broth.

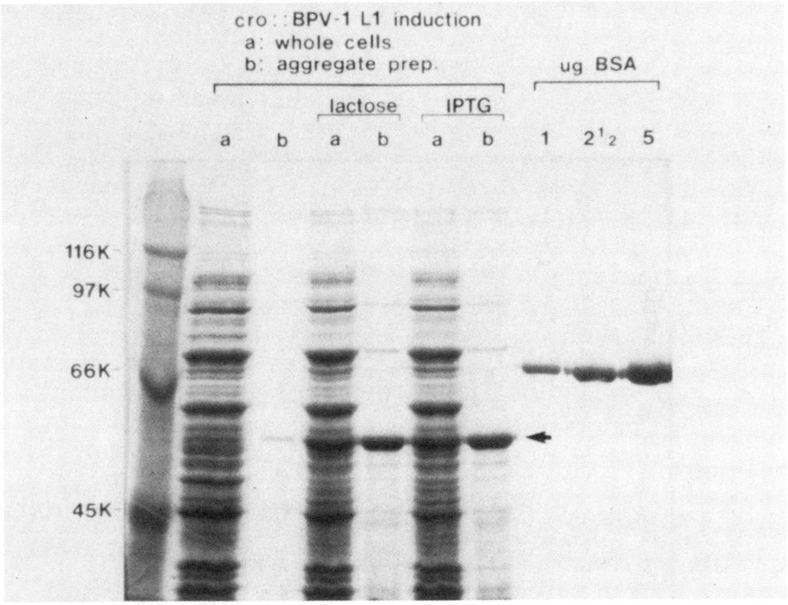


FIGURE 5. Coomassie-stained PAGE of induced and uninduced E. coli containing pBPT307 and of the purified λcro::BPV-1 L1 fusion protein from these cells. The

(Continued)

Fig. 5 (Continued)

fusion protein could be easily purified from lysed cells as an insoluble aggregate by low speed centrifugation. The position of the fusion protein is indicated by an arrow. BSA was added to three wells for a concentration standard.

Immunological Studies

The various BPV-1::β-gal fusion proteins were purified and used to immunize rabbits. Both purified aggregated protein as well as protein bands cut from PAGE were used along with either complete Freund's or an $Al(OH)_3$ adjuvant. More complete details of the immunizations are provided in (12).

The α-sera generated by the rabbits was used to IP $^{125}$I-labelled BPV-1 as shown in Figure 6. The λ-cro::BPV-1 L1::β-gal fusion proteins from both pFU323 and pC2V1 induced the production of α-sera which precipitated $^{125}$I-BPV-1 as did the positive controls, α-BPV-1 and α-P54. In all cases this reaction was specific, since contaminating $^{125}$I-BSA was not precipitated to a significant extent. Pre-immune sera was consistently negative. (A minor amount of contamination from the neighboring wells is observed in the pre-immune sera well for BPV-1.) There is considerable variation in the strength of the responses from animal to animal as can be seen with the two animals injected with the pFU323 fusion protein. As observed here, the cloned fusion proteins consistently elicited a weaker response than whole BPV-1.

The BPV-1 precipitating α-sera was also tested for its ability to inhibit the transformation of mouse C127 cells by BPV-1 in a type of in vitro viral neutralization assay. The results of one such assay are shown in Figure 7. Rabbit α-sera generated against the pC2V1 fusion protein prevented cell transformation when used to pretreat the infecting BPV-1 virions. This particular α-sera had a transformation inhibition titer of 36.

An enzyme linked immuno-sorbent assay (ELISA) was also developed to identify α-sera generated against BPV-1 proteins. It is described in more detail in (12). A compilation of the results obtained from ELISA and transformation inhibition experiments is presented in Table 1.

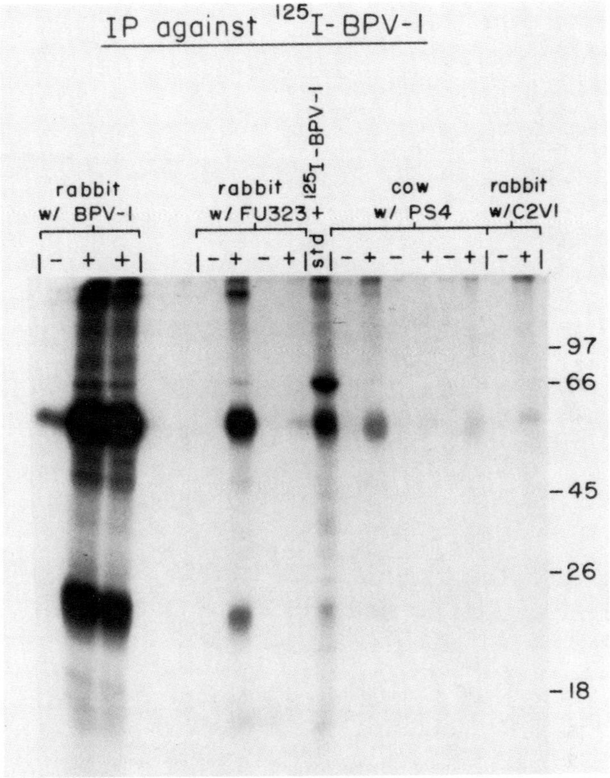


FIGURE 6. IP of $^{125}$Iodine labelled BPV-1 with various α-sera. "-" indicates pre-immune sera, "+", immune sera against the antigen indicated. FU323 and C2V1 are λcro::BPV-1 L1::β-gal fusions (see Figure 1) and rabbits were injected with purified aggregate protein. Controls included α-sera from a rabbit immunized with CsCl gradient purified BPV-1 and from a cow immunized with SDS-PAGE purified BPV-1 coat protein (P54). Some of the $^{125}$I-BPV-1 was added to the molecular weight standards in the middle well which shows the BPV-1 major coat protein band at about 54K along the minor viral proteins and also some contaminating BSA at about 66K.

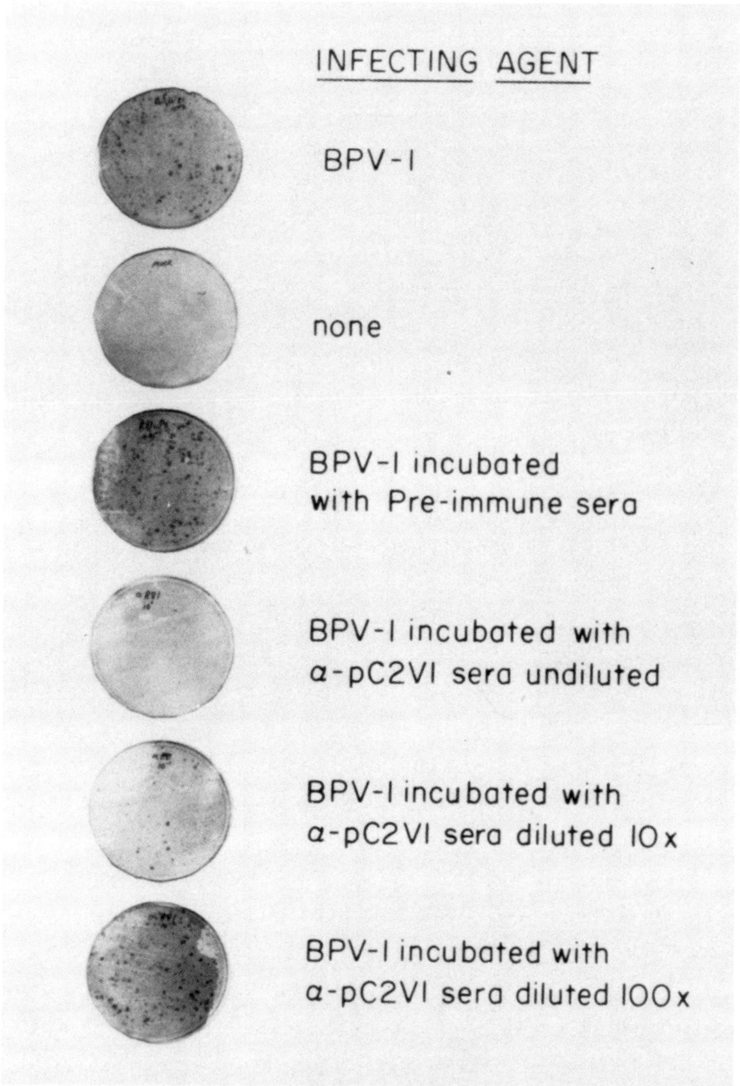


FIGURE 7. BPV-1 transformation inhibition by α-sera generated against pC2V1 fusion protein. C127 mouse cells were used in the assay developed by Dvoretyky et al (14). Each plate was inoculated with 100 focus forming units of BPV-1 from a crude wart grind.

TABLE 1
RESULTS FROM RABBIT IMMUNIZATIONS

| Antigen | ELISA[a] | Transformation inhibition[a] |
|---|---|---|
| whole BPV-1 | 4/4 | 4/4 |
| P54 protein | 3/3 | 0/2 |
| pC2V1 protein | 21/25 | 3/8 |
| pFU863 protein | 2/4 | 0/2 |
| pFU323 protein | 4/7 | 0/3 |
| pFU716 protein | 1/2 | 0/1 |
| pFU41 protein | 6/9 | 1/5 |
| pV1417 protein | 2/2 | 0/2 |

[a]results show # of different rabbits which showed positive serum results/total # of rabbits tested with this antigen.

Of the various BPV-1 constructions tested the pC2V1 fusion protein, containing most of the L1 ORF, showed the most consistent positive response by both ELISA and transformation inhibition.

Field Trials

In light of the positive results from the transformation inhibition assay, we initiated a field trial to test the use of the pC2V1 fusion protein as a vaccine for the prevention of warts in cattle. A subsequent field trial utilized the pBPT307 protein which contained more of the L1 product and was not fused to β-gal.

In the first field trial, 3 calves, three to four months old, were inoculated intramuscularly with 4.25 ml of heat inactivated, binary ethylene imine (BEI) treated, whole E. coli cells containing approximately 10 mg of the pC2V1 fusion protein with an $Al(OH)_3$ adjuvant. An identical inoculation was given 31 days later. Twenty-seven days after the boost these 3 animals along with 4 uninoculated calves were challenged intradermally with 1 X $10^{10}$ BPV-1 virions (as determined by EM) at each of 2 sites. The results of this trial are presented below.

TABLE 2
TRIAL 1 RESULTS

| | Week post challenge[a] 5 | 6 | 8 | % positive[b] |
|---|---|---|---|---|
| Vaccinates | 0/3 | 0/3 | 0/3 | 0 |
| Controls | 2/4 | 4/4 | 4/4 | 83 |

[a]results shown as # of animals with warts at challenge site/# of animals challenged
[b]averaged over the three examination times

In the second field trial, 10 calves, 2½ to 4½ months old, were inoculated intramuscularly with 5 ml of similarly treated E. coli cells containing approximately 5 mg of the pBPT307 fusion protein with an $Al(OH)_3$ adjuvant. Five animals were similarly inoculated with an

TABLE 3
TRIAL 2 RESULTS

| | Week post challenge 5 | 6 | 7 | % positive |
|---|---|---|---|---|
| Vaccinates | 1/10 | 1/10 | 1/10 | 10 |
| Placebos | 3/5 | 4/5 | 2/5 | 60[a] |
| Controls | 5/5 | 4.5/5 | 5/5 | 97[b] |

[a]significantly different from vaccinates at $p < 0.05$
[b]significantly different from vaccinates at $p < 0.01$

$Al(OH)_3$ plus buffer placebo. An identical inoculation was given 21 days later. Twenty-one days after the boost, the 15 inoculated animals, along with 5 uninoculated control calves were challenged as previously. The results of this trial are presented in table 3.

In both trials, there were significantly fewer animals that developed warts in the vaccinated group than in the control or placebo groups.

## DISCUSSION

The results presented show that a bacterin manufactured from E. coli cells expressing the BPV-1 L1 ORF can protect cattle from the development of warts due to BPV-1 infection. This is true even though a conservative method of data evaluation was used--averaging the results from three examination dates.

Examination of the results from the second trial also suggests a placebo effect, although the number of animals used was not large enough to show a statistically significant difference between the placebo and the uninoculated control group. A placebo effect was also suggested by the size of the warts in the various groups. The size of the warts in the placebo group averaged 12% smaller than those in the control group (but 44% larger than the single animal with warts in the vaccinated group; data not presented).

The relationship between level of expression and the stability of foreign proteins produced in E. coli is an interesting one. The observations we have made with the BPV proteins are similar to those with other foreign proteins expressed in E. coli. Generally, stable expression of a foreign protein from the E. coli lac promoter can only be observed when fused to a native E. coli protein such as β-gal. Even with β-gal protein fusions, cell samples obtained late in the growth cycle show preferential degradation of the foreign portion of the protein fusion. With expression from high level promoters, such as the trp/lac or $\lambda P_L$, most foreign proteins can be stably expressed unfused to a native protein; however, this level of expression is frequently lethal to the cell.

As mentioned in the Introduction, BPV-2 is also found in high percentage of warts in dairy and beef cattle within the U.S. Evidence from the literature suggests that BPV-1 and BPV-2 may cross protect (14). Additional field trials are planned to determine if our BPV-1 bacterin will protect cattle from challenge with BPV-2.

## REFERENCES


1. Orth G, Breitburd F, and Favre M (1978). Evidence of Antigenic Determinants Shared by the Structural Polypeptides of (Shope) Rabbit Papillomavirus and Human Papillomavirus Type 1. Virol 91:243-255.
2. Law M, Lancaster WD, and Howley PM (1979). Conserved Polynucleotide Sequences Among the Genomes of Papillomaviruses. J Virol 32:199-207.
3. Jenson AB, Rosenthal JD, Olson C, Pass F, Lancaster WD, and Shak K (1980). Immunologic Relatedness of Papillomaviruses from Different Species. JNCI 64:495-500.
4. Lancaster WD and Olson C (1978). Demonstration of Two Distinct Classes of Bovine Papilloma Virus. Virol 89:372-379.
5. Pfister H, Ling U, Gissmann L, Huchthausen B, Hoffmann D, and zur Hausen H (1979). Partial characterization of a new type of bovine papillomavirus. Virol 96:1-8.
6. Campo MS, Moor MH, Jarrett WFH, and Laird HM (1980). A new papillomavirus associated with alimentary cancer in cattle. Nature 286:180-182.
7. Jarrett WFH, Dept. of Vet. Path., Vet. Sch., Univ. of Glasgow, Scotland, unpublished results.
8. Chen EY, Howley PM, Levinson AD, and Seeburg PH (1982). The primary structure and genetic organization of the bovine papillomavirus type 1 genome. Nature 299:529-534.
9. Amtmann E, and Sauer G (1982). Bovine Papilloma Virus Transcription: Polyadenylated RNA species and Assessment of the Direction of Transcription. J Virol 43:59-66.
10. Engel LW, Heilman CA, and Howley PM (1983). Transcriptional Organization of Bovine Papillomavirus Type 1. J Virol 47:516-528.

11. Lowy DR, Dvoretzky I, Shober R, Law M, Engel L, and Howley PM (1980). In vitro tumorigenic transformation by a defined sub-genomic fragment of bovine papilloma virus DNA. Nature 287:72-76.
12. Pilacinski WP, Glassman DL, Krzyzek RA, Sadowski PL, Robbins AK (1984). Cloning and Expression in Escherichia coli of the Bovine Papillomavirus L1 and L2 Open Reading Frames. Bio/Technology 2:356-360.
13. Russell DR, Bennett GN (1982). Construction and Analysis of in vitro Activity of E. coli Promoter Hybrids and Promoter Mutants that Alter the -35 and -10 Spacing. Gene 20:231-243.
14. Dvoretzky I, Shober R, Chattopadhyay SK, and Lowy DR (1980). A quantitative in vitro Focus Assay for Bovine Papilloma Virus. Virol 103:369-375.

**Papillomaviruses: Molecular and Clinical Aspects, pages 273–276**


# THE SURGICAL TREATMENT OF LARYNGEAL PAPILLOMAS AND PAPILLOMAS OF THE AEROGASTRIC TRACT

C. D. Sooy and H. H. Dedo

Department of Otolaryngology, University of California, San Francisco 94143

## INTRODUCTION

The first description of laryngeal papillomas was "warts on the throat" [1] by Marcellus Donalus in the 17th century. The term laryngeal papillomas was introduced to the medical literature in 1871 by MacKenzie. [2] Before the development of effective laryngoscope papillomas first caused hoarseness and eventually became large enough to cause airway obstruction and death. Tracheotomy alone or occasionally laryngofissure and partial removal was occasionally done for respiratory obstruction.

Bruns reported the removal of a laryngeal polyp through through the mouth in 1862.[3] However, not until the direct laryngoscope was developed by Kirstan [4] could effective endoscopic surgery be performed. Since that time laryngeal papillomas treatment has closely paralleled the developing technology of laryngoscopy. By 1940 enough surgical removals had been done for Broyles [5] to advise that endoscopic removal was best for adults but not for children unless their disease was in remission. Apparently this was because the juvenile papillomas tended to be so extensive and recur so rapidly. With the improvement in illumination from candle and head mirror to rice grain light bulb, in the 1920's and finally fiber optic light sources in the 1960's, visualization improved. Also in the 1960's some surgeons, McCoy and Dekelboum, [6] advocated removal via direct laryngisciot every two months instead of waiting for papillomas to be visible on indirect laryngoscopy, hoarseness or marked airway obstruction in, as many advised, because of the rarity of cure with the old approach. The suspected viral etiology of papillomas led some surgeons to painting the raw areas after removal with tincture of resin of Podophyllum as adjunctive therapy to minimize local re-implantation,[7] since this substance had had some success in the 1930's when used on cutaneous and genital warts, but had less success as a primary therapy for laryngeal papillomas.[8]

After the introduction of the binocular microscope laryngoscopes, (Kleinsasser*, Jako ** and Dedo**) that would accommodate binocular magnified vision results improved enough that a few patients were cured even though resection was still done by removing the papillomas with cup forceps. The next big advance was the clinical introduction of $CO_2$ laser removal in 1971 by doctors Jako and Strong.[9] This allowed much more precise removal in a virtually bloodless field by vaporization with little or no spillage of virus particles in the larynx. With meticulous, regular $CO_2$ laser removals, they achieved remission in 34% of patients (no papillomas on exam for one year.). Because of the presence of virus particles in biopsies of normal appearing laryngeal tissue in these patients,[10] more effective methods are still being sought such as an effective vaccine or an antiviral substance. Interferon is now being tested as an adjunct to $CO_2$ laser removal every 8 weeks.

Papillomas are the most common laryngeal tumor occurring in children. They are histologically benign tumors although malignant transformation has been reported, usually in adults, occasionally after radiation therapy. Because of their location in the larynx or tracheobronchial tree, they are always potentially life-threatening and require treatment.

We feel laryngoscopy and laser removal should be done every 8 weeks for two reasons. First, the interval should not be much less because in our experience the new mucosa is too fragile to withstand instrumentation and can be too easily broken with subsequent re-implantation or web formation. Second, it is done whether there are any papilloma visible indirectly or not, because we have now found papillomas at microdirect laryngoscopy in 24 patients where none were visible on indirect laryngoscopy the day before. The best chance of cure is when there is only one little flat velvet patch of papilloma that can be removed before it has spread widely again. If and when a patient has no

---

* Wolf

** Pillings

papillomas visible through the microscope, we double the observation interval before the next direct laryngoscopy to 4 months, and if negative then to 8 months and then yearly times 3 and stop. We regard them as in remission if none for 5 years.

The individual laser resection is started by approaching the lesions as a benign but recurrent tumor by first marking around the rim of a lesion with the $CO_2$ laser going .5mm into normal mucosa and then down through the full thickness of the mucosa, eg, to Reinke's space on the true cord. All papillomata are removed except in potential areas of web formation, ie, if both sides of the anterior commissure at the true or false vocal cord level have papillomas, they are left on one side of the most anterior 3mm to prevent the raw surfaces adhering together. The resected areas are then painted with 25% tincture resin of Podophyllum. Should web formation occur, this is treated with endoscopic keel,[11] if in the anterior commissure or a microtrapdoor flap if in the posterior commissure.[12] Subglottic and tracheal stenosis stenosis is now handled in the same fashion as posterior commissure webs with laser submucosal scar removal and creation of a microtrapdoor flap.[12]

Our initial experience with the $CO_2$ laser for treatment of laryngeal papillomas in 109 consecutive patients reported in 1982.[7] Six of twelve tracheotomies present on arrival were removed. Forty one percent were in remission. There have been no deaths and tracheotomy was only necessary in 1.8%. This compares very favorably to mechanical removal where deaths ranged from 3.0% to 13.8%, and 4.4% to 64.3% required tracheotomies.

The $CO_2$ laser can also be used on other areas of the aerodigestive tract. Nasal papillomas are approached through a nasal speculum and nasopharyngeal papillomas by way of "cushion shots" off of a stainless steel mirror. Oral papillomas are handled with the help of a pharyngeal retractor while tracheobronchial papilloma are resected using the $CO_2$ laser bronchoscope.

In summary, the current surgical therapy provides dramatically better results for papillomatosis of the aerodigestive tract than previously. However, multiple surgeries are still required and there are still patients incurable with present methods. This suggests that a better adjunctive or primary medical (chemical) therapy is needed.

## REFERENCES


. Webb WW (1956). Papillomata of the larynx. Larynoscope 66: 871-918.
2. MacKenzie M (1821)."Essay on growths in the larynx." London: J and A Churchill.
3. Broyles EN (1948). History and development of laryngology. Trans Amer Acad Ophthal Otolaryngol 52: 247-253. [Brun reference cited therein]
4. Jako GJ ( ). Laryngeal endoscopy and micro-laryngoscopy. In Paparella and Shumrick,(eds) "Oto-laryngology" VIII, Phila: W. B. Saunders, pp. 2410-2430.
5. Broyles EN (1941). Treatment of laryngeal papilloma in children. South Med J 34: 239-242.
6. Dekelboum A (1965. Papillomatosis of the larynx. Arch Otolaryngol 81: 290-297,
7. Dedo, HH, Jackler RK (1982). Laryngeal papillomas: Results of treatment with the $CO_2$ laser and podophyllum. Ann Otol 91: 425-430.
8. Hollingsworth JB, Kohlmoos HW and McNaught RC (1950). Treatment of juvenile papilloma of the larynx with resin of podophyllum. Arch Otolaryngol 52: 82-87.
9. Jako G and Strong MS (1976). Recurrent respiratory papillomatosis-management with the $CO_2$ laser. Ann Otol 85: 508-516.
10. Steinberg BM, Topp WC and Schneider PS et al (1983). Laryngeal papilloma virus infection during clinical remission. New Engl J Med 308: 1261-1264.
11. Dedo HH (1979). Endoscopic Teflon keel for anterior glottic web. Ann Otol 88: 467-473.
12. Dedo HH and Sooy CD (1984). Endoscopic laser repair of posterior glottic, subglottic and tracheal stenosis by division of microtrapdoor flap. 94: 445-450.

# V. ANIMAL PAPILLOMAVIRUSES

Papillomaviruses: Molecular and Clinical Aspects, pages 279–297


# TRANSMISSIBLE ANIMAL PAPILLOMAS

Carl Olson and Robert O. Olson

Department of Veterinary Science
University of Wisconsin-Madison, WI

Cutaneous papillomas have been known and recorded for many years. The natural transmission from one animal to another is now recognized in about 24 species of animals. The experimental transmission of canine oral papillomas indicating a viral etiology was reported in 1898 by McFadyean and Hobday. Transmission of skin papillomas from horse to horse was reported by Cadeac in 1901.

The virus of animal papillomas have been generally regarded as species specific. In the 1930's, pioneer work of Shope demonstrated the cottontail papilloma virus capable of causing both papillomas and carcinomas in domestic rabbits as well as the native cottontail rabbits.

In most species, the papilloma viruses infect and transform sqaumous epithelium in which virions are formed. Papilloma virus of other species (cattle, deer, elk, and sheep) also transform fibroblasts of the species and of hamsters to a neoplastic state.

There are several bovine papilloma viruses. Types 1 and 2 cause fibropapillomas of the skin in cattle and fibromas of the skin in horses and mules. Progressive fibromas in hamsters and the brain of calves can be produced by bovine Types 1 and 2. Type 4 appears to be involved with alimentary adenocarcinoma. Types 3, 5, and 6 of the teats and so-called atypical skin papillomas involve only squamous epithelium.

Urinary bladder tumors (including fibromas, squamous and transitional cell carcinomas, adenocarcinomas, and mixed forms) pharyngeal carcinomas, and alimentary adenocarcinomas are associated with a low level ingestion of bracken fern growing in certain geographic regions. A plant-soil relationship appears necessary for development of the carcinogen. Bovine Types 1 and 2 will produce tumors in the urinary bladder. In one study, typical bovine papilloma virus were isolated from 6 cases of bladder tumors but the viral types are not known. Tropism for non-haired skin appears to be expressed by the bovine teat viruses.

For more detailed review see: Animal Papillomas: Historical Perspectives, C. Olson. In: N.P Salzman and P. Howley, editors, The Papavaviridae: The Papillomaviruses. Plenum Publishing Co., in press.

BOVINE PAPILLOMA VIRUSES

| | |
|---|---|
| TYPE-1 | FIBROPAPILLOMA OF SKIN |
| TYPE-2 | FIBROPAPILLOMA OF SKIN |
| TYPE-3 | PAPILLOMA OF SKIN |
| TYPE-4 | PAPILLOMA OF ALIMENTARY TRACT |
| TYPE-5 | FIBROPAPILLOMA OF SKIN |
| TYPE-6 | PAPILLOMA OF SKIN |

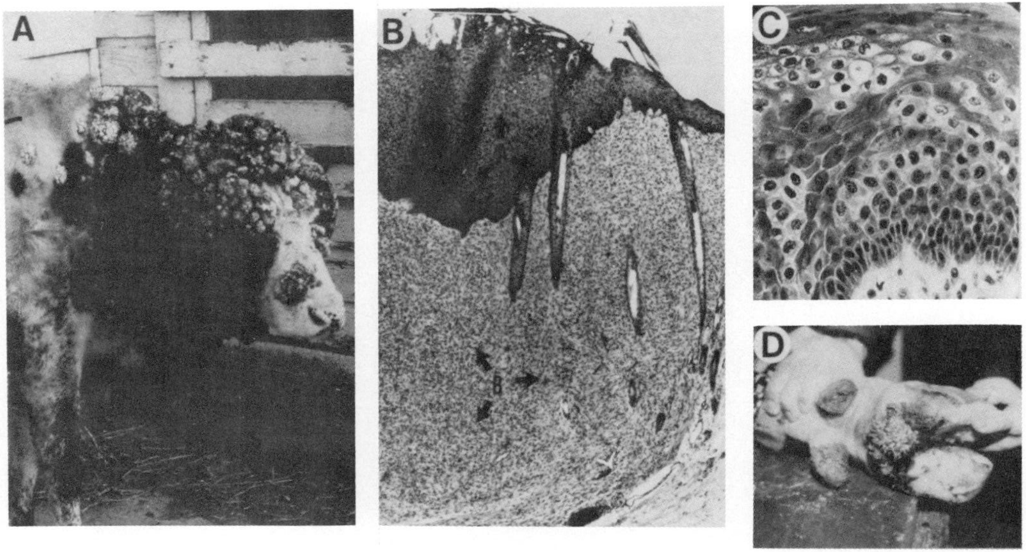


An unusually extensive natural case of bovine papillomatosis caused by BPV-1 in a calf (A). In the USA BPV-1 and 2 are associated with fibropapillomas of the head and neck of cattle. Figure B is a section of a bovine fibopapilloma demonstrating epithelial hyperplasia (arrow A) over the fibroma (arrow B). Figure C is higher magnification demonstrating pale cells in which virions are being produced. Figure D a natural case of BPV-1 between the claws of a cow.

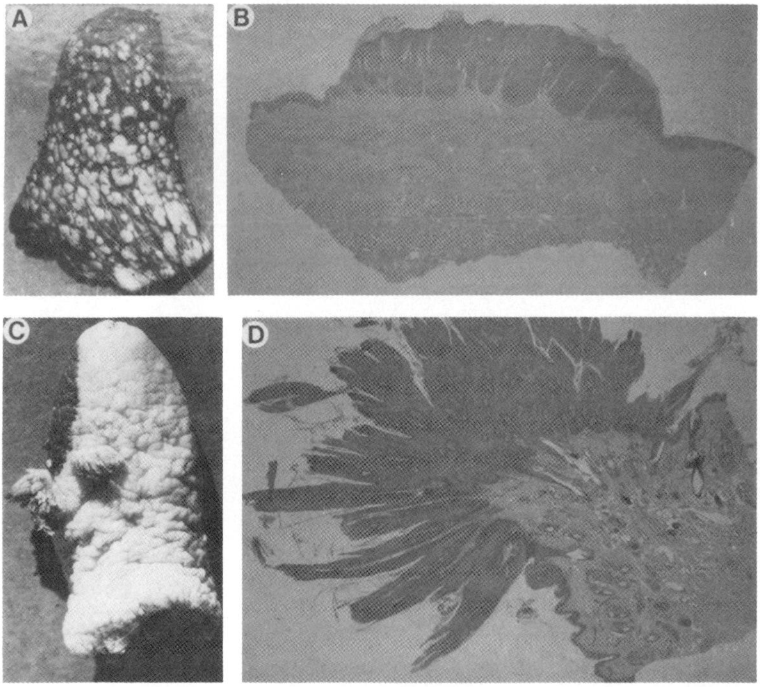


Flat teat papillomas (*fig A*) and filiform teat papillomas (*fig C*) as well as typical fibropapillomas are common in dairy cattle. Both flat and filiform teat papillomas (*fig B and D*) lack a fibromatous component. Virus isolated from flat and filiform teat papillomas are infectious in susceptible cattle.

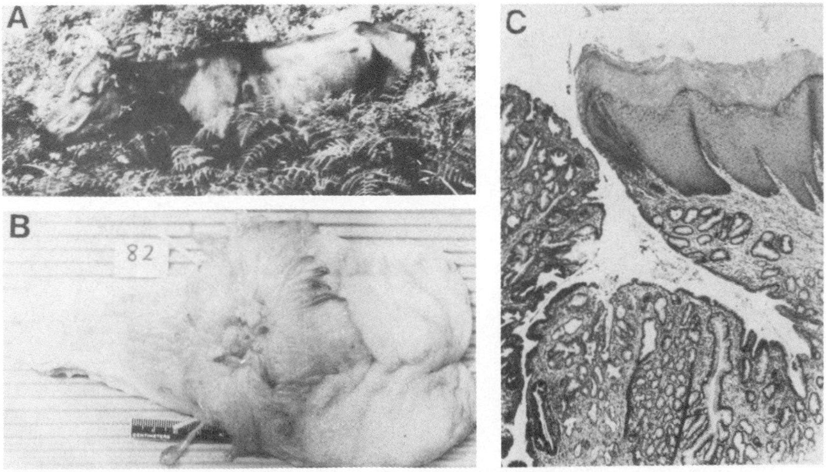


Some tumors of the bovine bladder are associated with a papilloma virus and the ingestion of a bracken fern carcinogen. Tumors can vary as fibromas, adenocarcinomas, transitional cell carcinoma or mixed. Bracken ferns with carcinogen seem to be restricted to certain soil conditions. Figure A, a cow eating bracken fern in an area of Brazil where tumors occur. When pastures are improved, cattle are no longer forced to eat bracken fern, tumors cease to occur. Figure B is a bladder tumor from a case of enzootic hematuria. Figure C, cystitis glandularis together with an area of squamous metaplasia of the bladder epithelium from which a bovine papilloma virus was isolated.

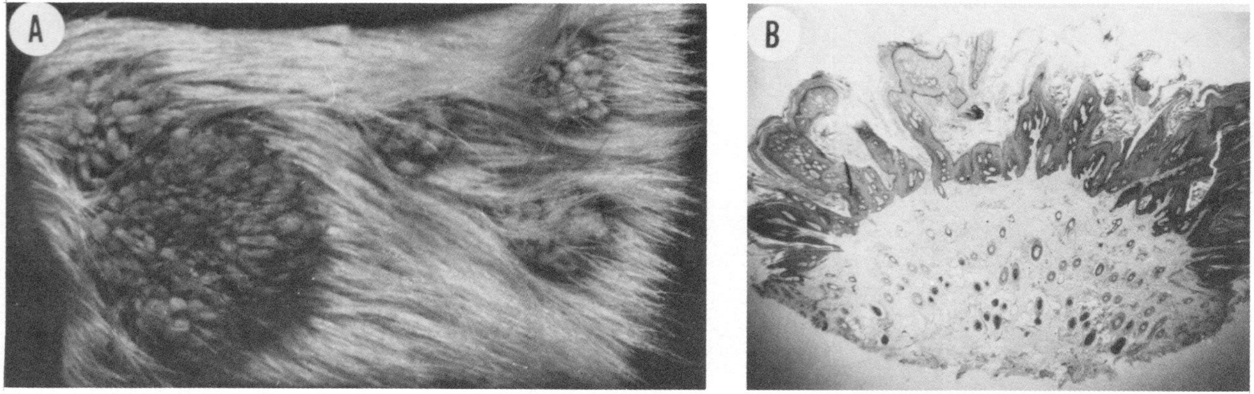


Atypical papilloma (figure A) which occurs on the skin of cattle. These lesions can persist and recur on the same animal. They are contagious but experimentally are poorly transmissible. Histological section of an atypical papilloma (figure B), note the normal dermis with hair follicles and lack of fibroma.

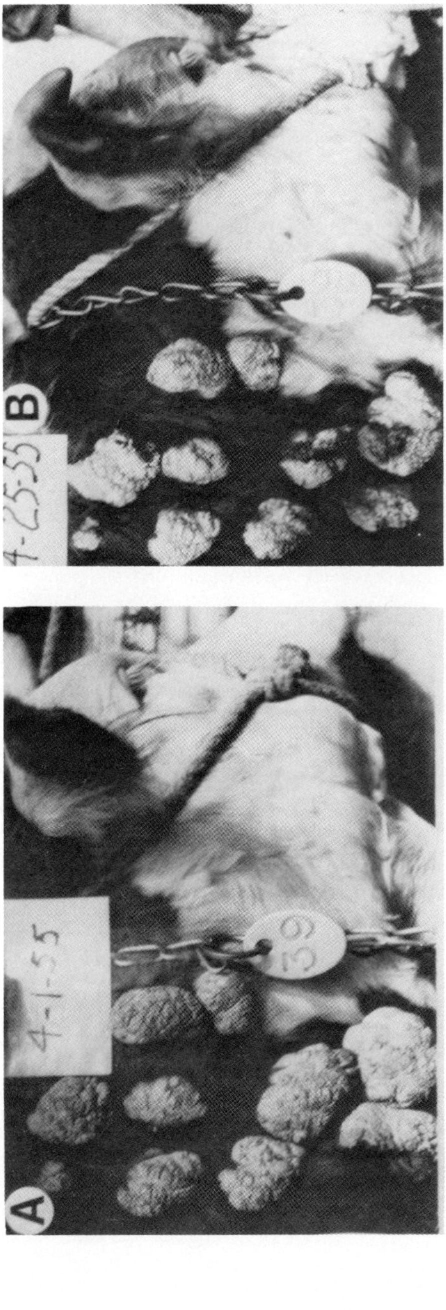


Figures A and B demonstrate the localized necrosis in beginning regression of experimentally induced BPV lesions.

# TRANSMISSIBLE ANIMAL PAPILLOMAS

A SELECTION OF ANIMAL PAPILLOMAS

| SPECIES AND PAPILLOMAVIRUS TYPE | LESION | TRANSMISSON TO OTHER SPECIES |
|---|---|---|
| Bovine | | |
| Type-1 | Fibropapilloma of skin | Yes |
| Type-2 | Fibropapilloma of Skin | Yes |
| Type-3 | Papilloma of Skin | Unknown |
| Type-4 | Papilloma of the Alimentary Tract | Unknown |
| Type-5 | Fibropapilloma of Skin | Unknown |
| Type-6 | Papilloma of Skin | Unknown |
| Deer | | |
| Whitetail | Fibroma of Skin | Yes |
| Mule | Fibroma of Skin | Unknown |
| Blacktail | Fibroma of Skin | Unknown |
| Reindeer | Fibropapilloma of skin | Yes |
| European Elk | Fibropapilloma of Skin | Yes |
| Sheep | Fibropapilloma of Skin | Yes |
| Horse | Papilloma of Skin | No Response |
| Rabbit | | |
| Cottontail | Papilloma of Skin | Yes |
| Domestic | Oral Papilloma | No Response |
| Canine | Oral Papilloma | No Response |
| Coyote | Oral Papilloma | Yes |
| Wolf | Oral Papilloma | Unknown |
| Pig | Genital Condyloma | Unknown |
| Elephant | Oral Papilloma | Unknown |
| Primates | | |
| Cebus | Papilloma of Skin | Unknown |
| Chimpanzee | Papilloma of Skin | Unknown |
| Chaffinch | Papilloma of Skin | Unknown |

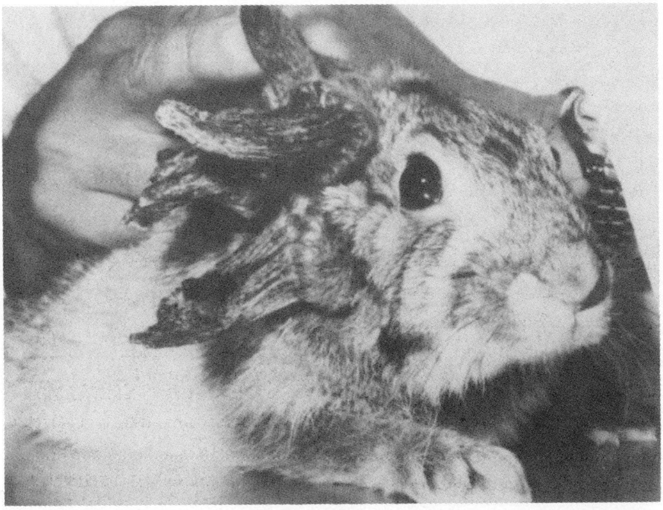

Cottontail rabbit papillomas, caused by a virus, CRPV. CRPV occurs in certain areas west of the Mississippi River. CRPV produces papillomas in both cottontail and domestic rabbits, but infectious virus is regularly produced only in the cottontail. After 6 months carcinoma develops in 25% cottontail and75% of domestic rabbits. Photo courtesy of Dr. Wm.C. Phelps.

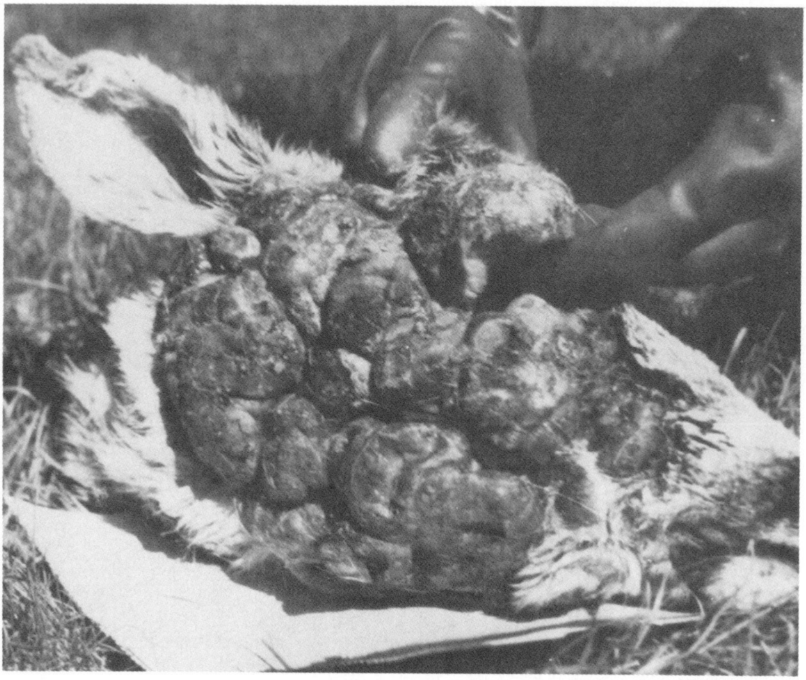

Extensive growth of fibromas on the face of a deer caused by deer fibroma virus (DFV). Experimental lesions can be readily produced by inoculation on scarified skin. Fibromas are first evident in 7 to 8 weeks. Deer fibroma virions are found in the thin epithelial cells covering the more massive growth of fibroma. Usually the lesions are small and regress.

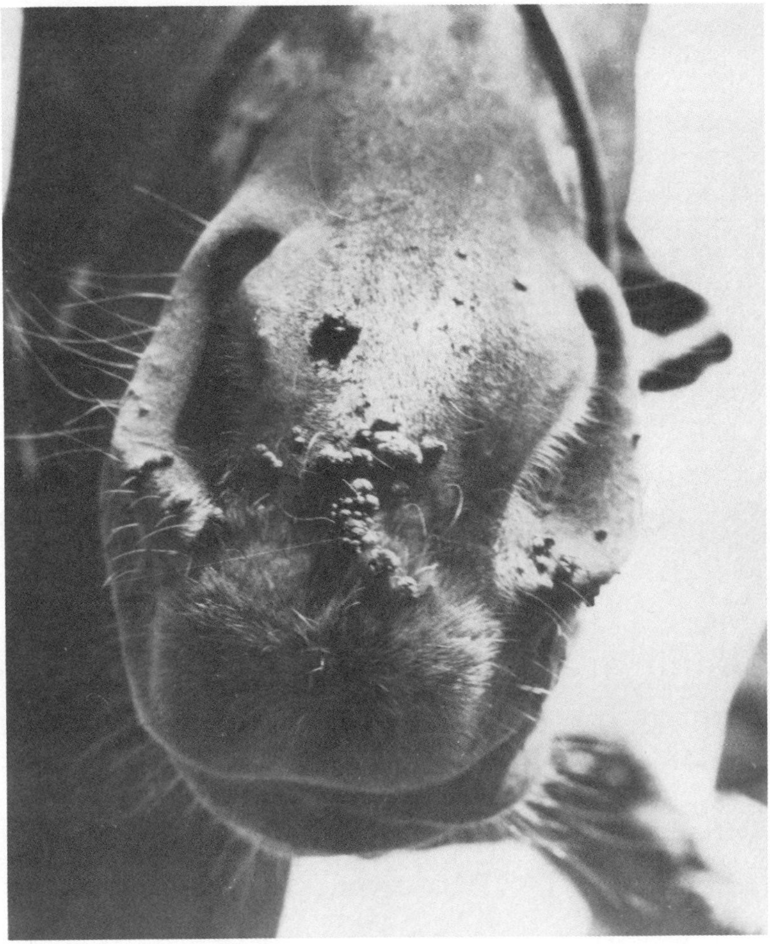

Equine papillomatosis usually affects young horses and ponies about the mouth, nose and head. These warts regress in a few weeks to several months.

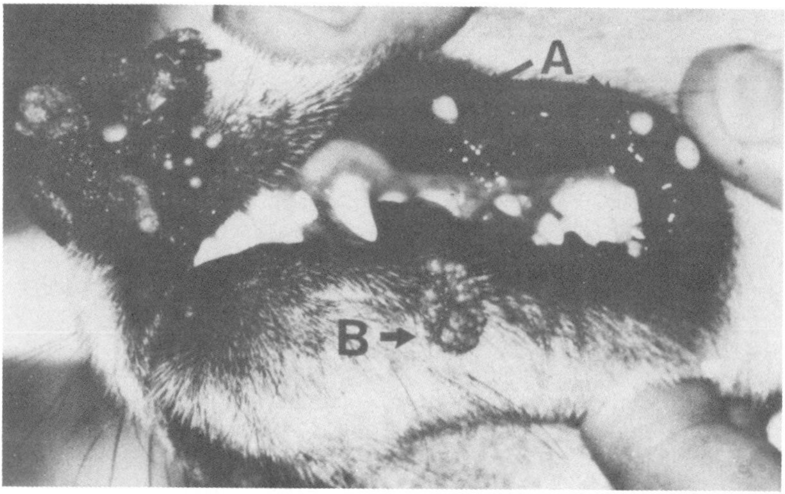


Canine oral papillomas (arrow A) caused by canine oral papilloma virus, COPV, are readily transmitted to susceptible dogs. The incubation period for COPV varies from 4 to 10 weeks and regression follows in 3 to 14 weeks. Occurrence of papillomas on the skin of the lower jaw and about the nose (arrow B) is unusual.

BOVINE PAPILLOMA VIRUS EXPERIMENTAL INFECTIONS

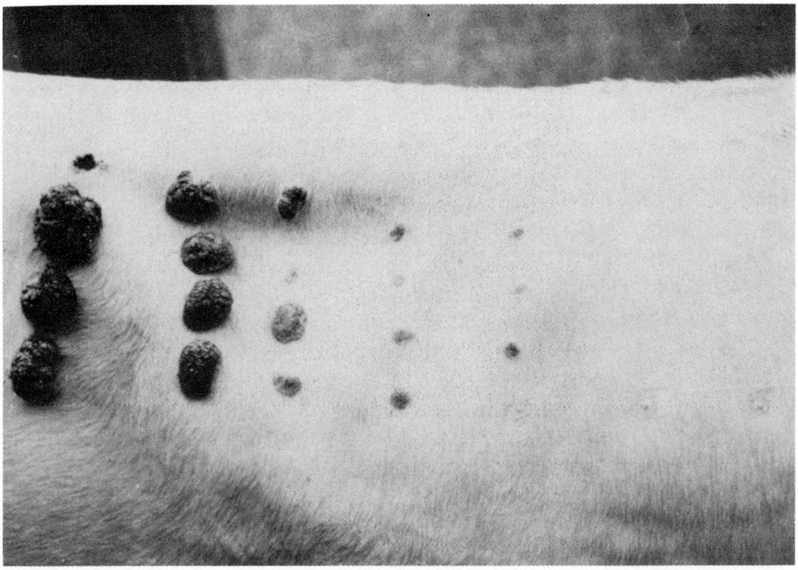

Titration of a BPV isolate in a 15% suspension on the skin of a susceptible calf 80 days after inoculation. Dilutions left to right: 1:10, 1:100, 1:1000, 1:10,000, 1:100,000 1:500,000 and 1:1,000,000 were inoculated at 4 vertical sites. Small growths are seen at one site of each of the 1:500, 000, and 1:,000,000 dilutions.

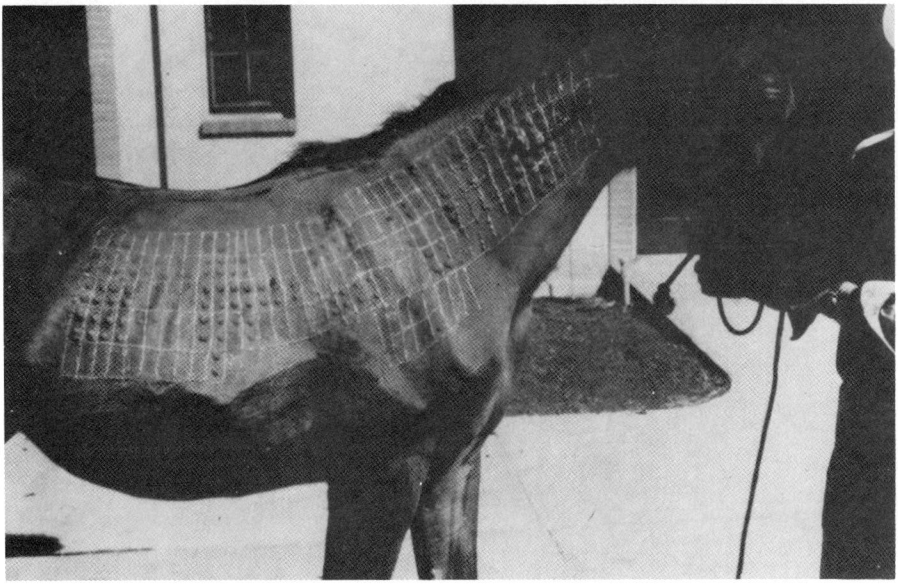

Skin test on a susceptible horse for neutralization of BPV mixed with serum from horses and cattle with experimental infections. Fibromas indicate no neutralization. The photo was taken 30 days post inoculation.

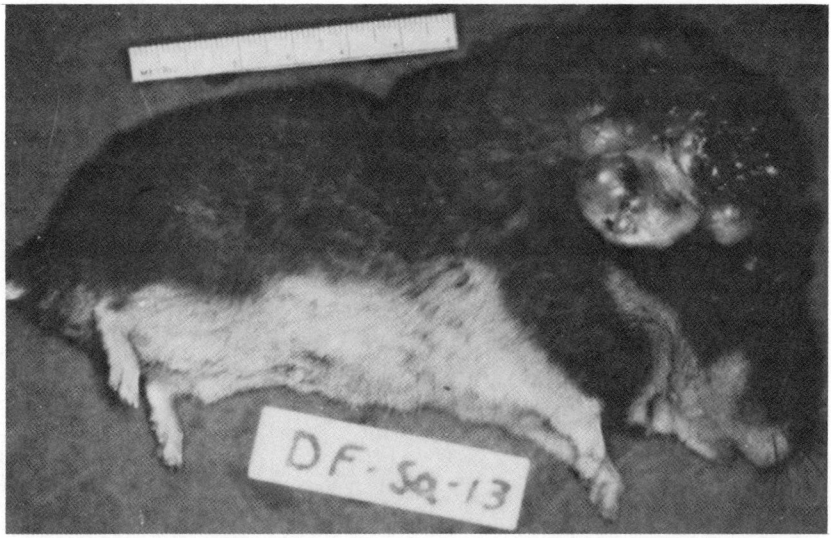


Fibroblastic tumors induced in a hamster by BPV. Such tumors are malignant in the hamster and may metastasize from the subcutis to the lungs, tail, and extremities of the leg. The lag time between inoculation of any age hamster and manifestation of tumor may be 6 months to 1 year.

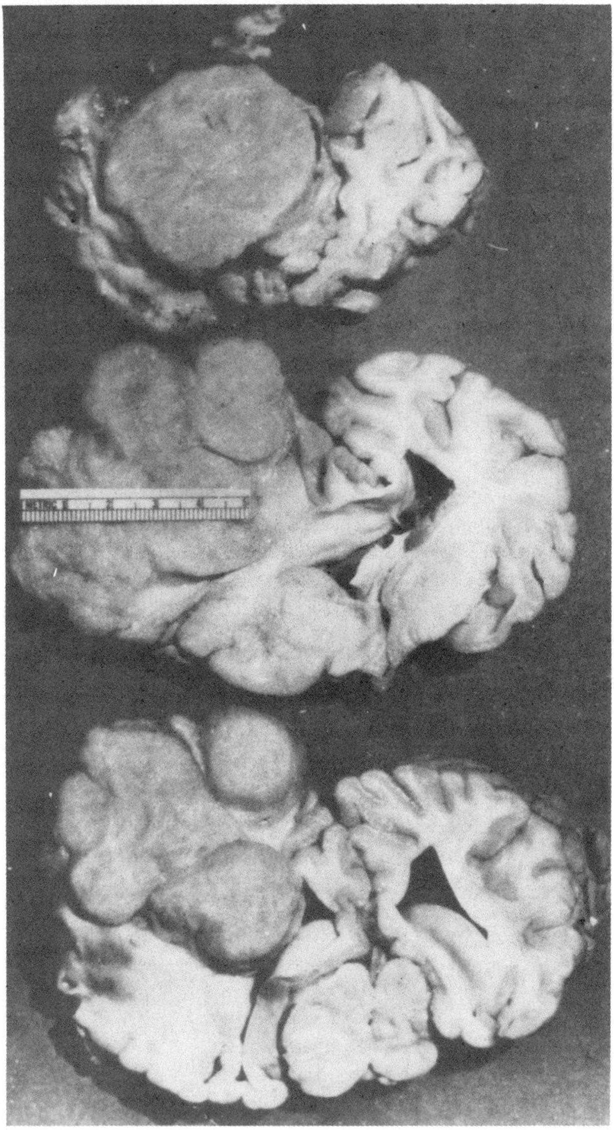

Cross section of the brain of a calf with fibroma compressing and replacing the cerebrum 105 days after local injection of BPV.

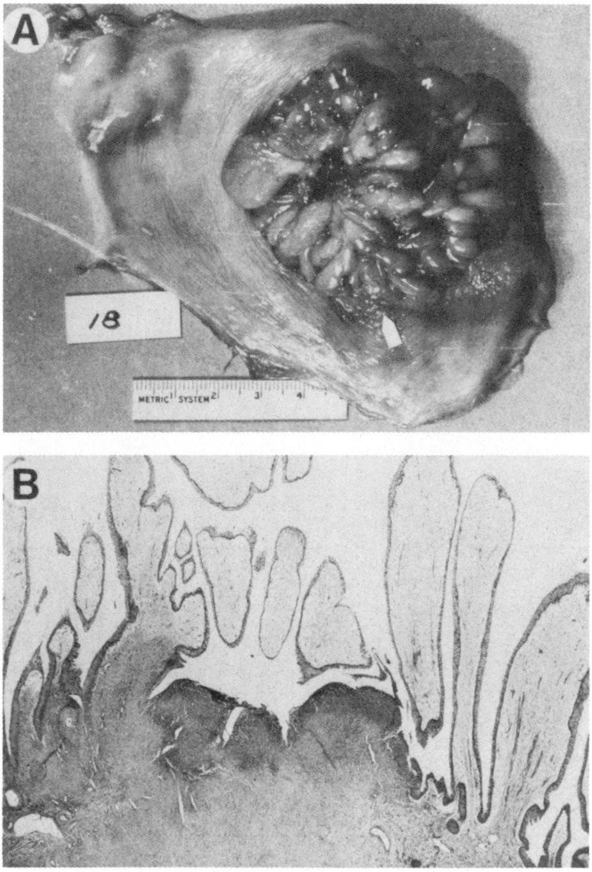


Figure A The mucosal aspect of a urinary bladder with a polyploid tumor overlaying a fibroma 374 days after injection of BPV into the submucosa. Figure B Section of a bovine urinary bladder tumor showing polyps and fibroma 48 days after inoculation with BPV.

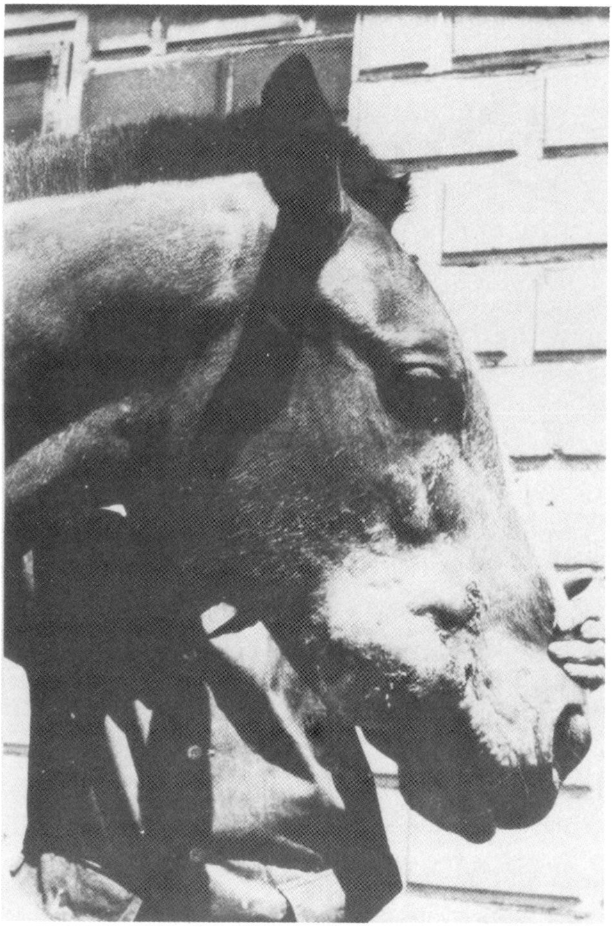

Equine sarcoid is a naturally occurring tumor in horses that contains DNA sequences of BPV-1 and or BPV-2.

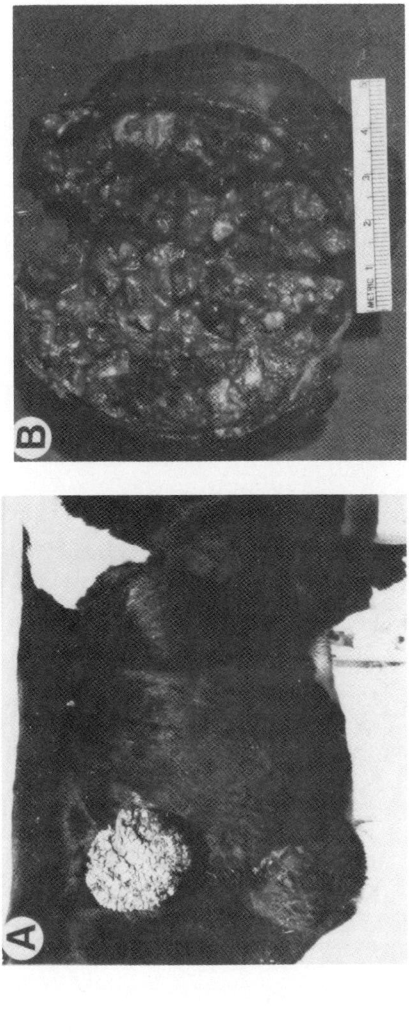


Subcutaneous papillomatous cysts (fig A) produced by implantation of bits of autologous skin bathed in a suspension of BPV. These implants were done 16 months previously. The cyst upper most left in figure A has been exteriorized at 10.5 months, continued growth of the papilloma is evident. The interior of a subcutaneous papillomatous cyst (fig B) demonstrating nodular hyperplastic epithelial lining surrounded by a thin fibromatous capsule. Cysts contain virions of BPV and also their antibodies.

**Papillomaviruses: Molecular and Clinical Aspects, pages 299–303**


# BIOLOGICAL CHARACTERISTICS OF BOVINE PAPILLOMAVIRUSES

W. F. H. Jarrett

University of Glasgow Veterinary School
Bearsden, Glasgow, Scotland, G61 1QH

ABSTRACT Bovine papillomaviruses (BPV) can be divided into two subgroups, one which causes fibropapillomas and the other epithelial papillomas. This is reflected in cell culture; only those of the first subgroup are capable of transforming fibroblasts *in vitro*. The subgroups can also be differentiated by genomic size, sequence homology, heteroduplex mapping and by the presence or absence of the so-called group specific antigen. BPV-2, as an example of subgroup A, has been shown, by infection of primary bovine fibroblasts at time of isolation, to possess all the genetic information required for both immortalization and transformation. Experimental infections have been made in groups of calves reared in isolation and studies have been carried out on the pathogenesis, virus replicative cycle and immunology of BPV 1, 2, 4, 5 and 6. Virus replication is only seen during the middle period of each developmental cycle. Cells which were cultured in the early phase of papilloma development of the squamous tumors of BPV-4 infection had a transformed phenotype *in vitro*, but did not contain any BPV genomes. In this type of fairly heavy artificial infection with BPV's none of the cattle responded to any of the viruses with a humoral immune response to virion structural proteins; this appears also to be true for the great majority of field infections also. However, it is possible to protect against tumor induction by immunizing with virion proteins. These experiments have also demonstrated that latency exists in BPV infections.

## INTRODUCTION

In the bovine, 6 papillomaviruses have been characterized and others have been isolated (1). These induce tumors which fall into 2 pathologic classes, (a) fibropapillomas and (b) epithlial papillomas. Table 1 shows the range of benign tumors induced specifically by each virus.

TABLE 1
VIRUS SPECIFIC TUMOR TYPES

| BPV | Papilloma |
|---|---|
| 1. | 1. Penile fibropapilloma |
| | 2. Teat frond fibropapilloma |
| | 3. Cutaneous fibropapilloma |
| 2. | 1. Cutaneous fibropapilloma |
| | 2. Alimentary fibropapilloma |
| 3. | Cutaneous epithelial papilloma |
| 4. | Alimentary epithelial papilloma |
| 5. | Teat "rice grain" fibropapilloma |
| 6. | Teat frond epithelial papilloma |

These tumor types have been described in detail in a recent review (1). It was of interest to compare those viruses which can transform both fibroblasts and epithilial cells and to contrast them with those which are only epitheliotrophic.

## RESULTS

Rabbit antisera to disrupted BPV-1 or 2 virions contain antibodies which react with epitopes on the major virion proteins of a wide range of PV's of other species (3); this has been thought to represent a group specific reaction. Using such antisera of high titre (1:500,000 against BPV 1 and 2) we found that these had a titer of 1:100 when reacted with rice-grain tumors which were replicating BPV-5 but did not react at all in immunoperoxidase or immunofluorescence on cryostat or paraffin sections with tissues containing BPV-4 or 6. Similar results were obtained in ELISA tests using highly purified viruses both intact and split (4). Using pairs of experimental calves we have recently shown that an animal which has undergone a full cycle of infection, tumor induction and rejection is immune to reinfection with the homologous virus but BPV-1 or 2 do not protect against BPV-4 or 6 or vice versa. DNA of BPV-6 was cross-hybridized in relaxed conditions to DNA restriction fragments of BPV-1 to 5. No hybridization was detected with DNA from BPV-1, 2 or 5, but a positive result was obtained with BPV-3 and 4 (4). Similar findings were obtained using cloned BPV-2 and 4 DNA as probes. Heteroduplex analysis gave similar relationships and indicated that the genomes of BPV-1, 2 and 5 were colinear as were those of BPV-3, 4 and 6. The molecular weights of the DNA's of the first subgroups were approximately $5 \times 10^6$ and of the second $4.5 \times 10^6$. These results results show that the distinctive biologic behavior and tissue-trophic transformation specificity of these 2 subgroups is reflected in a range of immunological and molecular parameters. It will be of considerable interest to see the relationship of each of these subgroups to the PV's of other species, particularly to their transformation potential. These results are summarized in Table 2.

TABLE 2
THE 2 SUBGROUPS OF BPV

| | | A | B |
|---|---|---|---|
| Tumors | | Fibropapillomas | Papillomas |
| Transformation in vitro | | + | - |
| Interspecies antigen | | + | - |
| DNA | MW | $5 \times 10^6$ | $4.5 \times 10^6$ |
| | kb | 7.2 | 7.9 |
| Colinearity to BPV-1 | | + | - |
| Colinearity to BPV-4 | | - | + |
| Sequence homology to BPV-1 | | 5-55% | 0 |
| Sequence homology to BPV-4 | | 0 | 20-50% |

Studies on in vitro Transformation.

We have carried out extensive studies on transformation of bovine fibroblasts by BPV-2 (so far no transformation has been accomplisedh with BPV's of subgroup B) (Watt, Leighton and Jarrett, in preparation). These may be summarized as follows. Cosnsistent results have been best achieved using cultures from the soft palate or conjunctiva of both late stage fetus or adults. Non-passaged primary cell cultures from these sites were infected with BPV-2. Morphologic alterations in the skin and palate cells were observed after 11.4 and 7.4 population doublings respectively, and consisted of piling up of the margins of adjacent cell whorls indicating loss of contact and density inhibition. Skin and palate cells were assessed for anchorage-independent growth at passages 5, 7 and 9 after infection. Both grew in soft agar at the seventh pass corresponding to 12.3 and 9.8 doublings respectively. The transformed cells were identical to those induced by this virus in established cultures from these sources. BPV-2 genomes were present in all of these cells. This demonstrates for the first time that BPV-2 can transform bovine fibroblasts that have not become adapted for short term growth in vitro nor developed the potential for indefinate subculture.

We have also used these methods for quantal assays of virus. These will be described in detail elsewhere (Watt, O'Neil, Laird and Jarrett, in preparation) but it was found that by comparison with EM virion counts the results were highly repeatable over 4 log 10 virus doses. This has allowed many previously unattainable determinations of experimental parameters to be made such as effect of time and temperatures of storage, effects of inactivating agents or genetic manipulations in vaccine studies and has enabled the devising of serum antibody neutralizing tests. The latter have been found to correlate well with results obtained by tissue immunoperoxidase, ELISA and complement fixation (see below).

Culture of BPV-4 papilloma cells. We have reported elsewhere that the squamous carcinomas which develop in cows feeding on bracken fern and which are often coincident with BPV-4 induced papillomas, do not contain persistent BPV-4 viral DNA. Cultures of transformed cells from these tumors are tumorogenic in nude mice but also are negative for viral genomes. We therefore attempted to culture cells from papillomas induced in the alimentary tract of calves by purified BPV-4. Infections were made by giving multiple closely spaced injection of virus to produce a packed mass of tumor. This allowed the very early and minute lesions to be sampled by biopsy. Only cells from this early stage would grow in culture and at 4-6 weeks after infection virus replication is barely perceptible. The cultured cells were obviously epithelial on EM showing desmosomes and typical keratinocyte morphology. Cellular DNA extracted at the 4th and 10th passages was negative for viral sequences. After pass 10 the cells grew in soft agar with a plating efficiency of 1%. Naturally, neither virions nor viral antigens were present in these cells. Tumorigenicity experiments are in progress. Cells from normal palate and those from all other stages of papilloma development failed to establish cultures under the same conditions. These facts raise interesting possibilities about the nature of epithelial transformation prior to the onset of the translation of virion proteins and the associated immune response.

The immune response of calves to BPV's. We have carried out a series of experimental infections and tumor inductions with BPV's 1, 2, 4, 5 and 6. These have been described in some detail (1). One surprising finding in all of these experiments, in which 100% "takes" were achieved, was that no single animal showed the production of antibodies to any virus despite fairly heavy tumor induction and the carrying on of the experiments until the tumors had been naturally rejected. Proven effective assays were used (ELISA, immunoperixidase, IFA and virus neutralization). These were controlled by hyperimmune bovine and rabbit serum. The tumors were not damaged in any way during the experiments. We have only found bovine antibody to BPV's in animals with massive and damaged tumors (such as may particularly happen in BPV-1 infections) or after parenteral immunization. This throws grave doubts on the use of serologic studies in epidemiology; and comparison of the virus dose required to immunize rabbits and cattle respectively with BPV points to the necessity to establish whether the PV's of any one species provoke a relatively poor response in that species as compared to others.

## REFERENCES


1. Jarrett WFH (1985). The natural history of bovine papillomavirus infections. In Klein G (ed): "Advances in Viral Oncology," New York: Raven Press, p 83.
2. Watt B, Leighton E, O'Neil BW, Laird HM, Campo, MS, Jarrett WFH. In preparation.
3. Jenson AB, Rosenthal JD, Olson C, Pass F, Lancaster WD, Shah K (1980). Immunologic relatedness of papillomaviruses from different species. J Nat Cancer Inst 64:495.
4. Jarrett WFH, Campo MS, O'Neil BW, Laird HM, Coggins LW. A novel bovine papillomavirus (BPV-6) causing true epithelial papillomas of the mammary gland skin: a member of a proposed new BPV subgroup. Virology 136:255.

Papillomaviruses: Molecular and Clinical Aspects, pages 305–326


# PRESENCE AND EXPRESSION OF BOVINE PAPILLOMAVIRUS TYPE 4 IN TUMOURS OF THE ALIMENTARY CANAL OF CATTLE AND ITS POSSIBLE ROLE IN TRANSFORMATION AND MALIGNANT PROGRESSION[1]

M.S. Campo[2], K.T. Smith, W.F.H. Jarrett
and M.H. Moar[3]

The Beatson Institute for Cancer Research and
Department of Veterinary Pathology,
Garscube Estate, Bearsden, Glasgow G61 1BD, U.K.

ABSTRACT BPV-4 induces papillomas of the upper alimentary canal, which can undergo malignant transformation and progression to squamous cell carcinomas. The carcinomas are often accompanied by adenomas and adenocarcinomas of the lower bowels. To elucidate the role of the virus in the transformation process we have analysed the expression of its DNA in the papillomas. We have identified seven viral mRNAs, varying in size from 4.2 kilobases (kb) to 1.0 kb, and have mapped them on the viral genome. All the RNA species are transcribed from the same DNA strand; are polyadenylated and, with the exception of the 1.0 kb RNA, internally spliced, and appear to share a common 5' leader sequence. We have identified the RNAs coding both for the structural and for the transforming proteins. We have also analysed several different malignancies of the alimentary canal and metastatic deposits for the presence of viral DNA. We have detected

[1]This work was supported by the Cancer Research Campaign, The Agricultural and Food Research Council and the National Institutes of Health.
[2]M.S. Campo is a Fellow of the Cancer Research Campaign.
[3]Department of Zoology, University of Edinburgh, West Mains Road, Edinburgh EH9 3JN, U.K.

the viral genome in only one transforming papilloma of the oesophagus and one carcinoma of the tongue. All the other cases were negative. Also, cell lines explanted both from papillomas and carcinomas did not contain the viral genome. We conclude that, although required for the induction of papillomas, the presence of the viral DNA is not necessary for the progression to, or the maintenance of, the transformed state.

## INTRODUCTION

Papillomaviruses are implicated in the aetiology of squamous cell carcinomas both in humans and in animals. The papillomavirus-associated cancers provide clear examples of the multifactorial nature of the disease: viral infection results in hyperproliferation of epithelial cells, with production of papillomas; some papillomas are stimulated to malignant progression to carcinomas by either genetic or environmental factors, or a combination or both (1-3). Despite their great multiplicity, only few papillomavirus types are associated with naturally occurring cancers. These include the human papillomaviruses (HPV) types 5,8,6,11,16 and 18 (3-7), the cottontail rabbit papillomavirus (CRPV) (8), and the bovine papillomavirus (BPV) type 4 (9).

BPV-4 induces epithelial papillomas of the upper alimentary canal, and in the Western Highlands of Scotland affected cattle are at much higher risk for the development of carcinomas than lowland animals. The geographical distribution of the cancer overlaps with that of the bracken fern, and strong circumstantial evidence has pointed to the fern as the environmental co-carcinogen (1). The cancers of the upper alimentary canal are often associated with adenomas and adenocarcinomas of the lower bowels (1). Whereas the papillomas produce large amounts of easily detectable mature virus progeny (10), no virus or viral antigens have been found in the carcinomas (9). BPV-4 has been isolated from productive papillomas (11) and subjected to detailed molecular and biological analysis (11-13). It is one of the members of subgroup B of bovine papillomaviruses (14), induces proliferation of epithelial cells only (14), has a smaller genome (11) and, although its transcription pattern and genome organization (15) show overall similarity with other PVs, is evolutionary distant from the viruses of subgroup A (11,16,17), all of which induce proliferation of both fibroblasts and keratinocytes (14). BPV-4 DNA transforms cells in vitro to the fully malignant phenotype: the transformed cells are anchorage-independent and, injected into nude mice, induce very aggressive fibrosarcomas (13).

The obvious association of BPV-4 with malignancies both naturally occurring and experimentally induced, has prompted us to investigate by which mechanism the virus transforms keratinocytes, and the nature of its role in the progression from a benign lesion to a fully malignant one. To this end we have analysed the expression of the viral genome in productive papillomas, and have screened large numbers of primary cancers and their metastases for the presence of the viral DNA.

## MATERIALS AND METHODS

### Papillomas and Cancers.

Routinely, papillomas were obtained from cattle in a large abattoir. Primary and metastatic cancers, and some papillomas, were obtained from diseased animals referred to the Veterinary School, Glasgow, by local farmers and veterinary doctors. All the specimens were frozen in liquid N2 as soon as possible after excision, and then stored at -70$^{o}$C until needed.

### Isolation and Purification of Tumour Nucleic Acids.

Nucleic acids were prepared by the method of Chirgwin et al. (18). Frozen tumours were ground in 4M guanidinium-thiocyanate solution and DNA and RNA were separated from cellular debris by centrifugation through equal volumes of 1.6 g/cc and 1.7 g/cc CsCl solutions. The DNA band at the interface between the two CsCl solutions was collected by needle aspiration, and precipitated with 3 vol. of 70% ETOH at 4$^{o}$C overnight. The final DNA pellet was dissolved in 10mM Tris pH 7.5, 1mM EDTA. The RNA pellet was resuspended in 7M guanidinium-hydrochloride and reprecipitated by adding 0.025 volumes of 1M acetic acid and 0.5 volumes of absolute ethanol. The solution was kept at -20$^{o}$C for at least 4h before centrifugation. The final pellet was resuspended in sterile water and stored at -20$^{o}$C. The polyadenylated RNA <poly(A)RNA> was purified by chromatography on oligo deoxythymidylate (oligo dT)-cellulose columns twice.

Molecular Cloning of Viral Fragments.

Subgenomic fragments of BPV-4 were prepared by the cleavage of the whole recombinant pBV4 plasmid (12) with appropriate restriction endonucleases. The digested DNA was electrophoresed in low melting point (LMP) agarose gels and the required fragment was eluted from the gel and purified (19). The DNA fragments were ligated to the vector pAT153 cleaved with the appropriate restriction nuclease, and recombinant plasmids identified as described previously (12). The subclones are referred to by the first letter of the restriction endonuclease sites bordering the fragments and by the size in kilobases (kb).

Restriction Enzyme Analysis of Tumour DNA and Southern Blot Hybridization.

Restriction endonucleases were purchased either from BRL England or Boehringer, Mannheim and used according to the manufacturer's specifications. The DNA fragments were electrophoresed in 1% agarose gels and transferred to Biodyne A nylon membranes (20). The blots were incubated with $P^{32}$-labelled nick-translated (21) recombinant BPV DNA, pBV4 and pBV1, (12) (sp.ac.$1x10^8$ cpm/µg) either overnight in 2xSSC at 65°C, or for 36 hours in 30% formamide, 5xSSC at 42°C (SSC = 0.15M NaCl, 0.015M sodium citrate, pH7). After extensive washing in 0.5xSSC at 55°C or 1xSSC at 37°C respectively, the blots were exposed to X-ray films at -70°C for different times.

Northern Blot Hybridization.

Total or polyadenylated RNAs were fractioned by electrophoresis in 1.4% agarose gels containing 2.2M formaldehyde (22). After electrophoresis rRNA markers were stained with 1 µg/ml ethidium bromide. The RNA was transferred directly to Pall Biodyne A nylon membranes in 20xSSC and hybridized to $^{32}P$-labelled nick translated BPV-4 DNA or subgenomic clones in 50% formamide, 5 x SSC at 42°C.

In situ Hybridization.

cRNA was transcribed in vitro from recombinant BPV-4 DNA by the use of Escherichia coli RNA polymerase and all four ribonucleotide triphosphates labelled with $H^3$. Cryostat sections of the tumours were fixed in 3:1 methanol-acetic acid, and the DNA was denatured with a brief heat treatment at 100°C for 15 sec. Thereafter, tissues were hybridized with 3 µg $H^3$-cRNA per ml for 16 hours at 60°C in 3xSSC. After hybridization, the sections were treated with 30 µg pancreatic RNAse per ml at 37°C for 30 min. followed by extensive washing in 2xSSC with a final rinse in an alcohol series (50-100%) and air drying. Autoradiography was performed by means of Ilford K2 emulsion, and autoradiographs were exposed at 4°C for several periods up to three months. After being developed, fixed and washed with distilled water, slides were stained in 6% Giemsa in phosphate buffer, pH 6.8.

## RESULTS

Transcriptional Map of BPV-4.

The number and sizes of BPV-4 specific RNAs in papillomas were determined by Northern blot hybridization of total papilloma RNA to the whole BPV-4 genome and to subgenomic fragments. When the entire viral genome was used, seven transcripts were detected (Fig. 1a). The 4.2, 2.8 and 1.0 kilobase (kb) transcripts were always the most abundant viral RNA species, whereas the 3.6 and 1.9 kb transcripts varied in amounts in different RNA preparations and were occasionally absent. All the viral RNAs were present in the polyadenylated fraction of papilloma RNA as shown by their retention on an oligo-dT cellulose column. Subgenomic viral DNA probes hybridized differentially to the several mRNAs (Fig. 1b-h), and DNA probes from widely separate regions of the viral genome hybridized to the same RNAs, indicating that many of the transcripts are spliced. Thus the 4.2 kb RNA appears to contain sequences complementary to all the subgenomic fragments (Fig. 1b-h), and, with the exception of probe P-P1.0 (Fig.1f), so does the 1.9 kb RNA. Conversely, the two major 2.8 and 1.0 kb RNAs hybridized only to fragments spanning two discrete contiguous regions of the genome (Fig. 1c,d,e,g,h). The transcribed regions of the viral genome were mapped more

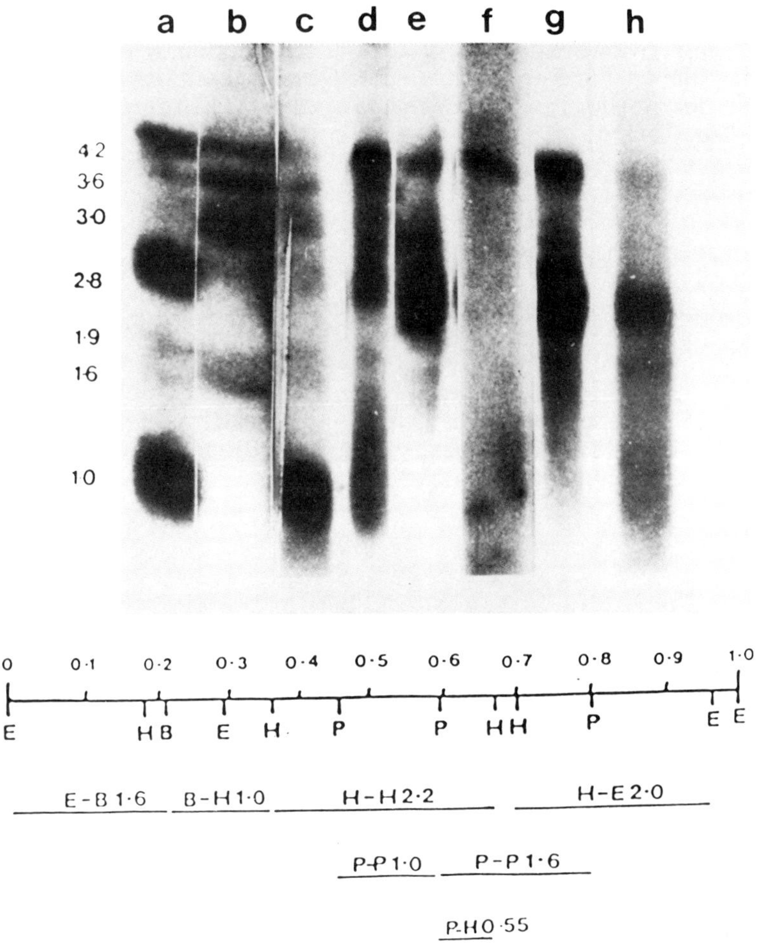


FIGURE 1. Mapping of BPV-4 specific transcripts in oesophageal papillomas. Total papilloma RNA was hybridized to the DNA probes shown diagramatically below the restriction map of BPV-4 DNA. The map positions of BamHI, Eco,RI, HindIII, and PstI restriction enzyme sites are shown as B,E,H, and P respectively and sizes are given in kb. a, pBV4; b, E-B1.6; c, B-H1.0; d, H-H2.2; e, dH-E2.0; f, P-P1.0; g, P-P1.6; h, P-H0.55. RNA sizes in kb are shown on the right-hand side of the diagram.

precisely using S1 nuclease digestion of RNA-DNA hybrids, formed between RNA and either unlabelled DNA fragments or 3'-end labelled and 5'-end labelled fragments (not shown; 15). This allowed the splicing pattern to be established (Fig. 2A). In addition, two major 3'-termini were identified by hybridizing short $P^{32}$-labelled cDNA to viral subgenomic fragments: one was located in fragment P-P1.0, and the other in fragment H-P0.63 (Fig. 2A). The transcriptional map of BPV-4 was constructed by assembling all the results obtained with the different techniques employed in this study (Fig. 2B).

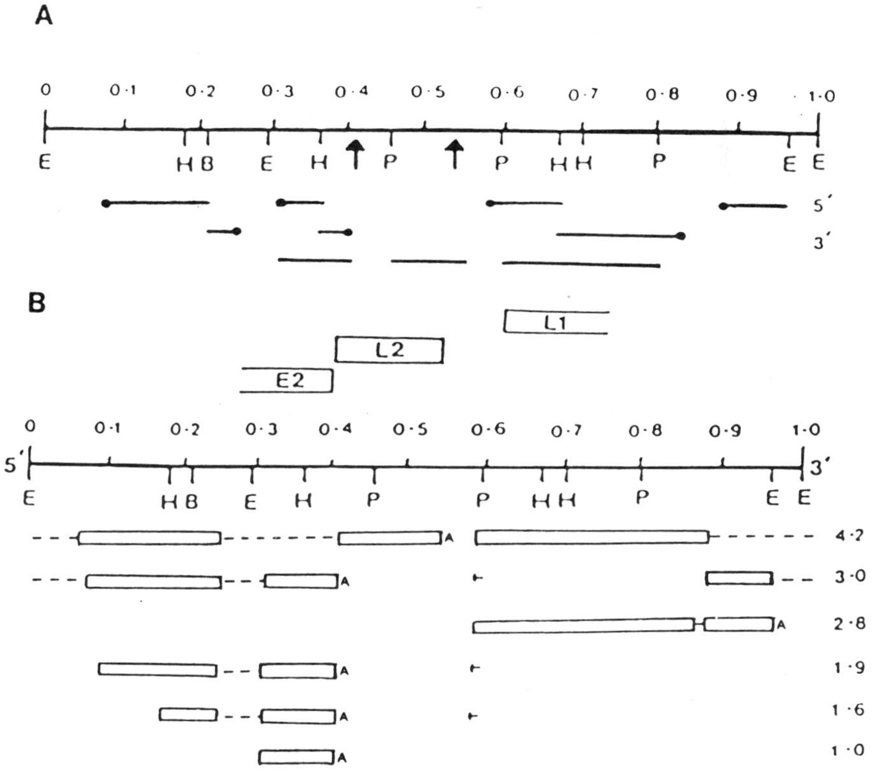


FIGURE 2. A, S1 protected fragments of BPV-4 DNA. The arrows indicate the two major 3'-termini. The 5' and 3' ends of the mRNAs are marked ( ). B, Transcriptional Map. The established open reading frames are shown above the restriction map of BPV-4 DNA.

The several RNAs, with the possible exception of the 1.0 kb species, may share a common 5' leader sequence as a DNA fragment from region 0.59-0.67 hybridizes to all of them (Fig.1,h). In agreement, two putative promoter elements have been identified in this region at approximately 0.59 map units (m.u.), each one containing a CAAT, a TATAA and and ACA box (Patel and Campo, in preparation).

The 4.2. kb and 2.8 kb RNAs share extensive coding regions. The 4.2 kb RNA is spliced twice and terminates at 0.56 m.u., where a polyadenylation site has been identified (Patel and Campo, in preparation), validating the cDNA hybridization to that region of the genome. The 2.8 kb RNA is most likely spliced once, since H-E2.0 was not entirely protected after S1 nuclease digestion, but gave rise to two fragments (not shown). A second polyadenylation site has been identified 110 bp downstream from H-E2.0 at map position 0.99 (Patel and Campo, in preparation), but as there is no hybridization of cDNA to this region of the genome, it is possible that alternative termination sites are used.

The 3.0, 1.9, 1.6 and 1.0 kb RNAs show extensive sequence overlap with each other; their main bodies have different 5' ends; the 3.0 kb RNA is spliced twice and the second splice is common to both the 1.9 kb and 1.6 kb RNAs; whereas the 1.0 kb RNA appears not to be spliced. The RNAs are co-terminus at their 3' end, at map position 0.4, where a third polyadenylation signal has been identified (Patel and Campo, in preparation), thus confirming the cDNA hybridization results.

The 3.6 kb RNA has been observed only sporadically and has not been mapped.

Analysis of the nucleotide sequence of the viral genome and of the amino acid sequence of the putative products has allowed the preliminary assignment of the functions to the several coding regions. There is a 1073 bp long open reading frame from 0.4-0.56 m.u. corresponding to the 3' end of the 4.2 kb RNA. The protein encoded by this open reading frame shows clear homology with the L2 protein of other papillomaviruses (Table 1). Therefore, the 4.2 kb RNA encodes the L2 structural protein of the virion (Fig. 2B). A second open reading frame is found downstream from L2 starting at 0.59 m.u. encompassing the 5' end of the 4.2 kb RNA and the 2.8 kb RNA. The amino-acid sequence of this region compares well with that of the L1 protein of other PVs (Table 1) and therefore, the 2.8 kb transcript encodes the L1 virion protein (Fig. 2B).

TABLE 1
AMINOACID HOMOLOGY BETWEEN THE PROTEINS
OF BPV-4 AND OTHER PVs

| | L2[a] | L1[a] | E2[a] |
|---|---|---|---|
| BPV-1 | 42 | 56 | 26 |
| HPV-1 | 48 | 60 | 36 |
| HPV-6 | 54 | 56 | 28 |
| CRPV | nd[b] | 36 | 48 |

[a]Percentage of homology in the first 50 N-terminus aminoacids of L2 and L1 and the last 50 C-terminus aminoacids of E2.
[b]not determined.

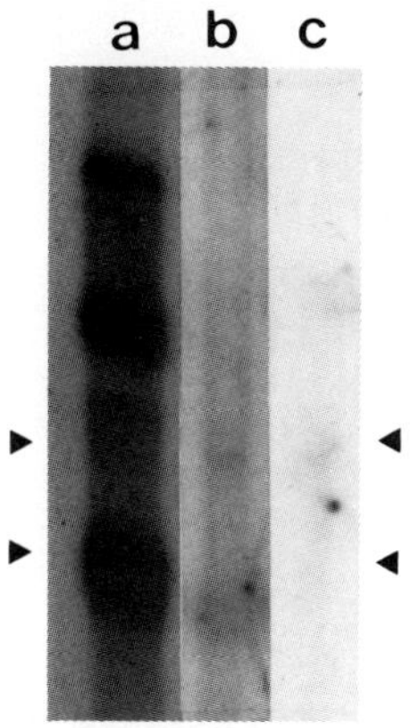


FIGURE 3. Blot hybridization of NIH3T3 transformed cell RNA to pBV4. a, 10 µg of total papilloma RNA; b, 20 µg and c, 10 µg of poly(A) RNA from a BPV-4 DNA transformed clone of NIH3T3 mouse fibroblasts. The arrows point to the positions of the 1.6 kb (top) and the 1.0 kb (bottom) RNA bands. Exposure to the X-ray film was for 3 days.

Interestingly, the 4.2 kb RNA may also encode the L1 protein. The C-terminus amino-acids derived from the nucleotide sequence corresponding to the 1.0 kb RNA and the overlapping 3' ends of the 3.0 kb, 1.9 kb and 1.6 kb RNAs show noticeable homology with the C-terminal amino-acids of the E2 open reading frame of other papillomaviruses (Table 1), thus indicating that this region of the genome codes for the E2 transforming protein (Fig. 2B).

The 1.0 kb RNA is not present in in vitro transformed mouse fibroblasts, where only the 1.6 kb and, occasionally, the 1.9 kb RNAs are found (Fig.3), suggesting that expression of the E2 open reading frame is specific for epithelial cells, and that the E2 protein is involved in keratinocyte transformation, and not needed for the in vitro transformation of fibroblasts. It has to be remembered that in vivo only epithelial cells are transformed by BPV-4.

## The Viral Genome is Not Present in Cancers.

We have analysed seventy cases of bovine primary and secondary tumours for the presence of BPV-4 DNA (Table 2).

TABLE 2
CANCERS OF THE ALIMENTARY CANAL AND THEIR METASTASES

| Upper Alimentary Canal | | Lower Bowels[a] | | Metastatic Deposits | |
|---|---|---|---|---|---|
| Transforming papillomas | 3 | Duodenum | 5 | Thyroid | 2 |
| Tongue | 3 | Colon | 6 | Salivary glands | 1 |
| Palate | 3 | | | Lymphnodes | 9 |
| Pharynx | 3 | | | Liver | 2 |
| Oesophagus | 9 | | | Kidneys | 1 |
| Cardia | 5 | | | | |
| Rumen | 18 | | | | |
| Total | 44 | Total | 11 | Total | 15 |

[a]Includes adenomas and adenocarcinomas.

The primary tumours include transforming papillomas and squamous cell carcinomas of the upper alimentary canal, and adenomas and adenocarcinomas of the lower bowels; the secondary cancers include metastatic deposits in the thyroid, liver, kidneys and lymphnodes. A transforming papilloma is a tumour at an intermediate stage between a benign papilloma and a carcinoma (23). Southern blots of cancer DNA were hybridized to in vitro labelled nick-translated BPV-4 DNA in 2xSSC at 65°C. Only one case of tongue carcinoma (Fig. 4a-d) and one case of transforming papilloma of the oesophagus (not shown) were positive for BPV-4 DNA. The viral DNA was episomal, showed the typical restriction enzyme pattern of BPV-4 DNA, and was present in approximately 5 copies per cell, as judged by a comparison with papilloma DNA hybridized in the same conditions (Figure 4e-g).

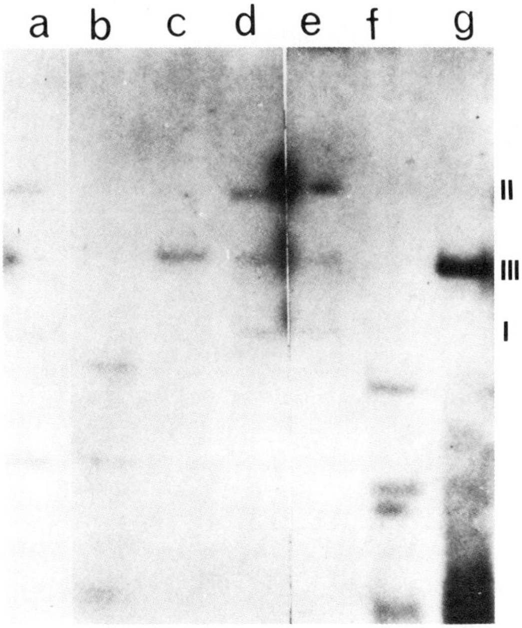


FIGURE 4. Blot hybridization of tumour DNA to pBV4. a-d, 10 µg of DNA from tongue carcinoma No. 67193; e-g, 0.5 µg of DNA from oesophageal papilloma; a,e, no enzyme; b.f, HindIII; c,g, BamHI; d, BglII. Hybridization was in 2 X SSC at 65°C, and exposure to x-ray film was for two days.

(Continued)

Fig. 4 (Continued)

I, II and III indicate supercoiled, relaxed and linear viral DNA, respectively. The lowest band in (a) is due to endogenous plasmid sequences hybridizing to the plasmid component of pBV4.

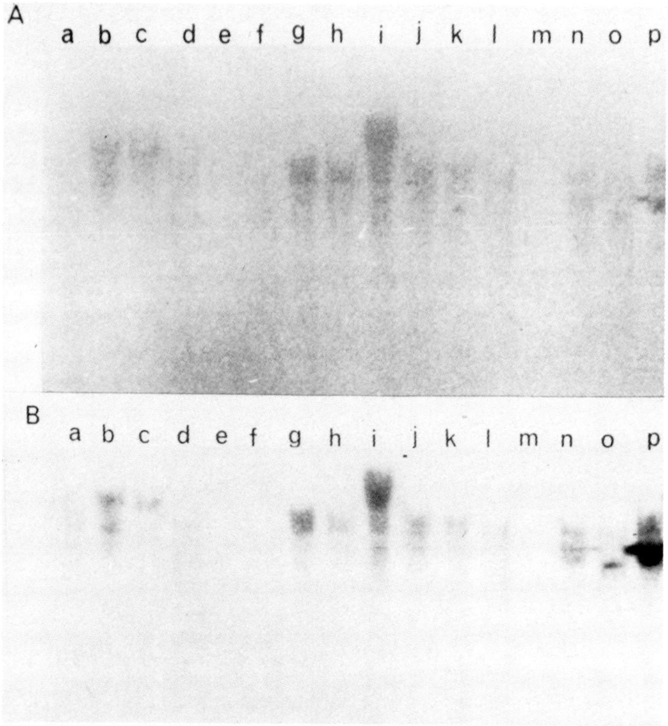


FIGURE 5. Blot hybridization of tumour DNA to recombinant BPV DNA. 10 µg of BamHI-digested tumour DNA were hybridized to (A), BPV-4 DNA, and (B), BPV-1 DNA. a,b, carcinomas of the oesophagus; d, carcinoma of the pharynx; c,e,g,h,i,m,n, carcinomas of the rumen; f, adenocarcinoma of the colon; j,k, metastases of lymphnodes from i; l, metastasis of the kidney from i; o, carcinoma of the palate; p, carcinoma of the cardia. c and d, f and g, and h and i are primary tumours at different sites from three animals. Hybridization was in 30% formamide-5 X SSC at 42°C. Exposure to x-ray film was for two days. Longer exposure times did not reveal any additional band.

To investigate the possibility that viral DNA sequences other than BPV-4 are present in the cancers, the DNAs were hybridized to recombinant BPV-4 and BPV-1 DNA in relaxed conditions at 40°C below Tm (30% formamide, 5xSSC, 42°C). BPV-1 and BPV-4 belong to papillomavirus subgroup A and B respectively (14) and, as there is extensive DNA sequence homology within the members of each subgroup (14, 16, 26), the two radioactive probes should easily detect related sequences from other viruses. No hybridization was observed with either probe even in relaxed conditions (Figure 5A and 5B) thus ruling out the involvement of other known papillomaviruses.

The possibility that multiple copies of BPV DNA are present only in very rare cells was eliminated by in situ hybridization experiments. A minimum of eight sections per cancer case were hybridized to BPV-4 or BPV-1 cRNA and each case proved negative, even after a 3-month long exposure (Figure 6A; BPV-1 hybridization not shown).

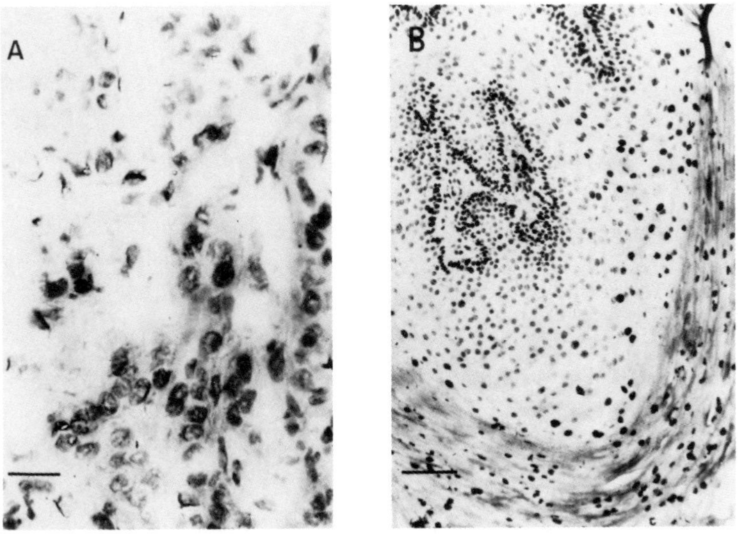


FIGURE 6. In situ hybridization of papilloma and carcinoma sections to BPV-4 cRNA. A. Oesophageal carcinoma; B. Oesophageal papilloma. Hybridization was performed in 3 X SSC at 60°C for 16 hr. Exposure time was three months for A, and three weeks for B. The bar is 3.5 μm in A and 7 μm in B.

In contrast, sections from papillomas always showed BPV-4 positive cells in all the layers of the tumour, from the deep layers to the keratinized outer layers (Figure 6B). However, if a single copy of the viral genome, or a portion of it, is present in very few cells, say one in $10^{-3}$-$10^{-4}$ or less, then this would be below the limit of detection both in our blot hybridization and in situ hybridization conditions.

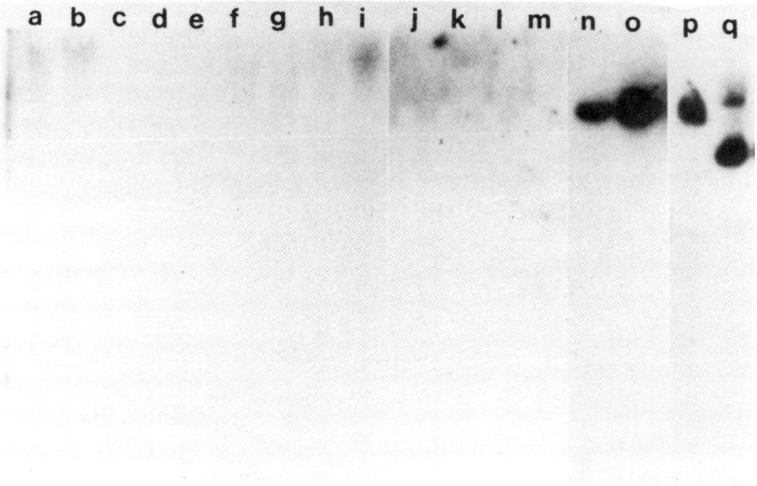


FIGURE 7. Blot hybridization of DNA from tumour cell lines to recombinant BPV-4 DNA. a, cell line from oesophageal papilloma AP3; b, cell line from oesophageal papilloma 50S; c, cell line from oesophageal papilloma 88529B; d-f, nude mouse tumours induced by 88529B cell line; g-i, cell lines explanted from d-f mouse tumours; j-k, cell line from oesophageal carcinoma 88529C; l-m, cell line from nude mouse tumour induced by 88529C cells; n,o, BPV-4 transformed NIH3T3 mouse fibroblasts; p,q, oesophageal papilloma; a-q, 10 µg of DNA; a-i,k,m-p, digested with BamHI; j,l,q, digested with BglII. BglII does not cut BPV-4 DNA. Papilloma 88529B and carcinoma 88529C are different tumours from the same animal. Hybridization was in 30% formamide, 5 X SSC at 42°C, and exposure to x-ray film was for 3 days except for p-q which was for 2 hours.

Recently we have successfully established epithelial cell lines both from papillomas and from carcinomas explanted in vitro (B. Watt, H. Laird, W.F.H. Jarrett, in preparation). These cells are capable of anchorage independent growth, induce tumours in nude mice and are therefore fully transformed. We have analysed three independently derived papilloma cell lines, three independently derived carcinoma cell lines, the tumours induced in nude mice by such cells, and cell lines explanted from the mouse tumours. We did not detect the BPV-4 genome in any of them (Fig. 7a-m) although in vitro transformed mouse fibroblasts contain multiple copies of BPV-4 DNA (Fig.7n,o; 13).

We conclude that the great majority of the alimentary canal cancers and their metastases do not harbour the viral genome and argue that, although BPV-4 is the causative agent of papillomatosis, and hence of keratinocyte transformation, the continuous presence and, therefore, expression of its genome are not required for the progression to, and the maintenance of, the transformed state.

## DISCUSSION

One of the aims of our long term investigation of the part played by BPV-4 in the stages of initiation, promotion and progression during carcinogenesis in cattle is the identification of the viral products responsible for epithelial cell transformation. Therefore we have analysed the expression of the viral genome in premalignant papillomas, and have identified both the structural and the transforming viral mRNAs. Here we shall limit ourselves to discussing only the transforming RNAs, as it is assumed that the structural RNAs do not play a significant part in cell transformation. However, the interesting observation that the L2 polypeptide of BPV-4 is more closely related to that of BPV-6 than to that of BPV-1 (Table 1) merits a brief comment. The L2 protein is thought to be involved in cell specificity (25,26); its C-terminus may be exposed on the surface of the virion and it could therefore interact with specific cell receptors. Both BPV-4 and HPV-6 infect mucous epithelium, and the close homology between the BPV-4 and HPV-6 L2 polypeptides may reflect the predilection of these viruses for the same type of epithelial cell.

The transcriptional organization of the putative

transforming region of the BPV-4 genome is similar to that of CRPV (27,28). All the transforming RNAs of BPV-4 span the E2 open reading frame, although the main bodies of the 3.0 kb, 1.9 kb and 1.6 kb RNAs have different 5' ends, and in addition are internally spliced. The 1.6 kb RNA is the only viral RNA present in NIH3T3 mouse fibroblasts transformed in vitro by BPV-4 DNA (13). In productive papillomas this RNA is spliced and includes part or all of E2, thus resembling the 1.3 kb RNA of CRPV (27,28). A similar pattern of splicing has been reported also for HPV-1 transcripts (29).

The 1.0 kb RNA covers the E2 region. It is by far the major viral transcript in papillomas, representing approximately 0.5% of the total polyadenylated RNA, and is not detected in BPV-4 transformed NIH3T3 cells. Interestingly, a similar RNA of 0.9 kb from the E2 open reading frame is found in productive CRPV tumours only (28). It is likely that the difference in transcription of E2 in papillomas and transformed fibroblasts reflects the difference in cell type and that transcription of the 1.0 kb RNA of BPV-4 and of the 0.9 kb RNA of CRPV is keratinocyte-specific. Moreover, the E2 polypeptide of BPV-4 is more closely related to that of the purely epitheliotropic CRPV, HPV-1 and HPV-6, than to that of BPV-1 which transforms both fibroblasts and epithelial cells (Table 1). This supports the hypothesis that this protein is implicated in cell-specific transformation.

Although the viral genome and its transcripts are always present in papillomas, only one transforming (malignant) papilloma of the oesophagus and one squamous cell carcinoma of the tongue, out of 70 cancer cases, harboured the genome of BPV-4, and moreover no other viral DNA sequences were detected using different BPV types in hybridization conditions that allow extensive cross-reaction. In addition, the lack of positive cells in in situ hybridization experiments ruled out the presence and replication of multiple copies of viral DNA in only a few cells. However, we cannot completely eliminate the possibility that a very short fragment of BPV-4 DNA is integrated into the cellular chromosome at a critical site, although such a situation has never been found in other papillomavirus-associated cancers. Moreover although remote, the additional possibility exists that the genome of a hitherto unknown, evolutionary unrelated virus is present in the cancers.

In other papilloma-carcinoma systems, the viral DNA

has been found to persist in some of the cancers (3-8), and the genome of BPV-1 or BPV-2 persists in equine sarcoids (30,31), in experimental tumours in hamster and derived cell lines (32,33) and in in vitro transformed cells (34,35).

Our results raise the question of why the genome of BPV-4 is absent in the bovine cancers and the answer depends on the role played by the virus in cell transformation, tumour induction and malignant progression.

The possibility that BPV-4 is not one of the factors involved in carcinogenesis, and that therefore the concurrence of time, geographical distribution, and anatomical sites between the benign and the malignant tumours is completely fortuitous, is unlikely, as all stages of direct transformation from papilloma to carcinoma have been observed and recognized, and viral DNA has been found in one case of transforming papilloma.

However, the great majority of cancers does not contain the viral genome, and this argues against the requirement for its presence and, therefore, its expression for the progression to, and the maintenance of, the transformed state. This conclusion is strengthened by the observation that cell lines explanted in vitro from alimentary canal papillomas and carcinomas, although capable of growth in agar and of tumour induction in nude mice, and therefore fully transformed, do not contain any viral DNA.

Several formal possibilities can account for the role of BPV-4 in carcinogenesis, but in all cases it has to be remembered that malignant progression in the natural hosts requires co-factors. Bracken fern not only contains a number of potent mutagens and carcinogens (36,37) but it is also immunosuppressive (38). The first possibility is that the virus is directly involved in cellular transformation and acts as an initiator by inducing one or more heritable changes (activation of proto-oncogenes?) in the cellular DNA at early stages of tumourigenesis; bracken supplies a promoter, a mutagen, or an immunosuppressant as one of several factors involved in later events. The transformed cell, no longer undergoing terminal differentiation, may be incapable of supporting the autonomous replication of the viral DNA, which is therefore lost.

The second possibility is that the virus acts indirectly in one or more of several ways. The virus-infected papilloma cells produce elevated amounts of growth factors, which in turn stimulate the expression of cellular proto-oncogenes (39-41) in non-infected cells. The ensuing cell proliferation increases the likelihood of a second transforming hit by the environmental co-carcinogens by increasing the target size. Alternatively, the virus acts as a promoter and the virus-induced proliferation leads to the clonal expansion of a cell already initiated by other agents. In all cases, the normal immunological reaction that mediates tumour rejection (42) is impaired and the transformed cell is allowed to proliferate. Whether induced by the virus directly or indirectly, cellular transformation is an early event in the papilloma-carcinoma transition, as indicated by the tumourigenic phenotype of the cell lines derived from "benign" papillomas.

Despite the absence of BPV-4 DNA in the cancers and in the explanted cell lines, the genetic make-up of the virus seems to be an important factor in the transformation process, since the BPV-2 induced fibropapillomas of the alimentary canal do not undergo malignant transformation and no connection with cancer has been observed (43). If BPV-4 specific genetic information were not required, there is no a priori reason why the dividing cells of the fibropapillomas should not provide an equally good target for the preceding or subsequent event(s) involved in neoplastic progression.

## ACKNOWLEDGMENTS

We wish to thank U.E. Loening, D.A.W. MacSorley, B.W. O'Neil, J. Murphy, M.L. Blaxter, F.A. Roe and M.L. Sartirana for their contribution to these studies; particular thanks go to J. Paul and N.M. Wilkie for their interest in, discussions of, and comments on our work. We are also grateful to the secretarial staff of the Beatson Institute and, in particular, to Miss Ruth Forbes, for their excellent assistance and to D. Tallach for skilful photographic work.

## REFERENCES

1. Jarrett WFH, McNeil PE, Grimshaw WTR, Selman IE and McIntyre WIM (1978). High incidence area of cattle cancer with a possible interaction between an environmental carcinogen and a papillomavirus. Nature 274: 215.

2. Kreider JW (1980). Neoplastic progression of the Shope rabbit papilloma. In Essex, Todaro and zur Hausen (Eds.) "Viruses in Naturally Occurring Cancers", Cold Spring Harbor Laboratory, p. 283.
3. Orth G, Favre M, Breitburd F, Croissant O, Jablonska S, Obolek S, Jarzabek-Chorzelska M and Rzesa G (1980). Epidermodysplasia verruciformis: a model for the role of papillomaviruses in human cancer. In Essex, Todaro and zur Hausen (Eds.) "Viruses in Naturally Occurring Cancers", Cold Spring Harbor Laboratory, pp. 259.
4. Ostrow RS, Bender M, Niimura M, Seki T, Kawashima M, Pass F and Faras AJ (1982). Human papillomavirus DNA in cutaneous primary and metastasized squamous cell carcinomas from patients with Epidermodysplasia verruciformis. Proc Natl Acad Sci 79: 1634.
5. Kremsdorf D, Jablonska S, Favre M and Orth G (1983). Human papillomaviruses associated with epidermodysplasia verruciformis. II. Molecular cloning and biochemical characterization of human papillomaviruses 3a, 8, 10 and 12 genomes. J Virol 48: 340.
6. Durst M, Gissman L, Ikenberg H and zur Hausen H (1983). A new type of papillomavirus DNA from a cervical carcinoma and its prevalence on cancer biopsies from different geographic regions. Proc Natl Acad Sci 80: 3812.
7. Boshart M, Gissmann, L, Ikenberg H, Kleinheinz A, Scheurlen W and zur Hausen H (1984). A new type of papillomavirus DNA, its presence in genital cancer biopsies and in cell lines derived from cervical cancer. EMBO J 3: 1151.
8. Wettstein FO and Stevens JG (1982). Variable-sized free episomes of Shope papilloma virus DNA are present in all non-virus producing neoplasms and integrated episomes are detected in some. Proc Natl Acad Sci USA, 79: 790.
9. Jarrett WFH, McNeil PE, Laird HM, O'Neil BW, Murphy J, Campo MS and Moar MH (1980). Papilloma viruses in benign and malignant tumours of cattle. In: Essex, Todaro and zur Hausen (Eds.), "Viruses in Naturally Occurring Cancers", Cold Spring Harbor Laboratory, p.215.
10. Jarrett WFH, Murphy J, O'Neil BW and Laird HM (1978a). Virus-induced papillomas of the alimentary tract of cattle. Int J Cancer 22: 323.

11. Campo MS, Moar MH, Jarrett WFH and Laird HM (1980). A new papillomavirus associated with alimentary tract cancer in cattle. Nature 286: 180.
12. Campo MS and Coggins LW (1982). Molecular cloning of bovine papillomavirus genomes and comparison of their sequence homologies by heteroduplex mapping. J Gen Virol 63: 255.
13. Campo MS and Spandidos DA (1983). Molecularly cloned bovine papillomavirus DNA transforms mouse fibroblasts in vitro. J Gen Virol 64: 549.
14. Jarrett WFH, Campo MS, O'Neil BW, Laird HM and Coggins LW (1984). A novel bovine papillomavirus (BPV-6) causing true epithelial papillomas of the mammary gland skin: a member of a proposed new BPV subgroup. Virology 136: 225.
15. Smith KT, Patel KR, MacSorley DAW and Campo MS (1985). Transcriptional organisation of bovine papillomaviruses type 4. J Virol (in press).
16. Campo MS, Moar MH, Laird HM and Jarrett WJF (1981). Molecular heterogeneity and lesion site specificty of cutaneous bovine papillomaviruses. Virology 113: 323.
17. Coggins LW, Ma JQ, Slater AA and Campo MS (1985). Sequence homologies between bovine papillomavirus genomes mapped by a novel low-stringency heteroduplex method. Virology (in press).
18. Chirgwin JM, Przybyla AE, MacDonald RJ and Rutter WJ (1979). Isolation of biologically active ribonucleic acid from sources enriched in ribonuclease. Biochemistry 18: 5294.
19. Weislander L (1979). A simple method to recover intact high molecular weight RNA and DNA after electrophoretic separation in low gelling temperature agarose gels. Anal Biochem 98: 305.
20. Southern EM (1975). Detection of specific sequences among DNA fragments separated by gel electrophoresis. J Mol Biol 98: 503.
21. Rigby P, Rhodes D, Dieckman M and Berg P (1977). Labelling deoxyribonucleic acid to high specific activity in vitro by nick translation with DNA polymerase I. J Mol Biol 113: 237.
22. Lehrach H, Diamond D, Wozney DJM and Boedtker DH (1977). RNA molecular weight determinations by gel-electrophoresis under denaturing conditions, a critical reexamination. Biochemistry 16: 4743.

23. Jarrett WFH (1981). Papillomaviruses and Cancer. In Anthony and MacSween (Eds.), "Recent Advances in Histopathology", Churchill Livingstone Publishers, p. 35.
24. Coggins LW, Hettich I, Smith KT, Slater AA, Roe FA, Pfister H and Campo MS (1983). The genomes of bovine papillomaviruses types 3 and 4 are colinear. J Gen Virol 64: 2771.
25. Danos O, Giri I, Thierry F. and Yaniv M (1984). Papillomavirus genomes: sequences and consequences. J Invest Dermatol 83: 7s.
26. Schwarz E, Durst M, Demankowski C, Lattermann O, Zech R, Wolfsperger E, Suhai S and zur Hausen H (1983). DNA sequence and genome organization of genital human papillomavirus type 6b. EMBO J 2: 2341.
27. Georges E, Croissant O, Bonneaud N and Orth G (1984). Physical state and transcription of the cottontail rabbit papillomavirus genome in warts and transplantable VX2 and VX7 carcinomas of domestic rabbits. J Virol 51: 530.
28. Nasseri M and Wettstein FO (1984). Differences exist between viral transcripts in cottontail rabbit papillomavirus-induced benign and malignant tumours as well as non-virus-producing and virus producing tumours. J Virol 51: 706.
29. Chow LT and Broker TR (1984). Human papilloma virus type 1 RNA transcription and processing in COS-1 cells. In Pearson and Steinberg (Eds.), "Gene Transfer and Cancer". Raven Press, New York, p. 125.
30. Lancaster WD (1981). Apparent lack of integration of bovine papillomavirus DNA in virus-induced equine and bovine tumours and virus-transformed mouse cells. Virology 108: 251.
31. Amtmann E, Muller H and Sauer G (1980). Equine connective tissue tumours contain unintegrated bovine papilloma virus DNA. J Virol 35: 962.
32. Pfister H, Fink B and Thomas C (1981). Extra-chromosomal bovine papillomavirus type 1 DNA in hamster fibromas and fibrosarcomas. Virology 115: 414.
33. Moar MH, Campo MS, Laird HM and Harrett WFH (1981). Unintegrated viral DNA sequences in a hamster tumour induced by bovine papillomavirus. J Virol 39: 945.

34. Moar MH, Campo MS, Laird HM and Jarrett WFH (1981). Persistence of nonintegrated viral DNA in bovine cells transformed in vitro by bovine papillomavirus type 2. Nature 293: 749.
35. Law M-F, Lowy DR, Dvoretsky I and Howley PM (1981). Mouse cells transformed by bovine papillomavirus contain only extrachromosomal viral DNA sequences. Proc Natl Acad Sci USA 78: 2727.
36. Evans A, Prorok JH, Cole RC, Al-Samani MH, Al-Samarrai AMH, Patel MC and Smith RMM (1982). The carcinogenic, mutagenic and teratogenic toxicity of bracken. In "Proceedings of the Royal Society of Edinburgh" 81B: p. 65.
37. Ushijima J, Matsukawa K, Yuase A and Okada M (1983). Toxicities of bracken fern in guinea pigs. Jpn J Vet Sci 45: 593.
38. Evans WC, Patel MC and Koohy Y (1982). Acute bracken poisoning in homogastric and ruminant animals. In "Proceedings of the Royal Society of Edinburgh" 81B: 29 .
39. Greenberg ME and Ziff EB (1984). Stimulation of 3T3 cells induces transcription of the c-fos proto-oncogene. Nature 311: 433.
40. Kruijer W, Cooper JH, Hunter T and Verma IM (1984). Platelet-derived growth factor induces rapid but transient expression of the c-fos gene and protein. Nature: 312: 711.
41. Muller R, Bravo R, Burkhardt J and Curran T (1984). Induction of c-fos gene and protein by growth factors precedes activation of c-myc. Nature 312: 716.
42. Pfister H (1984). Biology and biochemistry of papillomaviruses. Rev Physiol Biochem Pharmacol 99: 111.
43. Jarrett WFH, Campo MS, Blaxter ML, O'Neil BW, Laird HM, Moar MH and Sartirana ML (1984). Alimentary fibropapilloma in cattle: A spontaneous tumour, non-permissive for papillomavirus replication. J Natl Cancer Inst 73: 499.

**Papillomaviruses: Molecular and Clinical Aspects, pages 327–340**


# CHARACTERIZATION OF THE STRUCTURAL POLYPEPTIDES OF THE COTTONTAIL RABBIT (SHOPE) PAPILLOMA VIRUS BY SODIUM DODECYL SULFATE-POLYACRYLAMIDE GEL ELECTROPHORESIS AND TRYPTIC PEPTIDE MAPPING[1]

Mark A. Feitelson,[2] Felix O. Wettstein,[3] and Jack G. Stevens

Department of Microbiology and Immunology
UCLA School of Medicine
Los Angeles, California 90024

ABSTRACT Purified cottontail rabbit (Shope) papilloma virus (CRPV) was radiolabeled by direct iodination using chloramine T or by indirect iodination (acylation) using the Bolton-Hunter reagent. Structural polypeptides were then characterized by sodium dodecyl sulfate-polyacrylamide gel electrophoresis (SDS-PAGE) and tryptic peptide mapping. SDS-PAGE of these preparations showed a major polypeptide at 67,000 daltons, 5-7 bands between 20,000 and 60,000 daltons, and 3 bands below 20,000 daltons in size which comigrated with calf thymus histones. The peptide map of the major polypeptide shared 45% homology with the intermediate size polypeptides (20,000-60,000

---

[1]This work was supported by grant CA-18151 from the National Cancer Institute, National Institutes of Health, the California Institute for Cancer Research and the Cancer Research Coordinating Committee of the University of California. M.A.F. was a recipient of a National Research Service Award CA-9030.

[2]Present address: Fox Chase Cancer Center, Philadelphia, PA 19111.

[3]Present address: Department of Microbiology and Immunology, UCLA School of Medicine, Los Angeles, CA 90024; and Molecular Biology Institute, University of California, Los Angeles, CA 90024.

daltons), while the maps of these intermediate size components shared 70-75% homology among themselves. The results suggest that CRPV DNA possesses one gene coding for the major structural polypeptide and another coding for the family of intermediate size components. However, the apparent size of the major capsid polypeptide as well as its relationship to the intermediate size class of polypeptides suggest that some of its translated sequences are derived from the gene encoding these intermediate size components. These relationships could be the result of RNA splicing, post-translational modification, or both. Based upon this data, 40-50% of the virus genome encodes the major and intermediate size structural polypeptides of the Shope papilloma virus.

## INTRODUCTION

The cottontail rabbit (Shope) papilloma virus (CPRV) is a member of the family Papovaviradae (1). It is an unenveloped, 55 nm diameter icosahedron made up of 72 morphological units of structural protein (2), which surround a supercoiled molecule of DNA approximately 5 x $10^6$ daltons in size (4, 5, 7). In Eastern cottontail and domestic rabbits virus infection often results in the appearance of papillomas, some of which progress to carcinomas (21, 23). Two transplantable carcinomas, designated Vx2 and Vx7, derived from the metastatic tumors of CRPV infected domestic rabbits, have been passaged in vivo and in vitro for many years, providing models to study virus gene expression in the transformed state (3, 8). The association of CRPV with benign and malignant disease is also observed with several bovine papilloma viruses (BPVs) in cattle and human papilloma viruses (HPVs) in man (24, 34).

The gene products of CRPV and other related viruses responsible for replication, maturation as well as generation of both papillomas and carcinomas are poorly understood due, in part, to the lack of one or more tissue culture systems capable of supporting viral replication. These limits have partially been overcome by the cloning and sequencing of several papilloma virus genomes (14, 18, 19, 28, 31, 33), and with the characterization of viral transcripts obtained from papillomas and carcinomas mainly in the CRPV (30, 32) and BPV (24, 25, 29) systems.

Early studies directed toward the characterization of the CRPV protein from purified virus particles on polyacrylamide gels revealed a single polypeptide component (4) having a carboxy terminal theonine, a carboxy terminal sequence of tyr-leu-ala-thr, and an amino terminus which was probably blocked. Amino acid analysis revealed no special features, save that a higher proportion of acidic than basic residues was found (4). The CRPV polypeptide also required treatment with mercaptoethanol prior to SDS-PAGE for visualization within a separating gel (9). Later studies using SDS-PAGE revealed five to ten proteins (10, 11) ranging from 14,000 to 85,000 daltons in size. The major polypeptide was reported to have an apparent molecular weight of 60,000 daltons (11) or 54,000 daltons (10, 12). Two to 4 small proteins with molecular weights between 10,000 and 20,000 daltons were also found in CRPV (1, 10, 11), as well as in other papilloma viruses (10-13, 16, 22, 26, 27), and may be cellular histones. Minor polypeptide species both larger and smaller than the major components have also been observed in some studies (10-13, 16, 22, 26, 27). It is not known whether these are aggregates or breakdown products of the major polypeptide or whether one or more represent unique gene products of CRPV. Since the number and size of CRPV structural polypeptides vary among published studies (10-12) and it is not known whether one or both of the late genes are actually expressed in the virus as capsid components, purified CRPV was analyzed by SDS-PAGE and tryptic peptide mapping to ascertain the genetic organization of the CRPV late region.

## MATERIALS AND METHODS

Desert cottontails (<u>Sylvilagus audonboni</u>), Eastern cottontails and domestic rabbits were infected at multiple scarified sites on the back with 300 $ID_{50}$ of the Washington B strain of CRPV as described (17). For preparation of virions, 3-5 grams of papilloma tissue snap frozen in liquid nitrogen and stored at -70°C, were ground to a powder in a mortar cooled with dry ice. The sample was divided into 3-4 aliquots, each mixed with 3 ml of 0.02 M Tris-HCl, 0.002 M EDTA, pH 7.4, and then homogenized twice in an ice cooled homogenizer (Sorvall Omni Mixer) at 45,000 rpm for 5 minutes, followed by centrifugation at 5000 rpm for 5 minutes. Pellets were homogenized twice more and centrifuged as above. All of the supernatants were pooled, concentrated by Ficoll at 4°C, and finally clarified by centrifugation at 10,000 rpm, 15 minutes, 4°C. A small aliquot of this supernatant was labeled by chloramine T catalyzed iodination to follow the virus during subsequent purification. Virus was purified by centrifugation on 0.5-1.5 M sucrose gradients made up in 0.0067 M sodium phosphate buffer, pH 7.4, in a SW 27.1 rotor (Beckman) at 27,000 rpm, 3 hours, 4°C. Fractions containing the virus (confirmed by electron microscopy) were dialyzed for two days against phosphate buffer and then centrifuged to equilibrium with CsCl in an SW 50.1 rotor (Beckman), 40,000 rpm, 18-20 hours, 25°C. Virus-containing fractions were pooled, dialyzed, checked for purity and integrity by electron microscopy, and stored at 4°C. Two grams of three different control tissues (normal rabbit skin, DMBA induced papilloma and virus induced papilloma, all from domestic rabbits) were subjected to the same procedure. Virus samples were then radiolabeled either by direct iodination using chloramine T or by acetylation using the Bolton-Hunter reagent as described (20, except that SDS was not used during labeling), subjected to SDS-PAGE, and finally tryptic peptide mapping on thin layer cellulose plates (20).

## RESULTS

### Radiolabeling and Polypeptide Profile of CRPV on SDS Gels.

Samples of purified, intact CRPV were radiolabeled by direct iodination using chloramine T or by acylation using the Bolton-Hunter reagent. Chloramine T iodinated virus particles resolved into as many as 13 bands on 15% discontinuous SDS-polyacrylamide separating gels, although only 10 bands were consistently present among independent labelings and gel runs (Table 1). Radioacylation with the Bolton-Hunter reagent resulted in clearer profiles (having less background) with 9 reproducible bands, as shown in Figure 1. Both methods yielded a major band with an apparent molecular weight of 66,000-68,000 daltons (VP2, Table 1). In addition, the chloramine T iodinated profile showed a band at 72,000 daltons (VP1) and sometimes a band at 115,000 daltons (VP0) which were absent from the gel profiles of radioacylated CRPV components. The relationship of the components in this "high molecular weight group" (VP0, VP1 and VP2) to each other and the lower molecular weight polypeptides were further examined by tryptic peptide mapping as described below.

Table 1
SIZE DISTRIBUTION OF THE COTTONTAIL RABBIT (SHOPE) PAPILLOMA VIRUS STRUCTURAL POLYPEPTIDES

| Viral protein designation | Direct iodination[a] | Acylation labeling[b] |
|---|---|---|
| High molecular weight group | | |
| VP0 | 115[c,e] | |
| VP1 | 72 | |
| VP2 | 66[d] (underscored) | 68 (underscored) |
| Intermediate molecular weight group | | |
| VP3 | 56[e] | |
| VP4 | 51 | 53 |
| VP5 | 46 | 46.5 |
| VP6 | 42 | 41 |
| VP7 | 36 | |
| VP8 | 27 | |
| VP9 | 25 | 25 |
| VP10 | | 20.8 |
| Low molecular weight group | | |
| VP11 | 15.5 | 15.3 |
| VP12 | 14.2 | 13.7 |
| VP13 | 13 | 11.8 |

[a]Chloramine T iodinated CRPV polypeptides analyzed on 10% or 15% discontinuous SDS-polyacrylamide separating gels.

[b]Bolton-Hunter reagent acylated CRPV polypeptides analyzed on 15% discontinuous SDS-polyacrylamide separating gels.

[c]Molecular weights are reported in daltons x $10^{-3}$.

[d]Underscored molecular weight values indicate the major capsid polypeptide.

[e]Protein bands not evident in all preparations of chloramine T iodinated virus.

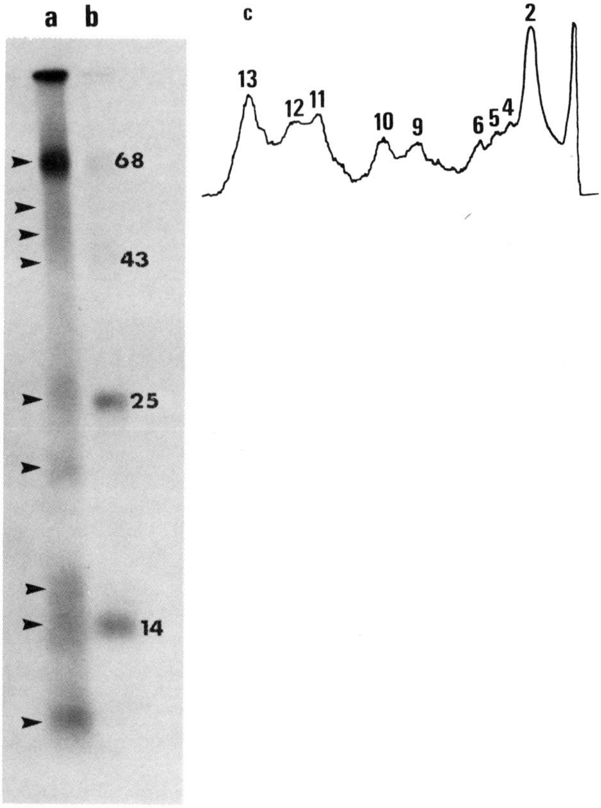


FIGURE 1. Discontinuous SDS-PAGE of acylated CRPV polypeptides. CRPV particles were labeled with freshly prepared Bolton-Hunter reagent. The polypeptides were further modified and resolved by SDS-PAGE exactly as described (20). The gels were then fixed, dried and autoradiographed (20). In (a) arrows indicate each of the radioacylated polypeptide bands. Molecular weight values were derived by comparison to the migration of (b) radioacylated marker polypeptides BSA (68K), ovalbumin (43K), chymotrypsinogen (25K), and hen egg lysozyme (14K). (c) Gel scan of the radioacylated CRPV associated polypeptides from the autoradiographic profile in (a). The top part of the vertical separating gel begins with the right side of the scan. Numerical designations above each peak indicate the viral polypeptide (VP) band seen on the autoradiogram in part (a) and recorded in Table 1.

An "intermediate molecular weight group" of polypeptides with apparent molecular weights from 20,000-60,000 daltons were resolved on 10% and 15% acrylamide slab gels following either labeling procedure. Here, iodination resulted in 7 minor bands while acylation revealed only 5. Both labeling procedures reproducibly demonstrated bands at 51,000-53,000 daltons (VP4), 46,000 daltons (VP5), 41,000-42,000 daltons (VP6), and at 25,000 daltons (VP9) (Table 1). Direct iodination also reproducibly showed bands at 36,000 daltons (VP7) and 27,000 daltons (VP8) which were not observed on any of the radioacylated gel profiles. In contrast, radioacylation reproducibly showed a band at 20,800 daltons (VP10) not seen by direct iodination. Either the consequences of direct iodination (oxidation by chloramine T or reduction by metabisulfite (6)) or the differential availability of the intact virion for radiolabeling may account for these differences.

Both labeling procedures also resulted in three polypeptides in the "low molecular weight group" (10,000-20,000 daltons; VP11, VP12 and VP13) which comigrated with calf thymus histones by SDS-PAGE (Figure 1, Table 1) and may represent these cell derived components.

Analysis of Bolton-Hunter reagent labeled polypeptides derived from control tissue extracts (normal skin, DMBA papilloma and domestic rabbit papilloma) by SDS-PAGE revealed faint bands in the region of the gel where the intermediate molecular weight group of proteins migrated (data not shown). The dissimilarities in gel profiles between control tissues and viral polypeptides combined with the absence of intense bands from the control tissues suggest that the components seen in the analysis are in fact viral polypeptides and not tissue contaminants. Further, peptide mapping of control tissue bands (where enough counts were present for such analysis) revealed maps which did not in any way resemble those of the CRPV polypeptides presented below.

Analysis of Individual CRPV Polypeptides by Tryptic Peptide Mapping.

Tryptic peptide mapping of chloramine T iodinated or radioacylated CRPV associated components was carried out to discern the structural relationships among them. Both labeling procedures yielded the same results. Figure 2 shows the autoradiograms of chloramine T iodinated VP2, VP4 and VP5 peptide maps presented with a composite diagram outlining the relationship between VP2 and the intermediate size polypeptides. From the composite in Figure 2d, approximately 31% of the peptide spots in VP2 are shared with all intermediate sized polypeptides and another 13% with some of the components in this group. The overall degree of relatedness, then, between VP2 and the intermediate molecular weight group is 45%. The intermediate size polypeptides share about 70-75% homology. Each component of this class, however, displayed several unique spots (up to 10% of the spots in each map), while the remainder of the spots were common to some but not all of these intermediate size polypeptides. Comparison of the maps of VP1 with VP2 demonstrated few differences, suggesting that the appearance of VP1 in the chloramine T iodinated profile may be due to oxidation and/or reduction of VP2 by direct iodination. Such damage could slightly alter the binding characteristics of VP2 with SDS, resulting in an artifactual doublet (data not shown, 6, 11). Direct iodination could also give rise to artifactual aggregation of one or more polypeptides on SDS gels. Indeed, comparative peptide mapping of VP0 with the other components in the high and intermediate molecular weight groups demonstrates virtual identify with VP4, suggesting dimerization (data not shown). Overall, the peptide mapping data suggest that all of the CRPV associated polypeptides are closely related to each other, except that the major component, VP2, also contains a large percentage of unique spots (55%) not found in the maps of any other CRPV associated polypeptide.

## DISCUSSION

As summarized in Table 1, the SDS-PAGE profiles of the CRPV associated structural polypeptides labeled by two different methods reproducibly demonstrated a single major viral component (VP2), a number of intermediate size components observed by both labeling procedures (VP4-6), and three low molecular weight components (VP11-13) comigrating with calf thymus histones. Recent sequence analysis of several papilloma virus genomes shows that the late region of each is composed of two open reading frames (L1 and L2) that alone or in some combination encode one or more structural polypeptides of these viruses (14, 18, 19, 24, 28, 31-33). Although L1 and L2 are in different translational reading frames in the different viruses, each appears capable of encoding a polypeptide roughly 50,000-55,000 daltons in size. While SDS-PAGE analysis of CRPV polypeptides have

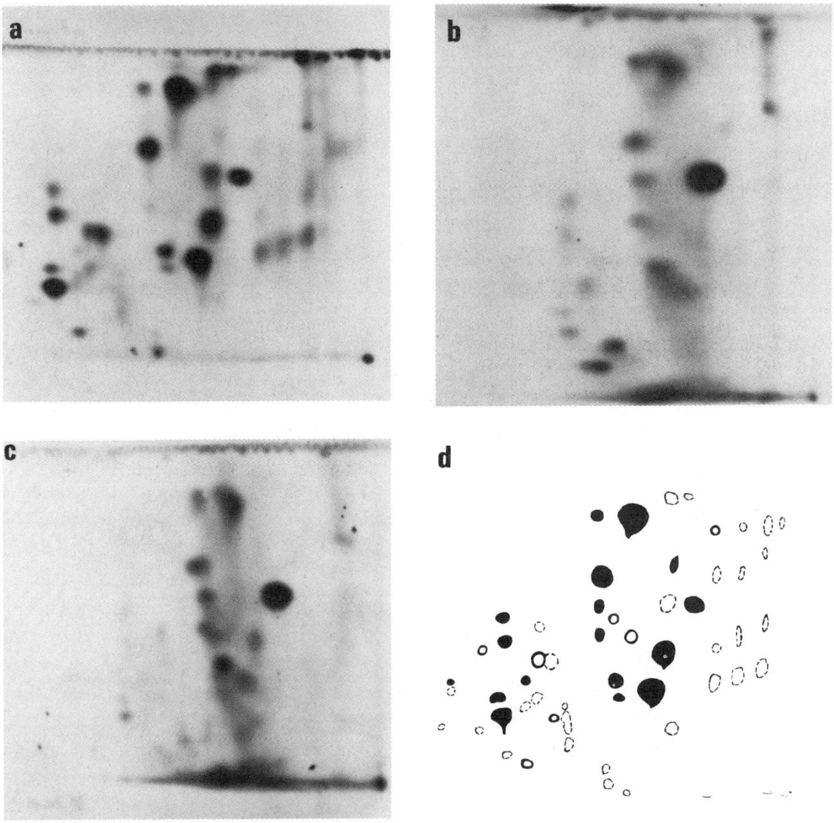


FIGURE 2. Tryptic peptide maps and peptide map composite of chloramine T iodinated CRPV polypeptides. Details of the methods used to iodinate CRPV particles, resolve individual polypeptides by SDS-PAGE, and generate tryptic peptide maps of each have already been described (20). In the autoradiograms, electrophoresis is from right to left and chromatography from bottom to top. Repetitive two dimensional peptide mapping of a given polypeptide from the same or different labelings demonstrated less than 5% variability in patterns due to differences between individual experiments. (a) VP2; (b) VP4; (c) VP5; (d) composite of VP2 and all intermediate sized polypeptides. Filled spots (●) are peptides common to VP2 and all intermediate sized polypeptides; empty spots (o) are common to more than one intermediate sized polypeptide; and dashed spots (◌) are unique to VP2.

demonstrated a single major component at about 54,000 daltons (10, 12) and similar results have been obtained with BPV (10, 13, 22) and HPV preparations (10, 12, 16, 22, 26, 27), the size of the CRPV major polypeptide has also been reported to be 60,000 daltons (11) and that of an HPV isolate approximately 63,000 daltons (11). In some HPV isolates a major doublet roughly between 50,000 and 60,000 daltons has been observed (16, 26, 27). Whether these results and the observation here that the CRPV major polypeptide is 66,000-68,000 daltons are due to strain variations is not known. However, the reported presence of several bovine and many human papilloma virus types in natural infections (23, 34) is consistent with there being variants on the molecular level.

The high degree of nucleic acid sequence homology noted among the L1 genes of the various papilloma viruses compared to the L2 regions (14, 19, 25, 33), the fact that the major polypeptide species of HPV and CRPV isolates share antigenic cross-reactivity (12), and the point that discrete wart specific RNA species mapping almost exclusively to L1 have been found (24, 25, 29, 32) suggest that the major capsid polypeptide of these viruses is encoded by L1. Comparison of the amino acid composition of the BPV-1 major structural polypeptide isolated from virions with the composition deduced from the nucleic acid sequences of BPV-1 L1 or L2 open reading frames indicates that the major polypeptide is more closely related to L1 than L2, but that there are still many differences between the predicted and actual amino acid compositions (19). In CRPV, some of the wart specific 4.8 kb RNAs mapping to the combined L1 and L2 regions have a small splice at the junction area of L1 and L2, removing a translation stop codon at the end of L2, suggesting that fusion polypeptides could be made from such RNAs. Polypeptides larger than the coding capacity of L1 have been reported in many papilloma virus preparations (10-13, 16, 22) and react with monoclonal antibodies (15) as well as sera from Vx7 tumor bearing rabbits (12), suggesting that these larger components are virus related and may be fusion products of L1 and L2. The characteristics of CRPV VP2 are consistent with it being a fusion product since by apparent molecular weight it exceeds the coding capacity of either L1 or L2 and that it contains many unique tryptic spots absent from each of the intermediate sized polypeptides. While it could be argued that the unique spots in VP2 represent a contaminant, it would have to bind very tightly to VP2 and not at all to any of the other polypeptide components even though they share a substantial amount of primary sequence homology. A contaminant migrating at 66,000-68,000 daltons (with VP2), further, must also migrate at 72,000 daltons (with VP1) after chloramine T iodination in order to generate the nearly identical peptide maps of VP1 and VP2. In addition, such a contaminant is not found in DMBA induced papillomas or normal tissue since no bands were found near these size values by SDS-PAGE. While these considerations do not prove the purity of the major CRPV polypeptide analyzed herein, they argue against the presence of such a contaminant.

There is considerable evidence suggesting the presence of one or more minor polypeptide species migrating like those in the intermediate size group presented above (10-13, 16, 22, 26, 27). Contributing to this variability may be partial proteolysis in situ prior to virus isolation. The use of trypsin in many of the isolation protocols used in papilloma virus work might also contribute, since it has been demonstrated that the major capsid polypeptide of HPV-1 is trypsin sensitive (27). The use of low temperature and EDTA to inhibit proteases during virus isolation here were chosen to limit proteolysis during purification. While limited evidence suggests that the major polypeptide in HPV isolates may be degraded to a component in the intermediate size group (26), it is not clear that this actually occurs post-translationally. Alternatively, the possibility exists that one or more intermediate size polypeptides may be generated from one of the late genes by differential splicing of the same transcript giving rise to the major capsid component. If this is so, and it seems by their structure that the late RNAs of BPV and CRPV are generated by differential splicing (15, 24, 32), then translation of the major component may derive from both of the late genes while translation of one or more of the intermediate sized polypeptides may derive exclusively from one of the late genes. The results here are consistent with the model that both late genes encode CRPV structural polypeptides, although alternative interpretations are certainly possible. Based upon the size and relationship of VP2 to VP4 (the largest of the intermediate group reproducibly found), some 40-50% of the viral genome would be required to encode these structural components. This is consistent with the size of the late regions of the papilloma virus genomes already published.

ACKNOWLEDGMENTS

The assistance by M. Cook with electron microscopy is gratefully acknowledged.

REFERENCES

1. Melnick JL, Allison AC, Butel JS, Eckhart W, Eddy BE, Kit S, Levine AJ, Miles JAR, Pagano JS, Sachs L, Vonka V. (1974). Papovaviridae. Intervirology 3:106.
2. Finch JT, Klug A. (1965). The structure of viruses of the papilloma-polyoma type. III. Structure of rabbit papilloma virus. J Molec Biol 13:1.
3. Osato T, Ito Y. (1967). In vitro cultivation and immunofluorescent studies of transplantable carcinomas Vx2 and Vx7. Persistence of a Shope virus-related antigenic substance in the cells of both tumors. J Exp Med 126:881.
4. Kass SJ, Knight CA. (1965). Purification and chemical analysis of Shope papilloma virus. Virology 27:273.
5. Watson JD, Littlefield JW. (1960). Some properties of DNA from Shope papilloma virus. J Molec Biol 2:161.
6. Hunter WM. (1967). The preparation of radioiodinated proteins of high activity. Their reaction with antibody in vitro: the radioimmunoassay. In Weir (ed): "Handbook of Immunology," Philadelphia: Davis, p. 608.
7. Kleinschmidt AK, Kass SJ, Williams RC, Knight CA. (1965). Cyclic DNA of Shope papilloma virus. J Molec Biol 13:749.
8. Kidd JG, Rous P. (1940). A transplantable rabbit carcinoma originating in a virus-induced papilloma and containing the virus in a masked or altered form. J Exp Med 71:813.
9. Kass SJ. (1970). Chemical studies on polyoma and Shope papilloma viruses. J Virol 5:381.
10. Favre M, Breitburd F, Croissant O, Orth G. (1975). Structural polypeptides of rabbit, bovine and human papilloma viruses. J Virol 15:1239.
11. Spira G, Estes MK, Dreesman GR, Butel JS, Rawls WE. (1974). Papovavirus structural polypeptides: Comparison of human and rabbit papilloma viruses with simian virus 40. Intervirology 3:220.
12. Orth G, Breitburd F, Favre M. (1978). Evidence for antigenic determinants shared by the structural polypeptides of (Shope) rabbit papillomavirus and human papillomavirus type 1. Virology 91:243.
13. Meinke W, Meinke GC. (1981). Isolation and characterization of the major capsid protein of bovine papillomavirus type 1. J Gen Virol 52:15.

14. Schwarz E, Durst M, Demankowski C, Lattermann O, Zech R, Wolfsperger E, Suhai S, zur Hausen H. (1983). DNA sequence and genome organization of genital human papillomavirus type 6b. EMBO J 2:2341.
15. Roseto A, Pothier P, Guillemin M-C, Peries J, Breitburd F, Bonneaud N, Orth G. (1984). Monoclonal antibodies to the major capsid protein of human papillomavirus type 1. J Gen Virol 65:1319.
16. Gissmann L, Pfister H, zur Hausen H. (1977). Human papilloma viruses (HPV): Characterization of four different isolates. Virology 76:569.
17. Stevens JG, Wettstein FO. (1979). Multiple copies of Shope virus DNA are present in cells of benign and malignant non-virus producing neoplasms. J Virol 30: 891.
18. Danos O, Katinka M, Yaniv M. (1982). Human papilloma-virus la complete DNA sequence: a novel type of genome organization among Papovaviridae. EMBO J 1:231.
19. Ahola H, Stenlund A, Moreno-Lopez J, Pettersson U. (1983). Sequences of bovine papillomavirus type 1 DNA-functional and evolutionary implications. Nucleic Acids Research 11:2639.
20. Feitelson MA, Wettstein FO, Stevens JG. (1981). Tryptic peptide mapping of picomolar quantities of protein labeled with the Bolton-Hunter reagent. Analytical Biochem 116:473.
21. Kreider JW. (1980). Neoplastic progression of the Shope rabbit papilloma. In Essex M, Todaro G, zur Hausen H (eds): "Viruses in Naturally Occurring Cancers," New York, Cold Spring Harbor Laboratory, p. 283.
22. Favre M, Breitburd F, Croissant O, Orth G. (1977). Chromatin-like structures obtained after alkaline disruption of bovine and human papillomaviruses. J Virol 21:1205.
23. Lancaster WD, Olson C. (1982). Animal papilloma-viruses. Microbiol Reviews 46:191.
24. Howley PM. (1983). The molecular biology of papillomavirus transformation. Am J Pathol 113:414.
25. Danos O, Yaniv M. (1983). Structure and function of papillomavirus genomes. Advances in Viral Oncology 3:59.
26. Pfister H, Gissmann L, zur Hausen H. (1977). Partial characterization of the proteins of human papilloma viruses (HPV) 1-3. Virology 83:131.
27. Pfister H, zur Hausen H. (1978). Characterization of proteins of human papilloma viruses (HPV) and antibody response to HPV 1. Med Microbiol Immunol 166:13.

28. Giri IO, Danos O, Yaniv M. Submitted for publication.
29. Engel LW, Heilman CA, Howley PM. (1983). Transcriptional organization of bovine papillomavirus type 1. J Virol 47:516.
30. Nasseri M, Wettstein FO. (1984). Cottontail rabbit papillomavirus-specific transcripts in transplantable tumors with integrated DNA. Virology 138:362.
31. Chen EY, Howley PM, Levinson AD, Seeburg PH. (1982). The primary structure and genetic organization of the bovine papillomavirus type 1 genome. Nature 299:529.
32. Nasseri M, Wettstein FO. (1984). Differences exist between viral transcripts in cottontail rabbit papilloma-virus-induced benign and malignant tumors as well as non-virus-producing and virus-producing tumors. J Virol 51:706.
33. Danos O, Engel LW, Chen EY, Yaniv M, Howley PM. (1983). A comparative analysis of the human type 1a and bovine type 1 papillomavirus genomes. J Virol 46:557.
34. Orth G, Favre M, Breitburd F, Croissant O, Jablonska S, Obalek S, Jarzabek-Chorzelska M, Rzesa G. (1980). Epidermodysplasia verruciformis: A model for the role of papilloma viruses in human cancer. In Essex M, Todaro G, zur Hausen H (eds): "Viruses in Naturally Occurring Cancers," New York: Cold Spring Harbor Laboratory, p. 259.

# VI. MOLECULAR BIOLOGY: TRANSCRIPTION, REPLICATION, AND GENOME ORGANIZATION

**Papillomaviruses: Molecular and Clinical Aspects, pages 343–361**


# IDENTIFICATION OF A NEW ENHANCER WITHIN THE NON-CODING REGION OF BPV-1 WHICH IS TRANS-ACTIVATED BY BPV-1 EARLY GENE PRODUCTS

Barbara A. Spalholz, Yu-Chung Yang, and Peter M. Howley

Laboratory of Tumor Virus Biology, National Cancer Institute, Bethesda, Maryland 20205

ABSTRACT We have mapped a transcriptional regulatory sequence within the 1.0 kb non-coding region (ncr) of the BPV-1 genome, using an enhancer dependent expression vector for chloramphenicol acetyltransferase (CAT). This transcriptional regulatory element works in a position and orientation independent manner, and its function is significantly augmented in BPV-1 transformed C127 cells. Using mouse C127 cells transformed by defined deletion mutants of the BPV-1 DNA or full-length viral cDNAs expressed from a SV40 early promoter, we demonstrate that the expression of this transactivating factor maps to the 3' open reading frames (ORFs) of the viral transforming region and specifically to the E2 ORF.

## INTRODUCTION

BPV-1, a papillomavirus, causes cutaneous fibropapillomas in cattle and can induce fibroblastic tumors in a variety of foreign hosts including hamsters and rabbits. Papillomaviruses have been difficult to study because they have never been successfully grown in tissue culture. BPV-1, however, is a member of a subgroup of papillomaviruses which is capable of transforming certain rodent cells *in vitro*. Transformation by these papillomaviruses has provided a biologic system for studying the latent, nonproductive infection of cells. In cell lines established from these tumors, and in rodent cell lines transformed in vitro by the virus or its cloned DNA, the viral genome is stably maintained as a multicopy nuclear plasmid (1). All of the detectable polyadenylated RNAs in BPV-1 transformed cells (2) as well as in productively infected cells of the viral induced fibropapillomas (3,4) are transcribed from a single strand. A region sufficient for transformation (5) as well as for stable plasmid maintenance (1) has been mapped to a 69% subgenomic fragment, from which all of the RNAs expressed in transformed cells are transcribed (2). This region of the genome contains eight open reading frames (ORFs) located on the same strand (the coding strand) (6,7) as well as important regulatory sequences. At the 5' end of these ORFs is a 1000 base non-coding region (ncr) which which contains transcription control elements (8), a DNAase I I hypersensitive site (9), the initiation site for plasmid DNA replication in rodent cells (10) and a plasmid maintenance sequence PMS 1 (11).

Lusky et al (12) have also characterized an element 3' to the polyadenylation site at base 4203, which has properties of a transcriptional enhancer in that it can function in an orientation and position independent manner to enhance the transcriptional activity of a heterologous promoter (12). However, recent studies from our laboratory in collaboration with that of J. Dahlberg's have been able to show that this distal enhancer element is not cis-essential for BPV-1 mediated transformation or for maintenance of the plasmid state in transformed cells as previously reported (Howley et al, manuscript in preparation). Currently the biologic function of this enhancer is not known.

To further identify and characterize other possible transcriptional control elements and factors involved in the regulated expression of BPV-1, we have subcloned segments of the viral genome into the $pA_{10}CAT$ vector described by Laimins et al (13) and analyzed its components for transcriptional enhancer function. This vector contains the gene for chloramphenicol acetyltransferase (CAT) behind the SV40 early promoter deleted of its 72 base pair repeat enhancer element. Expression of the CAT gene in this plasmid in mammalian cells is dependent upon the insertion of a functional enhancer to activate the SV40 promoter (14). In this study we show that the ncr of the BPV-1 genome can activate CAT expression from the SV40 promoter in an orientation and position independent manner, but that this enhancer functions only in BPV-1 transformed cells. This restricted activity indicates that this enhancer element is trans-activated by a BPV-1 gene product. Analysis of cell lines transformed by BPV-1 deletion mutants, maps the trans-activation function to the 3' ORFs of the transforming region. Further analysis of cell lines transformed by a series of full length cDNA clones functionally expressed behind the SV40 early gene promoter indicates that the E2 ORF expresses the diffusable factor responsible for the trans-activation of the ncr enhancer element.

## MATERIALS AND METHODS

### Cell Lines.

Mouse C127 cells (15), ID13 cells which are C127 cells transformed by BPV-1 virus (1), and African green monkey kidney CV-1 cells were maintained in Dulbecco's modified Eagle medium (DMEM, Gibco Laboratories) supplemented with penicillin (10 u/ml), streptomycin (100 ug/ml), and fetal bovine serum (10%). Bovine embryo fibroblasts (BEF) were grown from primary fetal bovine dermis for 5 to 8 passages and were maintained as above. Mouse C127 cells transformed by BPV-1 deletion mutants (plasmids, 620-7, 236-12, 327-25, 448-5 and 618-5) described by Sarver et al (8), or cells transformed by BPV-1 cDNAs (C58, C52, C59, C88 and C212) described by Yang et al (16), were also maintained as above.

Cotransformations of mouse C127 cells by the BPV-1 cDNAs, C23, C36, C48, C102 or C119, and pdMMTneo (a plasmid containing the bacterial gene for neomycin resistance within a mammalian transcriptional cassette consisting of the mouse metallothionein promoter, the SV40 small T splicing signals and the SV40 3' processing signals) were performed as described by Sarver et al (8).

### Construction of CAT Recombinant Plasmids.

The $pA_{10}CAT$ plasmid containing the CAT gene driven by the SV40 early promoter deleted of the functional SV40 enhancer and the pSV2CAT plasmid containing the SV40 early promoter with its functional enhancer 5' to the CAT, as shown in Figure 1, have been described previously (13,14).

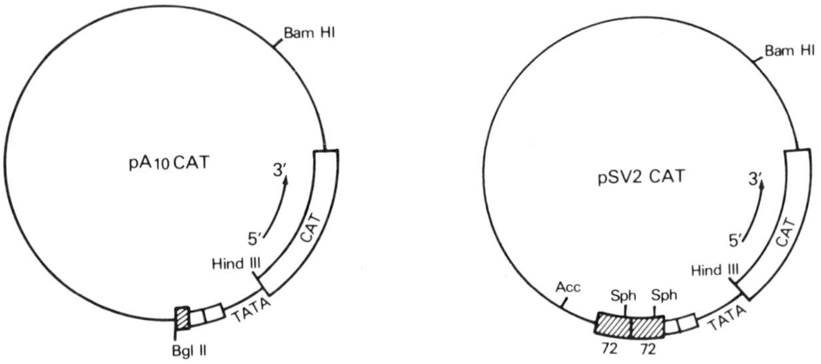


Figure 1. The plasmids $pA_{10}CAT$ and pSV2CAT.

Subgenomic fragments of BPV-1 were prepared by digesting the genome with the restriction endonucleases HindIII, HpaI and BamHI. The resulting fragments were separated by agarose gel electrophoresis and isolated by electroelution, followed by extraction with phenol and precipitation with ethanol. The 1 kb HpaI to HindIII fragment was modified at both termini with BamHI synthetic linkers. The 2.5 kb BamHI to HindIII fragment was modified with a BamHI linker at the HindIII site. Both fragments were cloned separately into the BglII and BamHI sites of $pA_{10}CAT$ in either orientation to generate plasmids p407-1, p407-2, p731-1, p732-1, p764-1, p765-1, p766-1 and p767-1 designated in Figure 2.

The 4.5 kb HpaI to BamHI fragment was further digested with either BglII or BclI and the subsequent 1.5 kb HpaI to BglII, 3.0 kb BglII to BamHI, and 0.6 kb BclI to BamHI frag- were purified as above. The HpaI site was modified with a BamHI linker. Each of these three fragments was cloned into the BglII site of $pA_{10}CAT$ in either orientation to generate the plasmids p405-1, p405-2, p408-1, p408-2, p409-1 and p409-2. Transformation of *Escherichia coli* K-12 HB101 (17), screening of bacterial transformants (18) and propagation of recombinant plasmids (19,20), as well as the molecular manipulations described above, were performed by conventional methods (21).

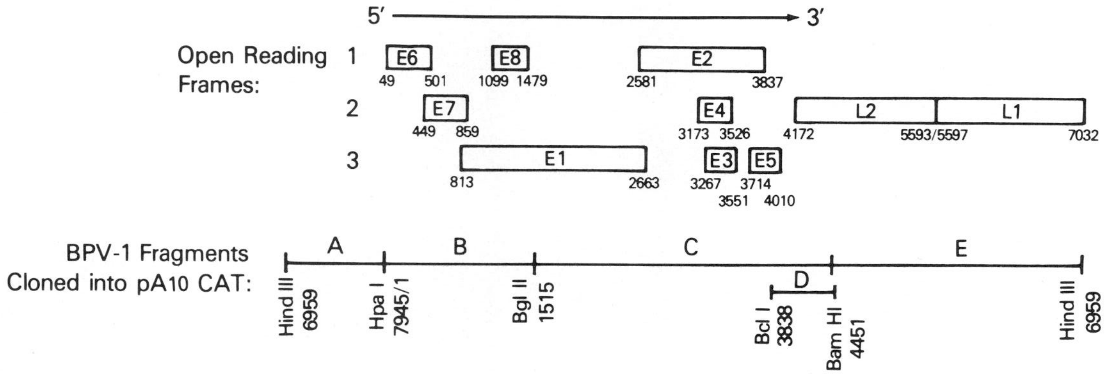


| Position Relative to CAT | Orientation Relative to CAT | Plasmid Number A | B | C | D | E |
|---|---|---|---|---|---|---|
| 5′ | sense | 407-1 | 408-1 | 409-1 | 405-1 | 764-1 |
| 5′ | antisense | 407-2 | 408-2 | 409-2 | 405-2 | 765-1 |
| 3′ | sense | 731-1 | — | — | — | 766-1 |
| 3′ | antisense | 732-1 | — | — | — | 767-1 |

Figure 2. BPV-1 restriction fragments cloned into $pA_{10}CAT$: Plasmid number designation for position and orientation of the BPV-1 fragment relative to the CAT gene. Fragments are shown in reference to BPV-1 open reading frames.

Mammalian Cell Transfections and CAT Assays.

DNA transfections were performed by calcium phosphate coprecipitation (22). The cells were treated with 15% glycerol (23) for 1 minute, four hours after transfection. After washing, the cells were incubated in complete media with 5 mM sodium butyrate for 48 hours (24).

CAT assays were performed on crude cell extracts as described by Gorman et al (14) and Laimins et al (13).

## RESULTS

Generation of BPV-1/CAT Recombinants and Rationale.

Subgenomic fragments of BPV-1 were cloned into $pA_{10}CAT$ as diagrammed in Figure 2. All the fragments were cloned 5' to the CAT gene at the BglII site of $pA_{10}CAT$ in either possible orientation. The HindIII to HpaI fragment and the BamHI to HindIII fragment, representing the ncr and the late transcription ORFs respectively, were also cloned in either orientation 3' to the CAT gene at the BamHI site. Four plasmids, p405-1, p405-2, p409-1 and p409-2, contain the 60 bp distal enhancer element previously described (12,25).

A functional enhancer must be supplied in *cis* to the SV40 promoter in order to activate the CAT expression in these plasmids. The transient expression of the CAT gene is measured 48 hours after transfection into competent mammalian cells, by incubating the crude cellular extract with $[^{14}C]$-labelled chloramphenicol and acetyl CoA and determining the amount of chloramphenicol which is acetylated. Previous studies have established that the level of CAT activity measured is proportional to the extent of RNA transcription of the gene.

Analysis of BPV-1/CAT Recombinant Plasmids for CAT Expression.

In this initial experiment the possibility of species specificity of a BPV-1 enhancer element was tested by assaying each of the BPV-1/CAT recombinant plasmids shown in Figure 2 for CAT expression in CV-1 cells (a monkey kidney cell line); bovine embryo fibroblasts (BEF) isolated from primary bovine embryo dermal tissue; and C127 cells (a mouse cell line).

The results from this experiment are presented in Table 1. Each cell line was tested with $pA_{10}CAT$ which contains

TABLE 1
CAT EXPRESSION FROM CAT RECOMBINANT PLASMIDS IN CELL LINES FROM VARIOUS SPECIES

| Plasmid | CAT ACTIVITY[a] | | | |
|---|---|---|---|---|
| | CV-1 | BEF | C127 | ID13 |
| $pA_{10}CAT$ | - | - | - | - |
| pSV2CAT | ++ | +++ | ++ | +++ |
| p405-1 | - | - | - | - |
| p405-2 | - | - | - | - |
| p407-1 | - | +/- | +/- | ++ |
| p407-2 | - | - | +/- | ++ |
| p731-1 | - | ND | - | + |
| p732-1 | - | ND | - | + |
| p408-1 | - | - | - | - |
| p408-2 | - | - | - | - |
| p409-1 | - | - | - | +/- |
| p409-2 | - | - | - | - |
| p764-1 | - | ND | - | - |
| p765-1 | - | ND | - | - |
| p766-1 | - | ND | - | - |
| p767-1 | - | ND | - | - |

[a] CAT activity was quantitated by measuring the amount of ($^{14}C$) chloramphenicol which was acetylated by the cellular extract in the presence of 4 mM Acetyl CoA after 30 minutes at 37°.

(-) 0-3% Chloramphenicol acetylated
(+) 3-10 % " "
(++) 10-50% " "
(+++) 50-100% " "
(+/-) < 3% but greater than the negative control for that cell line.
(ND) Not done.

no enhancer and serves as a negative control for the expression of CAT, and with pSV2CAT which contains the intact SV40 enhancer and serves as a positive control for CAT expression. The bovine, monkey, and mouse cells transfected with pSV2CAT produced significant quantities of the CAT enzyme indicating that each of the cell lines is competent for the uptake and expression of the CAT gene. None of the BPV-1/CAT recombinant plasmids, however, show any significant CAT expression in these lines, indicating that none of the BPV-1 DNA fragments were capable of activating CAT expression from the SV40 early promoter in any of these three cell lines. Even the DNA fragments containing the distal enhancer element previously described by Lusky et al (12) contained in p405-1 and p405-2 as well as p409-1 and p409-2 were negative in this assay.

We also tested whether any of the BPV-1 fragments cloned into $pA_{10}$CAT could act as an enhancer for CAT expression in ID13 cells (mouse C127 cells stably transformed by BPV-1). This experiment would test whether BPV-1 might encode a diffusable factor that would activate a viral specific _cis_-regulatory element in _trans_. In general, the levels of CAT activity from all CAT plasmids were slightly higher in the ID13 cells than in nontransformed C127 cells, however, CAT expression from the four plasmids containing the BPV-1 ncr p407-1, p407-2, p731-1 and p732-2 was greatly increased. This dramatic increase of CAT activity was most pronounced with the ncr fragment cloned at the 5' _BglII_ site of $pA_{10}$CAT in either transcriptional orientation (p407-1 and p407-2), but was also significantly elevated with the ncr cloned in either orientation at the 3' _BamHI_ site (p731-1 and p732-1). As the ncr fragment can activate the CAT gene from the SV40 promoter in an orientation and position independent manner, we concluded that the ncr contains a classical enhancer element. This activity, however, can only be demonstrated in ID13 cells suggesting that a viral gene product expressed in BPV-1 transformed cells is required in _trans_ to activate this enhancer element.

To determine whether the transcriptional enhancer function of the ncr was specific for BPV-1 transformed cells or was a general property of transformed C127 cells, we tested the levels of CAT expressed by p407-1 in C127 cells which were transformed by polyoma virus middle T antigen using the plasmid pPyMT1 (26) in comparison to the levels expressed in untransformed C127 cells. The pSV2CAT control plasmid is transcriptionally active in this cell line indicating susceptibility to the uptake and expression of the exogenous CAT gene. Using p407-1, however, no significant level of CAT expression could be detected (data not shown). Trans-activation of the BPV-1 ncr enhancer element is, therefore, not a general property of transformed C127 cells and appears to be due to a BPV-1 specific function.

Mapping of the Trans-activation Function.

To determine the region of the BPV-1 genome responsible for the activation of the ncr enhancer, C127 cell lines transformed by various deletion mutants of the BPV-1 genome were transfected with the positive and negative control CAT expression vectors, pSV2CAT and $pA_{10}CAT$, as well as the pBPVncrCAT vector, p407-1. Cell lines which had been transformed by different mutants with deletions mapping in different regions within the early region were chosen so as to investigate the role of defined regions and functions of the genome on the trans-activation of the ncr enhancer (Table 2). The cell lines NS620-7 and NS236-12 were transformed by mutants with deletions which affect the E1 ORF, a region required in trans for plasmid maintenance and replication (8,27). The cell lines NS327-25, NS448-5 and NS618-5 were transformed by mutants which contain deletions of the 3' early region 5' from the BclI site at base 3838 but leave the E1 ORF intact (8). For each of the mutant transforming DNAs, three independent transformed cell lines were assayed and the results are presented as an average in order to randomize any variability in BPV-1 expression due to variables between cell lines such as viral DNA copy number or site of integration.

Each of these cell lines is capable of the uptake and expression of the CAT gene as seen by the $pA_{10}CAT$ and pSV2CAT, negative and positive controls (Table 2). The expression of CAT from p407-1, however, varies depending on the cell line and the specific BPV-1 deletion mutant used for the transformation. In this experiment, CAT expression from p407-1 was increased approximately 5 fold in ID13 cells as compared to the untransformed parent line, C127. Since the ncr also contains PMS 1 (11), a region required in cis for plasmid maintenance and replication, it was important to show that the increased CAT expression from p407-1 in transfected ID13 cells could not be explained by amplification of the plasmid DNA.

TABLE 2

CAT EXPRESSION FROM CAT RECOMBINANT PLASMIDS IN C127 CELLS TRANSFORMED BY BPV-1 DELETION MUTANTS

| Cell Line | BPV-1 Deletion in Transforming DNA[b] | ORFs Affected | CAT Activity[a] | | |
|---|---|---|---|---|---|
| | | | $pA_{10}CAT$ | pSV2CAT | p407-1 |
| C127 | ---- | ---- | 0.7 | 37.5 | 1.6 |
| ID13 | none | none | 0.8 | 34.5 | 8.5 |
| NS620-7 | 2113-2405 | E1 | 0.6 | 26.7 | 17.5 |
| NS236-12 | 1-2405 | E6,E7,E8,E1 | 0.7 | 48.1 | 17.2 |
| NS327-25 | 3737-3838 | E2,E5 | 0.6 | 33.7 | 1.4 |
| NS448-5 | 3456-3838 | E2,E3,E4,E5 | 1.1 | 26.2 | 3.1 |
| NS618-5 | 2775-3838 | E2,E3,E4,E5 | 1.7 | 29.7 | 3.3 |

The data represent the average from three isolates of each cell line. The cellular extract in each assay was normalized for protein content before incubation.

[a] CAT activity is measured as the percent of chloramphenicol which is acetylated by the cellular extract in 30 minutes at 37°.

[b] Deletions are given in terms of the nucleotide number on the BPV-1 genome.

The cell lines NS620-7 and NS236-12 which were transformed by deletion mutants affecting the E1 ORF provide the trans factor required for the the activation of the ncr enhancer. Since the E1 ORF is required for plasmid maintenance and replication (8,27), this result indicates that the increased expression of CAT in ID13 cells is not due to a plasmid replication. The high level of CAT expression from p407-1 in NS236-12 cells which were transformed by a BPV-1 DNA deleted of the E1, E6, E7, and E8 ORFs indicates that the E6, E7 and E8 ORFs are also not responsible for the trans-activation of the ncr enhancer.

In contrast, cells transformed by BPV-1 mutants with deletions in the 3' ORFs did not provide this trans-activation factor. Even cell lines transformed by the mutant deleted of bases 3737 to 3838 represented by NS327-25 abolishes the expression of CAT from p407-1, as do the larger deletions of the mutants used in transforming the NS448-5 and NS618-5 cell lines. The NS327-25 deletion removes 101 nucleotides from the 3' terminus of the E2 ORF and from the 5' terminus of E5. However, this deletion leaves the remainder of E5 intact, including the first AUG for this ORF at base 3879 (16). These initial results strongly suggest that the E2 ORF is the region responsible for the enhancer activation.

To more definitively assign the region of the genome responsible for the enhancer trans-activation, the pBPVncrCAT vector (p407-1) was assayed in C127 cells transformed by BPV-1 cDNAs. The expression of specific cDNAs within cells allowed a direct correlation between a specific putative BPV-1 gene product and functional trans-activation. The cDNA library was prepared from ID13 cells and was cloned into an Okayama and Berg expression vector as described by Yang et al (16) and individual isolates can be functionally studied since it is cloned into a functional mammalian cell transcriptional cassette. C127 cells transformed by cDNAs, C52, C58, C59, C88 and C212 were selected by BPV-1 morphological transformation while lines expressing C23, C36, C48, C102 and C119 were cotransfected with pdMMTneo and selected for resistance to G418. Table 3 shows the CAT expression from $pA_{10}CAT$, pSV2CAT and p407-1 in each of the cDNA cell lines. The CAT expression from the positive control, pSV2CAT, was substantially lower in cell lines selected by G418 resistance than in those selected by morphological transformation. As the cell extracts were normalized for protein concentration prior to assaying for CAT

TABLE 3

CAT EXPRESSION FROM CAT RECOMBINANT PLASMIDS IN C127 CELLS TRANSFORMED BY BPV-1 cDNAs.

| Trans-fected cDNA | cDNA Primary ORF[a] | Other Intact ORFs | % Chloramphenicol Acetylated | | |
|---|---|---|---|---|---|
| | | | $pA_{10}CAT$ | pSV2CAT | p407-1 |
| None | ---- | ----- | 0.6 | 18.0 | 0.7 |
| C23[f] | E1/E4-truncated | E3,E5 | 0.1 | 4.2 | 0.3 |
| C36[f] | E2-shortened | E3,E5 | 0.1 | 4.8 | 0.4 |
| C48[f] | E7 | E3,E5 | 0.1 | 1.8 | 0.3 |
| C58[g] | E6 | E7,E6/E7,E3,E5 | 0.2 | 16.1 | 1.0 |
| C102[f] | E6/E7 | E3,E5 | 0.1 | 2.9 | 0.3 |
| C119[f] | E6/E4 | E3,E5 | 0.1 | 2.6 | 0.2 |
| C52[g] | E2[b] | E3,E4,E5 | 0.1 | 17.1 | 1.8 |
| C59[g] | E2[c] | E3,E4,E5 | 0.1 | 16.2 | 4.9 |
| C88[g] | E2[d] | E3,E4,E5 | 0.1 | 24.3 | 6.0 |
| C212[g] | E2[e] | E3,E4,E5 | 0.4 | 27.3 | 22.3 |

[a] Primary ORF is defined as the first large ORF initiated by an AUG methionine codon.
[b,c,d,e] The 5' terminus is at base 1889, 2360, 2440, 2534, respectively.
[f] Cell line selection was by resistance to G418
[g] Cell line selection was by BPV-1 morphological transformation

activity it is unlikely that differences in the growth rate of these cells account for the lowered expression. Also, as in in the case of the deletion mutants, these data represent an average of three independent cell lines for each cDNA. The lowered CAT expression, therefore, seems to be a general characteristic of these cells.

The data in Table 3 demonstrate that the cDNAs representing the E2 ORF are those which provide the ncr enhancer trans-activation function. C127 cells transformed by C59, C88 and C212 clearly activate CAT expression from p407-1. The level of CAT expression from the C212 transformants is considerably higher than that from those transformed by either C88 or C59, and the level from the C52 transformants is barely above background. These four E2 cDNAs differ in their 5' flanking sequences. C212 has the shortest 5' extension from the E2 ORF while C52 extends an additional 645 nucleotides upstream. If this variability is due to altered expression of E2, it could suggest that the different 5' segments in the cDNA clones could result in differences in transcription, quantitatively or qualitatively, or could result in different translational efficiencies.

Further examination of the data in Table 3 confirms that the E1, E6 and E7 ORFs as well as the E1/E4 and E6/E7 spliced ORFs are not responsible for the transactivation function. The data also further suggest that E3 and E5 are not involved since they are present in all the cDNAs, even those which do not trans-activate. This fact is particularly evident in the lack of CAT expression from p407-1 in C127/C36 cells. C36 is a member of a particularly abundant class of cDNA (16). It can encode only the COOH half of the E2 ORF as well as E3 and E5 intact. Correlating this evidence with that from the deletion mutant cell line NS327-25 leads to the conclusion that the entire E2 ORF is required for the activation of the ncr enhancer.

## DISCUSSION

Many elements controlling the transcription of eukaryotic genes have been described yet the mechanisms of the regulation of gene expression through these elements is still largely unknown. The most recent addition to the list of transcriptional control elements is the enhancer sequence. Unlike promoters, enhancers can function over long distances and function in an orientation and position independent manner with respect to the direction of transcription of the gene (28). In this paper we have identified a new transcriptional enhancer in the BPV-1 genome. It is located within the 1 kb ncr of the genome and is distinct from the BPV-1 enhancer previously described by Lusky et al (12).

The BPV-1 ncr is an integral part of the 69% fragment which is sufficient for BPV-1 transformation (1). It is located 5' to a series of eight overlapping ORFs which may be expressed in BPV-1 non-productively infected cells. The ncr contains no translational ORFs but does contain cis-regulatory elements involved in plasmid DNA replication and viral transcription. A major DNAase I hypersensitivity site is located in the ncr (9) and the origin of plasmid DNA replication has been mapped to this region (10). Lusky and Botchan (11) have also mapped a plasmid maintenance sequence (PMS-1) to the Cla C fragment contained in the ncr. Deletion studies have indicated that a transcriptional promoter necessary for expression of the early genes is located at least in part in the ncr (8). The presence of a transcriptional enhancer within this region is not surprising and suggests that it may be crucial in the regulation of the transcription of the early ORFs.

The major finding of this paper is that this BPV-1 ncr enhancer element functions only in cells expressing BPV-1 gene products indicating that it is activated in trans by a BPV-1 gene product. The increased transcriptional activity of plasmids containing the ncr is not due to replication of the input plasmid since it is independent of the trans plasmid replication function of the E1 ORF (8, 27). By assaying for the enhancer function of the ncr in mouse cells transformed by defined BPV-1 deletion mutants or by BPV-1 cDNAs whose expression is under the control of the SV40 early promoter, we concluded that the E2 ORF gene product is required for the trans-activation of the ncr enhancer. Additional studies in which BPV-1 cDNAs and BPV-1 subgenomic fragments under the control of the SV40 early promoter were acutely cotransfected with the CAT recombinant plasmids into monkey CV-1 cells and then assayed after transient expression for CAT activity confirm that E2 encodes the ncr transactivation factor (Spalholz, Yang and Howley, manuscript submitted).

Trans-activation of viral transcriptional control elements has been described in a number of other systems. The E1a gene product of the human adenovirus type 5 can activate a regulatory sequence upstream from the E2 transcription unit which functions in a position and orientation independent manner (29,30,31,32). In SV40 infected cells, large T antigen activates expression from the late promoter (33,34). The human T-cell leukemia virus types 1 and 2 also each encode a gene product (px) from a long ORF which trans-activates a transcriptional regulatory element in the long terminal repeat of the provirus (35). Herpes virus regulatory genes which act in trans on transcriptional regulatory elements have also been characterized (29,36).

Although some enhancers, like the SV40 enhancer, function in most cells examined, other viral and cellular enhancers exhibit species or tissue specificity, or both. Presumably, this specificity is based on the cell type's ability to express a factor required in trans to activate the enhancer. Examples of such specificities include the cellular enhancers for the immunoglobulin heavy and light chain genes, insulin and chymotrypsin genes (37,38,39,40,41). The inducibility of these enhancer elements by factors supplied in trans is likely related to cellular transcriptional regulatory factors expressed during differentiation or in response to specific stimuli. Activation of cellular or viral enhancer elements may result from an interaction with either cellular factors or from particular viral trans-acting factors.

In the case of BPV-1, how the E2 ORF gene product activates the ncr enhancer and what role this activity may play in either transformation or lytic infection remains unknown. There are two general mechanisms by which this type of activation could occur. The first is that the E2 gene product may interact directly with the enhancer sequence to bring about an increase in transcription. The second possibility is that the E2 gene product may act indirectly through some cellular factor which then activates the enhancer sequence. This type of host-viral interaction has already been postulated for the activation of the adenovirus E2 transcription unit by adenovirus E1a gene product and by a variety of other similar acting viral and cellular genes (4,29,30,42).

In terms of how this interaction between the E2 gene product and the ncr enhancer work within the viral life cycle, one hypothesis involves the recent evidence from Yang et al (16) and Stenlund et al (43). Their studies indicate that there are two promoter sites within the early region of BPV-1.

The first is 5' of the eight early ORFs. The 5' ends of mRNAs from this promoter map near base 89, 31 bases downstream from a TATAAA sequence at base 58. The second promoter element is upstream from the first AUG of the E2 ORF in the vicinity of base 2440 (16). It is postulated that these two promoters transcribe two sets of genes. A model in which there is an ordered and controlled expression of BPV-1 RNAs in transformed cells would allow the promoter element around nucleotide 2440 to direct the expression of the E2 gene. The product of E2 could then activate the ncr enhancer which would subsequently turn on the upstream promoter leading to the expression of the 5' ORFs. This mechanism in all probability is very much simplified. Other cis-acting sequences or trans-acting products could further modulate the transcription from either promoter in either a positive or negative manner, perhaps dependent on the accumulation of a viral gene product. Experiments are in progress to test whether expression of the BPV-1 gene is ordered and controlled as predicted in this model, and to test whether the 5' ORFs encode a gene product which modulates the expression of the 3' ORFs.

ACKNOWLEDGEMENTS

We would like to thank Ellen Cheung for technical assistance and Nan Freas for preparation of this manuscript. This work was supported in part by a Damon Runyon-Walter Winchell Cancer Fund Fellowship, DRG-028, to B.A.S.

REFERENCES

1. Law M-F, Lowy DR, Dvoretzky I, Howley PM (1981). Mouse cells transformed by bovine papillomavirus contain only extrachromosomal viral DNA sequences. PNAS 78:2727.
2. Heilman CA, Engle L, Lowy DR, Howley PM (1982). Virus-specific transcription in bovine papillomavirus-transformed mouse cells. Virology 119:22.
3. Amtmann EG (1982). Bovine papilloma virus transcription: polyadenylated RNA species and assessment of the direction of transcription. J Virol 43:59.
4. Engel, LW, Heilman CA, Howley PM (1983). Transriptional organization of the bovine papillomavirus type 1. J Virol 47:516.
5. Lowy DR, Dvoretzky I, Shober R, Law M-F, Engel L, Howley PM (1980). In vitro transformation by a defined subgenomic subgenomic fragment of bovine papillomavirus DNA. Nature 287:72.

6. Chen EY, Howley PM, Levenson, AD, Seeburg PH (1982). The primary structure and genetic organization of the bovine papillomavirus type 1 genome Nature (London) 229:529.
7. Danos O, Engel LW, Chen EY, Yaniv M, Howley PM (1983). Comparative analysis of the human type 1a and bovine type 1 papillomavirus genomes. J Virol 46:557.
8. Sarver N, Rabson MS, Yang Y-C, Byrne JC, Howley PM (1984). Localization and analysis of bovine papillomavirus type 1 transforming functions. J Virol 52:377.
9. Rosl F, Waldeck W, Sauer G (1983). Isolation of episomal bovine papillomavirus chromatin and identification of a DNase-I hypersensitive region. J Virol 46:567.
10. Waldeck W, Rosl R, Zenfgraf H (1984). Origin of replication in episomal bovine papillomavirus type 1 DNA isolated from transformed cells. EMBO 3:2173.
11. Lusky M, Botchan MR (1984). Characterization of the bovine papillomavirus plasmid maintenance sequences. Cell 36:391.
12. Lusky M, Berg L, Weiher H, Botchan M (1983). Bovine papilloma virus contains an activator of gene expression at the distal end of the transcriptional unit. Mol Cell Biol 3:1108.
13. Laimins LA, Khoury G, Gorman C, Howard B, Gruss P (1982). Host-specific activation of transcription by tandem repeats from simian virus 40 and Moloney murine sarcoma virus. PNAS 79:6453.
14. Gorman CM, Moffat LF, Howard BH (1982). Recombinant genomes which express chloramphenicol acetyltransferase in mammalian cells. Mol Cell Biol 2:1044.
15. Dvoretzky I, Shober R, Lowy D (1980). Focus assay in mouse cells for bovine papillomavirus. Virology 103:369.
16. Yang Y-C, Okayama H, Howley PM (1985). Bovine papillomavirus contains multiple transforming genes. PNAS 82:1030.
17. Hutchinson KW, Halvorson HO (1980). Cloning of randomly sheared DNA fragments from a 105 lysogen of Bacillus subtilis--identification of prophage-containing clones. Gene 8:267.
18. Holmes DS, Quigley M (1981). A rapid boiling method for the preparation of bacterial plasmids. Anal Biochem 114:193.
19. Clewell DB (1972). Nature of the Col $E_1$ plasmid replication in Escherichia coli in the presence of chloramphenicol. J Bacteriol 110:667.

20. Wesnik PC, Finnegan DJ, Donelson JE, Hogness DS (1974). A system for mapping DNA sequences in the chromosomes of Drosophila melanogaster. Cell 3:315.
21. Maniatis T, Fritsch EF, Sambrook J (1982). Molecular cloning: A laboratory manual. In Maniatis T, Fritsch EF (eds). Cold Spring Harbor Laboratory, Cold Spring Harbor, New York.
22. Graham FL, van der Eb AJ (1973). A new technique for the assay of infectivity of human adenovirus 5 DNA. Virology 52:456.
23. Frost E, Williams J (1978). Mapping temperature-sensitive and host-range mutations of adenovirus type 5 by marker rescue. Virology 91:39.
24. Gorman CM, Howard BH, Reeves R (1983). Expression of recombinant plasmids in mammalian cells is enhanced by sodium butyrate. Nuc Acids Res 11:7631.
25. Weiher H, Botchan MR (1984). An enhancer sequence from bovine papilloma virus DNA consists of two essential regions. Nuc Acids Res 12:2901.
26. Treisman R, Novak U, Favaloro J, Kamen R (1981). Transformation of rat cells by an altered polyoma virus genome expressing only the middle-T protein. Nature 292:595.
27. Lusky M, Botchan MR (1985). Genetic analysis of the bovine papillomavirus type 1 trans acting replication factors. J Virol 53:955.
28. Khoury G, Gruss P (1983). Enhancer elements. Cell 33:313.
29. Imperiale MJ, Feldman LT, Nevins JR (1983). Activation of gene expression by adenovirus and herpes virus regulatory genes acting in trans and by a cis-acting adenovirus enhancer element. Cell 35:127.
30. Imperiale MJ, Nevins JR (1984). Adenovirus 5 E2 transcription unit: An E1A-inducible promoter with an essential element that functions independently of position or orientation. Mol Cell Biol 5:875.
31. Jones N, Shenk T (1979). An adenovirus 5 early gene function regulates expression of early viral genes. PNAS 76:3665.
32. Jones NC, Richter DJ, Weeks DL, Smith LD (1983). Regulation of adenovirus transcription by an E1a gene in microinjected Xenopus laevis oocytes. Mol Cell Biol 3:2131.
33. Brady J, Khoury G (1985). Transactivation of the SV40 late transcription unit by T-antigen. Mol Cell Biol (in press).

34. Keller JM, Alwine JC (1984). Activation of the SV40 late promoter: Direct affects in the absence of viral DNA purification. Cell 36:381.
35. Sodroski JG, Rosen CA, Haseltine WA (1984). Trans-acting transcriptional activation of the long terminal repeat of human T lymphotropic viruses in infected cells. Science 225:381.
36. Feldman LT, Imperiale MJ and Nevins JR (1982). Activation of early adenovirus transcription by the herpes virus immediate early gene: evidence for a common cellular control factor. PNAS 79:4951.
37. Banerji J, Olson L, Schaffner W (1983). A lymphocyte-specific cellular enhancer is located downstream of the joining region of immunoglobulin heavy chain gene. Cell 33:729.
38. Gillies SD, Morrison SL, Oi VT, Tonegawa S (1983). A tissue-specific transcription enhancer element is located in the major intron of a rearranged immunoglobulin heavy chain gene. Cell 33:717.
39. Picard D, Schaffner W (1984). A lymphocyte-specific enhancer in the mouse immunoglobulin Kappa gene. Nature 307:80.
40. Queen C, Baltimore D (1983). Immunoglobulin gene transcription is activated by downstream sequence elements. Cell 33:1958.
41. Walker M, Edlund T, Boulet A, Rutter W (1983). Cell-specific expression controlled by the 5' flanking region of insulin and chymotrypsin genes. Nature 306:557.
42. Imperiale M, Kao H-T, Feldman L, Nevins J, Strickland S (1984). Common control of the heat shock and early adenovirus genes: Evidence for a cellular E1A-like activity. Mol Cell Biol 4:867.
43. Stenlund A, Zabielski J, Ahola H, Moreno-Lopez J, Pettersson U (1985). The messenger RNAs from the transforming region of bovine papilloma virus type 1. J Mol Biol (in press).

**Papillomaviruses: Molecular and Clinical Aspects, pages 363–377**


# STRUCTURAL ANALYSIS OF VIRAL cDNAs FROM BOVINE PAPILLOMAVIRUS TRANSFORMED MOUSE CELLS

Yu-Chung Yang,[1] Hiroto Okayama[2] and Peter M. Howley[1]

[1]Laboratory of Tumor Virus Biology, National Cancer Institute, Bethesda, Maryland 20205; and [2]Laboratory of Molecular Genetics, National Institute of Child Health and Development, Bethesda, Maryland 20205

ABSTRACT Previous studies have identified several mRNA species from BPV-1 transformed cells and have shown that these transcripts share a common 3' end. To further define the structure of these viral transcirpts, we constructed a cDNA library with mRNA from BPV-1 transformed mouse cells using the Okayama and Berg method designed to select for full-length cDNA clones. 200 BPV-1 specific cDNA clones were isolated from a library of $10^5$ independent clones. Sequence analysis of these cDNA clones has provided structural information which defines the 5' and 3' ends, the splice donor and acceptor sites, and the coding exons for the mRNA species present in BPV-1 transformed cells. In conjunction with the open reading frames (ORFs) deduced from BPV-1 DNA sequence, it is possible to predict the structure of the putatively encoded proteins.

## INTRODUCTION

Papillomaviruses are members of the papovavirus family and induce benign squamous epithelial tumors in a wide variety of higher vertebrates. The molecular genetics of papillomaviruses have not been well understood, mainly due to the lack of a permissive tissue culture system suitable for virus propagation. This difficulty has recently been partially circumvented by the molecular cloning of the genomes of several different papillomaviruses.

Bovine papillomavirus type 1 (BPV-1) has been extensively studied and has served as a model for the study of the molecular biology and genomic organization of the papillomaviruses.

BPV-1 causes benign fibropapillomas (warts) in cattle and also induces fibrosarcomas in heterogenous hosts. The virus and its molecularly cloned DNA can transform mouse C127 cells in vitro and the viral DNA persists as an extrachromosomal multicopy plasmid in the transformed cells (1). A 69% subgenomic fragment ($BPV_{69T}$) bounded by the unique HindIII and BamHI sites is sufficient for BPV-mediated transformation (2) as well as for autonomous replication (3).

The genomic organization of BPV-1 has been well established because the complete DNA sequence (4) and the transcription data from both BPV-1 transformed cells (5) and productively infected bovine fibropapillomas (6,7) are available. All the detectable mRNA species from transforming or productive infection systems are transcribed from a single strand and all the (ORFs) greater than 400 base pairs are located on the same strand. Several mRNAs from BPV-1 transformed mouse cells have been mapped in the 69% transforming region where eight of the ORFs (E1 through E8) are located. These viral transcripts have a common 3' end at 0.53 map units (5). It appears that these transcripts are generated by differential splicing, however, no splicing was detected in these earlier studies. Due to the low abundance of viral RNAs present in transformed cells, transcriptional analysis have been limited and little is known about the functional proteins encoded by any papillomavirus.

In order to assign transforming or replication functions to different portions of the BPV-1 genome, several laboratories have engineered mutants containing deletions or insertions within the BPV-1 genome or have analyzed the function of specific fragments of BPV-1 under the control of mammalian cell transcriptional regulatory signals (8-12). Although these studies localized regions on the viral genome important for cell transformation or plasmid replication, interpretations have sometimes been difficult due to the lack of transcriptional data indicating how the various ORFs are spliced together as exons at the level of RNA. It was, therefore, critical to understand the basic structure of viral transcripts and their encoded proteins.

In order to further define the structure of mRNA in transformed cells and to identify functional proteins encoded by individual viral transcripts, we constructed a cDNA expression library using an Okayama and Berg plasmid vector with mRNA from BPV-1 transformed mouse cells. Sequence analysis of the viral cDNA clones has provided structural information which defines the 5' and 3' ends, the splice donor information which defines the 5' and 3' ends, the splice donor and acceptor sites, and the coding exons from the mRNA species present in BPV-1 transformed cells. In conjunction with the ORFs for BPV-1, it is possible to predict the structure of the virally encoded proteins which could, therefore, potentially be translated in BPV-1 transformed cells. The plasmid vector used for cDNA cloning contains the simian virus 40 (SV40) early promoter, the SV40 late region introns and the SV40 late region polyadenylation site, allowing expression of cDNA clones in mouse cells for functional analysis (13).

In this manuscript, we present data on the detailed structural analysis of viral mRNAs from BPV-1 transformed mouse cells. The potential coding capacities of each of the viral transcripts will be discussed.

## METHODS AND RESULTS

### Construction of cDNA Library with pCD Expression Vector.

BPV-1 transformed mouse C127 cells (ID13) were grown to half confluency and total RNA was obtained by lysis of cells in 4M guanidinium isothiocyanate, sedimentation through a CsCl cushion and ethanol precipitation (14). Polyadenylated RNA was obtained by two cycles of oligo(dT) cellulose chromatography (15). A cDNA library was constructed from this RNA with the plasmids pCDV1 and pL1 using the plasmid primer method described by Okayama et al (13) except that the bacterial transformation was performed using E. coli strain DH1 (16).

### Screening of cDNA Library for BPV-1 Sequences.

A library of 100,000 independent clones was made from 0.5 ug of the polyadenylated RNA from ID13 cells. Using a BPV-1 specific radiolabeled probe (specific activity $10^8$ cpm/ug), the library was screened by colony hybridization (17,18) and 200 BPV-1 specific clones were isolated. Positive clones were then hybridized with subgenomic fragments of BPV-1 DNA to provide preliminary mapping data and information on which to design a sequencing strategy. The insert sizes of viral cDNA clones ranged from 0.2 to 2.8 kb. Since viral RNAs in BPV-1 transformed cells range in size from 1 to 4 kb (5), only clones that contained inserts 1 kb or larger were analyzed by detailed restriction enzyme mapping and were sequenced by Maxam and Gilbert techniques (19).

Structural Analysis of BPV-1 Specific cDNA Clones.

Several classes of cDNA clones can be distinguished based on their insert size and splicing pattern and the representative structure of each cDNA class is shown in Figure 1.

The 5' ends of several of the spliced messages map to base 89 and these cDNA sequences are shown in Figure 2A. This agrees with the data of Ahola et al (20), who mapped base 89 as a major 5' end of the mRNAs present in transformed cells. There is a TATAAA sequence at base 58, 31 bases upstream from base 89. The "TATA"-like sequence has been shown in many systems to be part of a RNA polymerase II transcriptional promoter and to function in positioning the 5' ends of the mRNAs (21). Many of the cDNAs have 5' ends mapping downstream from base 89. Although some of these may represent copies of truncated viral RNAs, some could be representative of full-length RNA generated from an additional viral promoter. In particular, class V cDNAs and one of the class VI cDNAs (C88) have 5' ends mapping to base 2440, the sequence TAATATT is located at base 2414, 27 nucleotides upstream from base 2440. As shown in Figure 2B, the cDNA sequences around base 2440 are stretches of As' instead of the authentic BPV-1 genomic sequences. This difference might be due to staggering by reverse transcriptase in a region with high secondary or tertiary structure or may be due to the frequent occurrence of the particular corresponding RNA in transformed cells. S1 mapping and primer extension techniques have confirmed that base 89 and 2440 are major 5' ends in BPV-1 transformed mouse cells (data not shown). The class III cDNA clone (C58) has a 5' end that maps upstream from base 89, indicating that promoter sequences other than those with the "TATA" box at nucleotide 58 and 2414 function in BPV-1 transformed cells although at lower frequency.

In most of the cDNAs characterized, spliced messages were identified. Splice donor sites were identified at bases 304, 864 and 2505. Splice acceptor sites were found at bases 527 and 3224. Fig. 3 shows the actual sequences of each of the viral splice junctions within different classes of cDNA clones. These sequences, as indicated in Figure 4, are in fairly good agreement with the consensus splice donor and acceptor sequences found in eukaryotic cells (22).

In addition to spliced messages, we also identified several unspliced cDNA clones (Class VI) with sizes ranging from 1.9 to 2.5 kb and 5' ends mapping from base 1889 to base 2534.

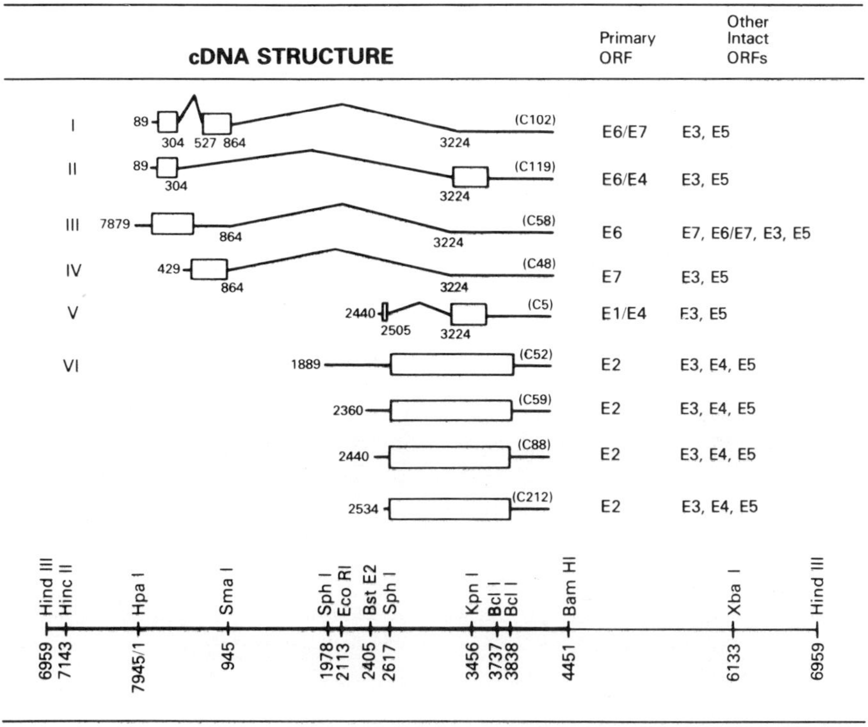


Figure 1. Representative structures of classes of BPV-1 cDNA clones isolated from BPV-1 transformed mouse C127 cells. The structures of various cDNA clones are indicated with the most 5' coding region following an AUG indicated by open box. The class V clone could be a truncated E1/E4 clone although there is no AUG located in the boxed segment. The downstream potentially non-translated regions are indicated by the solid line, and the intervening sequences are shown by the slanted lines. Numbers outside the primary coding region represent 5' ends and splice junctions. Primary ORFs and other ORFs present in each individual cDNA clones are designated on the right. A restriction map is at the bottom of the figure for orientation. This schematic representation of the cDNA structure has been published previously (28) and is reproduced with permission.

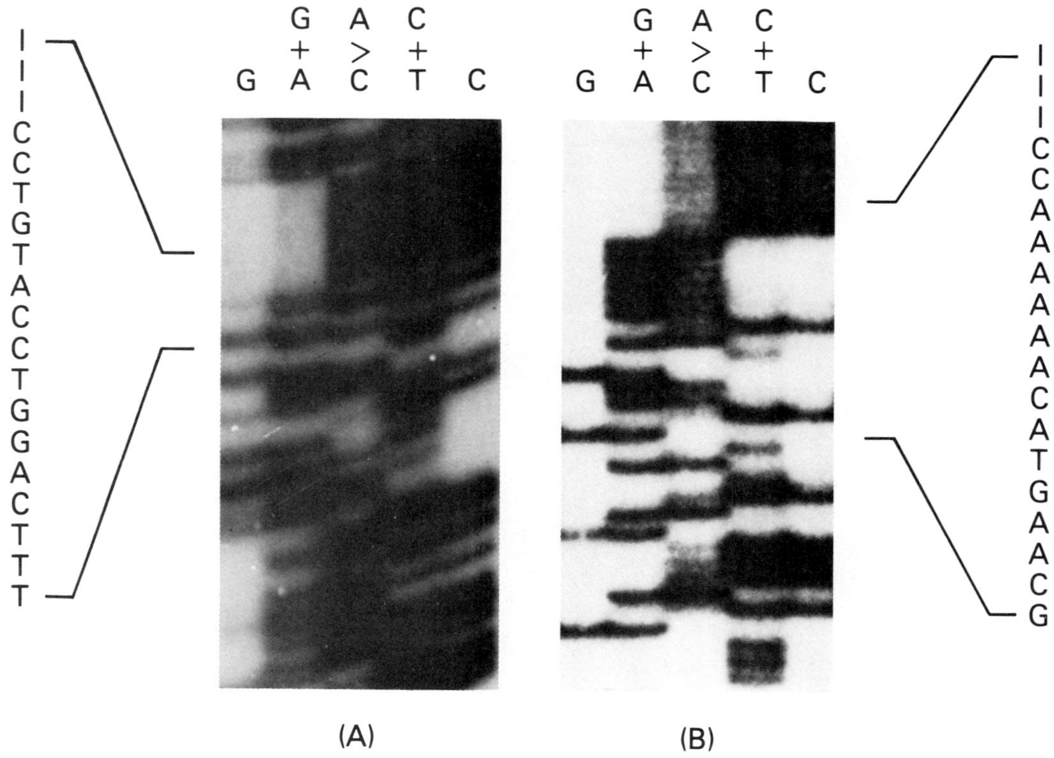


Figure 2. DNA sequences around the two major 5' ends of cDNA clones from BPV-1 transformed mouse C127 cells. (A) 5' end structure at base 89; (B) 5' end structure at base 2440.

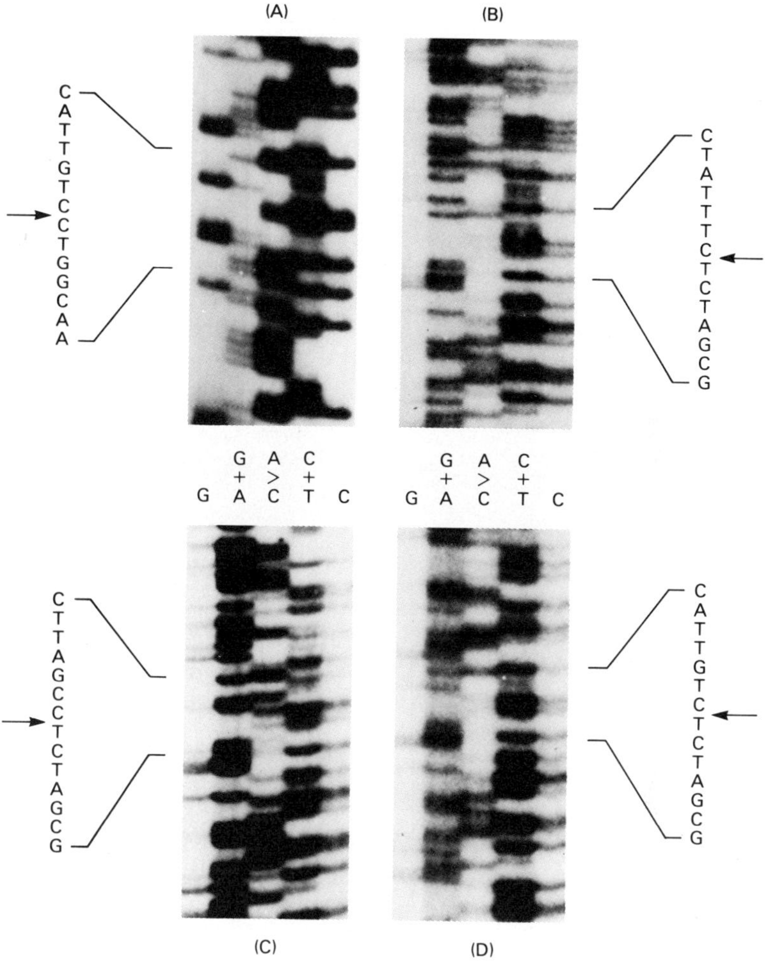


Figure 3. DNA sequences around the splice junctions of various cDNA clones from BPV-1 transformed mouse C127 cells: (A) Splice junction between base 304 and base 527; (B) Splice junction between base 864 and base 3224; (C) Splice junction between base 2505 and base 3224; (D) Splice junction between bae 304 and base 3224.

**COMPARISON OF BPV-1 SPLICE JUNCTIONS WITH CONSENSUS ACCEPTOR AND DONOR SITES**

| Base no | Viral donor site | Base no | Viral acceptor site |
|---|---|---|---|
| 304 | CAG↓**GT**GAGG | 527 | TCACCTGC**AG**↓GA |
| 864 | AAG↓**GT**AGCA | 3224 | CTGATTTT**AG**↓AG |
| 2505 | CGG↓**GT**GAGC | | |

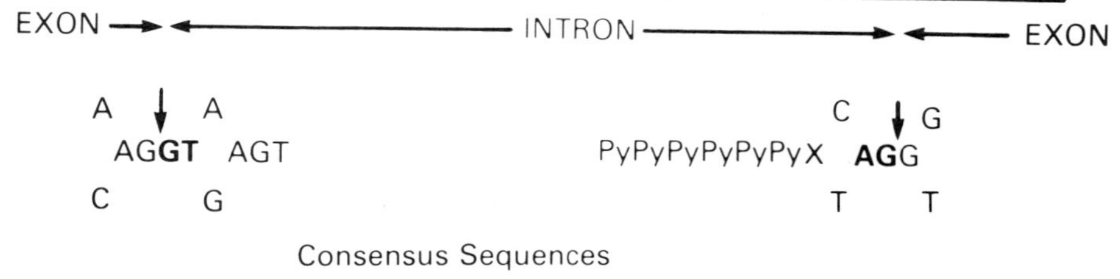


Figure 4. Comparison of BPV-1 splice junctions with consensus acceptor and donor sites. This schematic representation of viral splice junction and consensus sequences has been published previously (28) and is reproduced with permission.

Previous transcriptional analysis of the mRNAs present in BPV-1 transformed cells has indicated that the different viral transcripts have a common 3' end at 0.53 map units. Sequence analysis of several cDNAs indicates that mRNA is polyadenylated at base 4203, 24 bases 3' to the first A of the polyadenylation recognition site AATAAA (Fig. 5). The 3' ends of most RNA polymerase II transcripts in mammalian cells are found to be polyadenylated at sites 10-25 nucleotides 3' to the AAUAAA signal (23).

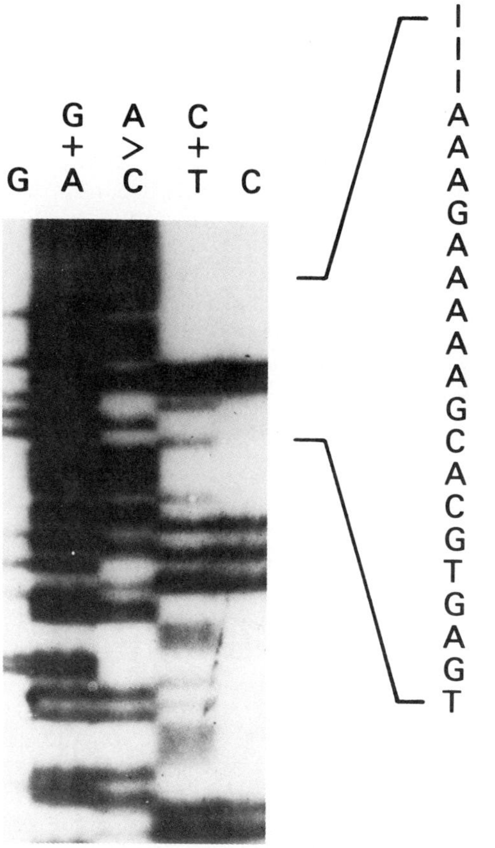


Figure 5. DNA sequences around the 3' end of cDNA clones from BPV-1 transformed mouse C127 cells.

Potential Coding Capacities for Individual cDNA Clones.

Potential coding sequences for each cDNA class are presented in Fig. 1. Since no viral protein has yet been identified in BPV-1 transformed cells, the putative protein encoded by each of the cDNA classes was predicted based on the general rules for protein translation in eukaryotic cells (24).

In Fig. 1, listed adjacent to the cDNA structures are the primary ORFs that would be predicted to be expressed by the cDNAs, assuming that mRNAs are functionally monocistronic. The class I cDNA clone (C102) splices E6 and E7 ORFs together in frame and could direct the synthesis of a 21-K Da protein using the initiation codon AUG at bases 91-93 and the termination codon UAA at bases 860-862. This class of cDNA contains a second splice from base 864 to base 3224; however, these sequences are likely to represent non-coding regions of the mRNA molecule because they are located 3' to the termination codon. The class II clone (C119) could direct the synthesis of a 20-K Da protein that is derived from in frame splicing of the E6 and E4 exons and uses base 91-93 (AUG) and 3527-3529 (UGA) for the initiation and termination codons. The class III cDNA (C58) has a 5' end upstream from base 89 and splice donor and acceptor sites at bases 864 and 3224. C58 could direct the synthesis of a 15.5-K Da E6 protein with an AUG initiation codon at bases 91-93 and the termination codon UAG at bases 502-504. The class IV cDNA (C48) with a 5' end at base 429 could be a truncated class III cDNA or, if expressed in transformed cells, could direct the synthesis of a 15.5-K Da E7 protein using the initiation codon AUG at base 479-481 and the termination codon UAA at bases 860-862.

The class V cDNA clones are the copies of the most abundant mRNA species in BPV-1 transformed cells. These each had a 5' end at base 2440 and were spliced from base 2505 to base 3224. The splice results in the fusion of the E1 and E4 ORFs, however, there is no methionine initiation codon in this fused ORF. We could assign E1/E4 as the major ORF for this particular class of cDNA, assuming that it is a truncated copy of viral mRNA molecule. However, Pettersson and his group have obtained evidence by heteroduplex analysis of a class of RNA molecules with 5' ends that map to this region (25). It is, therefore, possible that the cDNAs represented by the class V structures are faithful copies of RNAs within cells that have been modified in the sequences at their 5' ends as a result of some specific RNA cleavage process.

Alternatively, if base 2440 is the true cap site for this species of mRNA molecule, the major ORF of this particular cDNA class would be E5 ORF.

The class VI cDNA clones were unspliced and could direct the synthesis of a 48 K Da E2 protein with initiation codons at 2608-2610 and 3838-3840, respectively.

Although most of the eukaryotic mRNAs are functionally monocistronic, there is growing evidence that polycistronic messages exist inside the cell (see 24). Therefore, the downstream ORFs in each cDNA clone cannot be dismissed at this point. Indicated in Fig. 1, right column, are the other ORFs which are left intact within these cDNAs which might be expressed if these cDNAs represented polycistronic messager RNAs.

## DISCUSSION

BPV-1 transformed cells contain multiple viral transcripts which vary in size from approximately 1000 to 4000 bases (5). Precise mapping of the viral RNAs has been difficult because of the low abundance of viral transcripts in these transformed cells. The structural analysis of the cDNA clones from BPV-1-transformed cells presented in this study indicates that the viral RNAs are generated by differential splicing. Splice donor sites map to bases 304, 864 and 2505 and splice acceptor sites map to bases 527 and 3224. Previous studies have indicated that the viral mRNAs have a 3' coterminus at 0.53 map units (5). Direct sequence analysis of cDNA clones indicates that the site of polyadneylation is at the guanine residue at base 4203, located 24 bases downstream from the polyadenylation recognition sequence AAUAAA at 4180.

We map two major 5' ends to bases 89 and 2440. A TATAAA sequence at base 58 and a TAATATT sequence located at base 2414 may represent the "TATA" boxes of transcriptional promoters for these transcriptional start sites. The presence of 165 base pairs of sequences upstream from base 89 in one cDNA clone sequenced indicates that there can be upstream start sites and that there is an additional promoter functional in BPV-1 transformed cells.

The different classes of RNA detected in this study and their splice junctions are in good agreement with the studies of Stenlund et al (25) who mapped the polyadenylated viral RNA species present in BPV-1 transformed cells by heteroduplex analysis. However, in neither study was message containing E1 ORF intact detected. The E1 gene product has been shown by genetic studies to be important for stable plasmid replication and maintenance (11,26). The inability, thus far, to detect the E1 mRNA is probably due to its low abundance inside the cell or its synthesis under cell cycle control.

Recent studies from our laboratory and others have identified several regions of the BPV-1 genome that influence the expression of the viral transforming functions. Deletion mutants affecting the E2 ORF are reduced in their ability to transform mouse C127 cells, suggesting that the putative E2 protein is important in the transformation process (8-12; DiMaio, personal communication). Several groups have shown that mutation at the BstXI site within E5 ORF significantly affect the transformation efficiency. However, the expression of E2 and/or E5 alone is not sufficient for the fully transformed phenotype. Deletion mutagenesis studies map an additional function that is critical for the fully transformed phenotype to the region between the HpaI site (base 1) and the SmaI site (base 945)(8).

In addition to assigning transformation function to E2, E5 ORFs and sequences between HpaI and SmaI sties, Spalholz et al (27) have recently mapped a transcriptional regulatory sequence within the 1.0 kb non-coding region of the BPV-1 genome that can be transactivated by a gene product encoded by the 3' ORFs of the viral genome.

Since each of the cDNA inserts was cloned in an expression vector containing SV40 transcriptional regulatory elements, it was possible to assay biological functions directly. We have identified two classes of cDNA clones (Class III and Class VI) that can independently transform mouse C127 cells. These two classes of cDNAs contain E2 or E6 as the primary ORF (Fig. 1). The putative viral functions encoded by each of these cDNA classes appear to act synergistically in transforming mouse C127 cells (28). We have also established that Class III cDNA clones containing E2 as the primary ORF can provide transactivation functions in a transient assay (27).

Our interpretation that the transformation and transactivation functions are due to these putative proteins, however, must be tempered because of our current inability to directly define the viral proteins present in cells transfected with vairous cDNA clones. Due to the complexity of eukaryotic translation system, the potential role of the downstream ORFs present in these cDNA clones (i.e., E3, E4, or E5) cannot be ruled out at this time. Mutagenesis studies using cDNA molecules described in this paper and attempts to overproduce viral protein products encoded by each of the cDNA clones are underway. These studies should provide answers and reagents to permit our further understanding of the viral functions expressed in BPV-1 transformed cells.

ACKNOWLEDGEMENT

We are grateful to Nan Freas for the preparation of this manuscript.

REFERENCES

1. Law M-F, Lowy DR, Dvoretzky I, Howley PM (1981). Mouse cells transformed by bovine papillomavirus contain only extrachromosomal viral DNA sequences. PNAS 78:2727.
2. Lowy DR, Dvoretzky I, Shober R, Law M-F, Engel L, Howley PM (1980). In vitro transformation by a defined subgenomic subgenomic fragment of bovine papillomavirus DNA. Nature 287:72.
3. Sarver N, Gruss P, Law M-F, Khoury G, Howley PM 1981. Bovine papilloma virus deoxyribonucleic acid: a novel eucaryotic cloning vector. Mol Cell Biol 1:486.
4. Chen EY, Howley PM, Levenson, AD, Seeburg PH (1982). The primary structure and genetic organization of the bovine papillomavirus type 1 genome Nature (London) 229:529.
5. Heilman CA, Engle L, Lowy DR, Howley PM (1982). Virus-specific transcription in bovine papillomavirus-transformed mouse cells. Virology 119:22.
6. Amtmann EG (1982). Bovine papilloma virus transcription: polyadenylated RNA species and assessment of the direction of transcription. J Virol 43:59.
7. Engel, LW, Heilman CA, Howley PM (1983). Transriptional organization of the bovine papillomavirus type 1. J Virol 47:516.
8. Sarver N, Rabson MS, Yang Y-C, Byrne JC, Howley PM (1984). Localization and analysis of bovine papillomavirus type 1 transforming functions. J Virol 52:377.
9. Lusky M, Berg L, Weiher H, Botchan M (1983). Bovine papilloma virus contains an activator of gene expression at the distal end of the transcriptional unit. Mol Cell Biol 3:1108.
10. Nakabayashi Y, Chattopadhyay SF, Lowy DR (1983). The transforming function of bovine papillomavirus DNA. PNAS 80:5832.

11. Lusky M, Botchan MR (1984). Characterization of the bovine papillomavirus plasmid maintenance sequences. Cell 36:391.
12. Schiller JT, Vass WC, Lowy, DR (1984). Identification of a second transforming region of bovine papillomavirus. PNAS 81:7880.
13. Okayama H, Berg P (1983). A cDNA cloning vector that permits expression of cDNA inserts in mammalian cells. Mol Cell Biol 3:280.
14. Chirgwin JM, Przybyla AE, MacDonald RJ, Rutter WJ (1979). Isolation of biological active ribonucleic acid from sources enriched in ribonuclease. Biochem 18:5294.
15. Aviv H, Leder P. (1972). Purification of biological active globin messenger RNA by chromatography on oligothymidylic acid-cellulose. PNAS 69:1408.
16. Hanahan D (1983). Studies on transformation of Escherichia coli with plasmids. J Mol Biol 166:557.
17. Rigby PD, Rhodes MD, Berg P (1977). Labeling deoxyribonuclei acid to high specific activity in vitro nick translation with DNA polymerase. J Mol Biol 113:237.
18. Grunstein M, Hogness DS (1975). Colony hybridization: a method for the isolation of cloned DNAs that contain a specific gene. PNAS 72:3961.
19. Maxam A, Gilbert W (1980). Sequencing end-labeled DNA with base-specific chemical cleavages. Methods Enzymol 65:499.
20. Ahola H, Stenlund A, Moreno-Lopez J, Pettersson U (1983). Sequences of bovine papillomavirus type 1 DNA: functional and evolutionary implications. Nucl Acids Res 11:2639.
21. Benoist D, Chambon P (1981). In vivo sequence requirements of the SV40 early promoter region. Nature (London) 290:304.
22. Seif I, Khoury G, Dhar R (1979). BKV splice sequences based on analysis of preferred donor and acceptor sites. Nucleic Acid Res 6:3387.
23. Fitzgerald M, and Shenk T (1981). The sequence 5'-AAUAAA-3' forms part of the recognition site for polyadenylation of late SV40 mRNAs. Cell 24:251.
24. Kozak M (1983). Comparison of initiation of protein synthesis in prokaryotes, eucaryotes, and organelles. Micro Reviews 47:1.
25. Stenlund A, Zabielski J, Ahola H, Moreno-Lopez J, Pettersson U (1985). The messenger RNAs from the transforming region of bovine papilloma virus type 1. J Mol Biol (in press).

26. Lusky M, Botchan MR (1985). Genetic analysis of the bovine papillomavirus type 1 trans-acting replication factors. J Virol 53:955.
27. Spalholz, BA, Yang Y-C, Howley PM (1985). Transactivation of a bovine papillomavirus transcriptional regulatory element by the E2 gene product. Submitted for publication.
28. Yang Y-C, Okayama H, Howley PM (1985). Bovine papillomavirus contains multiple transforming genes. PNAS 82:1030.

**Papillomaviruses: Molecular and Clinical Aspects, pages 379–390**


# CHARACTERIZATION OF TRANSCRIPTION CONTROL REGIONS OF THE COTTONTAIL RABBIT PAPILLOMAVIRUS

Isabelle Giri+, Olivier Danos+, Françoise Thierry+
Elisabeth Georges++, Gerard Orth++ and Moshe Yaniv+

+Unité des Virus Oncogènes
Département de Biologie Moléculaire
++Unité des papillomavirus, Département de Virologie
Institut Pasteur, 25 rue du Docteur Roux
75724 Paris Cedex 15, FRANCE

ABSTRACT The 5' ends of the viral mRNAs present in the VX2 transplantable carcinoma induced by CRPV (cottontail rabbit papillomavirus) were mapped by S1 and primer extension techniques. Two initiation sites for the RNA were localized in the non coding region and after the first ATG of the E6 open reading frame respectively. A third one was found 5' to the E7 open reading frame. To test the promoter activity of the viral sequences, we cloned the entire non coding region of CRPV upstream of the bacterial chloramphenicol acetyl transferase (CAT) gene in a promoter-less eucaryotic expression vector. This DNA fragment functions as a cell specific promoter being expressed only in VX2 derived cell lines.

## INTRODUCTION

In recent years, rapid progress have been made in our understanding of papillomavirus gene structure and function. Although it is still far from complete, we have now a picture of what can be the essential cis or trans acting elements required for the transcription and replication of the viral genome. Much of our knowledge came from determinations of the genome structures of several papillomavirus by DNA sequencing[1] and from studies on the transformation of murine fibroblasts by Bovine Papillomavirus type 1 (BPV1)[2,3,4]. Our own interest has been focused on the Cottontail Rabbit

Papillomavirus (CRPV), as the whole process of papilloma-to-carcinoma progression can be studied on laboratory animals[5], thus providing a convenient system for examining the role of papillomavirus gene expression in tumor formation. Moreover, transplantable carcinoma lines that have been maintained for decades in domestic rabbits still contain actively expressed CRPV genomes suggesting that the viral transcripts are of some importance for the maintenance of the tumorigenic state. More recently, cell lines have been derived from these carcinomas[6,7] hopefully providing a permissive cellular system for papillomavirus gene expression.

We have determined the pattern of viral mRNA expression found in the VX2 transplantable carcinoma of the rabbit. This allows us to identify putative promoter elements both in the non coding and the coding sequences of CRPV. By using chimeric CAT plasmids, we show that the non coding region of the virus functions as an active promoter only in VX2 cells which already express the viral genome. It does not express in any other rabbit or non rabbit cell lines that we tested.

## GENOME STRUCTURE AND EXPRESSION

We have established the complete nucleotide sequence of the CRPV DNA[8]. The genome is 7868 base pairs long and as for other papillomaviruses only one strand of DNA contains significant large open reading frames susceptible to represent viral genes or exons. By analogy to other papillomaviruses[1,9], the viral genome (figure 1a) can be divided into two regions : early (E) and late (L). Transcripts from the E region are found in the CRPV associated benign and malignant tumors[6,10,11,12]. The E open reading frames are believed to encode viral proteins involved in genome replication and in tumor formation and maintenance. The L region contains two open reading frames coding for the viral structural proteins (L1 and L2). Transcription of these genes seems to require specific factors provided by the infected terminally differenciating keratinocyte as **L** mRNA are only found in the virus producing papillomas and in the VX7 transplantable carcinoma which still exhibits some of the keratinocyte differenciated properties[12]. The two coding regions are bordered on their 3' side by a polyadenylation signal and separated by a non coding region of 678 nucleotides.

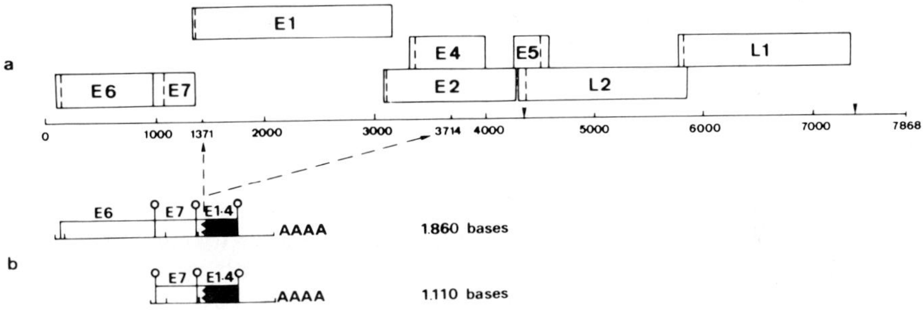


FIGURE 1. CRPV genome organization and structure of the major transcripts found in the VX2 transplantable carcinoma.

a) The reading frames of the CRPV genome are shown. The dotted lines indicate the first ATG codon. The arrowheads show the position of the polyadenylation sites.

b) The structure of the 1860 and 1110 bases mRNAs is depicted ( ⚲ ): stop codon. The first codon is indicated by a vertical bar. The positions of the donor (1371) and acceptor (3714) sites are indicated.

The refined analysis of the E mRNA present in the VX2 carcinoma[11] allowed to deduce the nature of the viral proteins that should be present in the transformed cell. The two major transcripts (1860 and 1110 bases) are formed of two exons corresponding to the E6/E7 and E2/E4 coding regions (figure 1). Yet the splicing event does not lead to a fusion of proximal (E6/E7) and distal (E2/E4) open reading frames, as the donor site is located 5' to the E7 stop codon. Instead, the two messages have the following structure : (i) the 1860 bases species contains 5' to 3', the open reading frames E6, E7 and E1-4 ; (ii) the 1110 bases species contains E7 and E1-4 (see figure 1b for the detailed coordinates). Considering the general rules of mRNA translation in eucaryotic cells[13], it is likely that only the first open reading frame will be translated from these polycistronic mRNAs. Yet, we cannot exclude the possibility of translation reinitiation which could lead to the production of an E1-4 polypeptide. In addition, the 1860 bases mRNA population is heterologous at its 5' end and could thus lead to the syntheis of two versions, full-length and truncated of the E6 protein depending on which ATG initiation codon is used for translation. Three minor mRNA species present at about 1 copy/cell were also detected in the E2/E4 region but their 5' ends have not been precisely characterized.

## IDENTIFICATION OF PROMOTER ELEMENTS

The combination of nuclease S1 and primer extension analysis on the CRPV mRNAs in the VX2 tumor allowed us to define their 5' extremities (cap site). A first group of microheterogenous 5' ends was found upstream of E7 and corresponds to the 1110 bases long transcripts. A second set of cap sites was observed upstream of E6 (1860 bases transcripts). In each case, a suitable TATA box around position -30 relative to the start point of transcription is found, arguing for the presence of two different regions with promoter activity (figure 2). The analysis of DNA sequence in the non coding region (i.e. upstream of E6) reveals typical structures for eucaryotic upstream promoter enhancer elements. The sequence immediately upstream of the two potential E6 TATA boxes is shown in figure 2a. It includes a palindromic sequence (position 7825) followed by a CAAT box like element, and this feature is remarkably conserved in every sequenced papillomavirus genome . The CRPV non coding region (figure

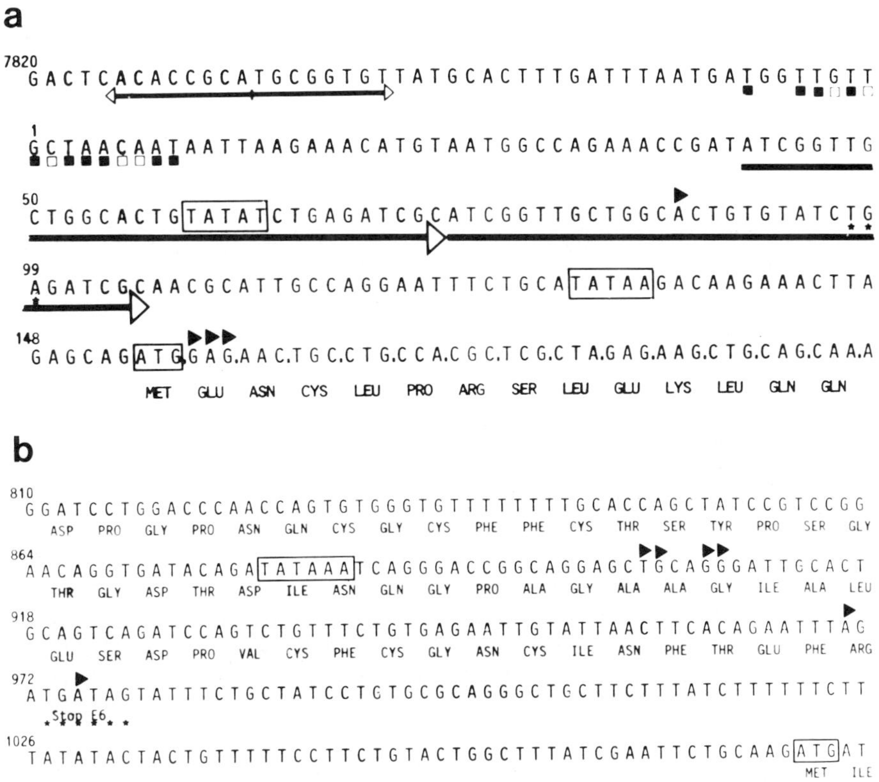

FIGURE 2. Start point for the transcription of the CRPV major mRNAs in the VX2 carcinoma.

a) The E6 open reading frame starts at position 100 and its first ATG codon is framed. Arrowheads above nucleotides 87, 157, 158 and 159 indicate 5'ends of the 1.860 bases species. The 32 bp repeat and the palindromic stucture at position 7825 are underlined. Nucleotides marked with squares are conserved in all sequenced papilloma virus genomes. The two TATA boxes, corresponding to the two set of 5' ends are framed.

b) The E7 open reading frame starts at position 979 and its first ATG as codon is framed . Arrowheads above nucleotides 903, 904, 907, 908, 970 and 975 indicated 5' ends of the 1110 bases species. A potential TATA box at position 879 is framed.

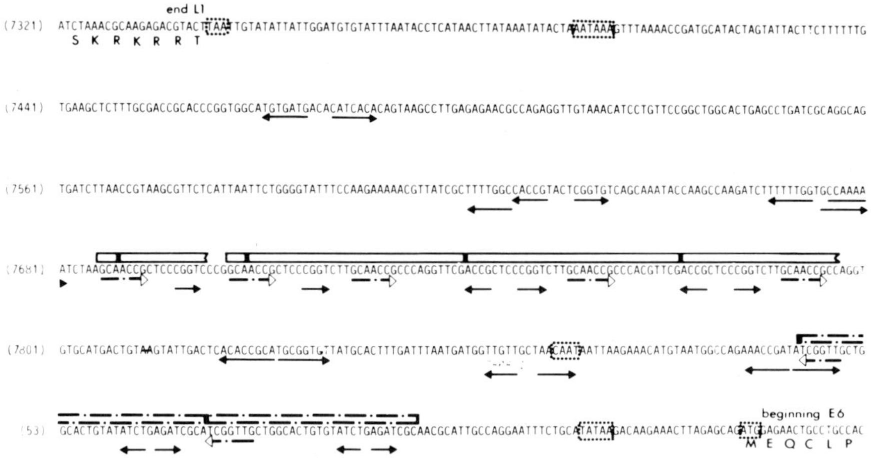


FIGURE 3. The non coding region of the CRPV genome. The sequence between the end of the L1 open reading frame and the beginning of the E6 one is shown. The putative late polyadenylation signal in the middle of the AT rich region is boxed. The main inverted repeats found in this region are indicated by arrows. Two perfect palindromes of 8 and 7 bp are found at positions 7825 and 35 respectively. The direct repeats are shown by boxes, the first series with bold lines, the second one with dotted lines. The seven base pairs sequence (GCAACCG) common to the two repeats is underlined with dashed arrows. Small inverted repeats inside of the main ones are also shown. The small motive AAAGA or its complementary sequence TCTTT is repeated ten times all along the region.

3) also presents a striking set of repeated sequenced : shown in figure 2a is a 32 bp repeat, which is preceded further upstream in the control region by a different 32 bp unit repeated twice. Both repeats share a common 7 bp sequence (GCAACCG or the complementary CGGTTGC). The upstream repeat is also surrounded by truncated versions of itself. The constant length of these repeated elements is intriguing and suggests that they are the site of action for some transcription factors provided by the host cell or the virus itself. Other clues for binding of regulatory molecules in these regions come from the frequent occurance of short inverted repeats (5 to 7 bp). One of these repeats (5'ACCGNNNNCGGT3') is found seven times and is common to all papillomavirus non coding regions : it is observed once in HPV1 and four time in BPV1 and HPV6. These potential signals may also be involved in the control of viral DNA replication which is very likely coordinately regulated with transcription.

## TEST OF PROMOTER ACTIVITY

The analysis of mRNA mapping data and of the nucleotide sequence prompted us to examine the promoter activity of the CRPV non coding region. For this purpose, we used the chloramphenicol acetyl transferase (CAT) transient expression assay of Gorman et al.(14). This system permits a rapid quantitative test of the promoter activity of any DNA fragment placed 5' to the bacterial chloramphenicol acetyl transferase (CAT) gene and introduced in a variety of eucaryotic cells.

The Pst I fragment of CRPV DNA spanning the entire non coding region and the N-terminal extremity of E6 open reading frame coding for the first 12 amino-acids (position 7106 to 187) was inserted in the HindIII site of pSB1(15) (see figure 4 and legend for details). Three constructions differing in the linker region between E6 and CAT were tested fo their ability to induce CAT activity after transfection of various recipient cells. The same cells were also transfected with the promoter-less pSB1 vector or with pSVECAT, a plasmid containing the SV40 early promoter upstreamm of the CAT gene(14) ; the first gives a very low level of CAT activity whereas the second is active in all the cell lines that we ever tested. After transfection with CRPV-CAT plasmids, no activity was detected in extracts from cells of murine (FR3T3, C127) or human (Hela, 293) origin (data not

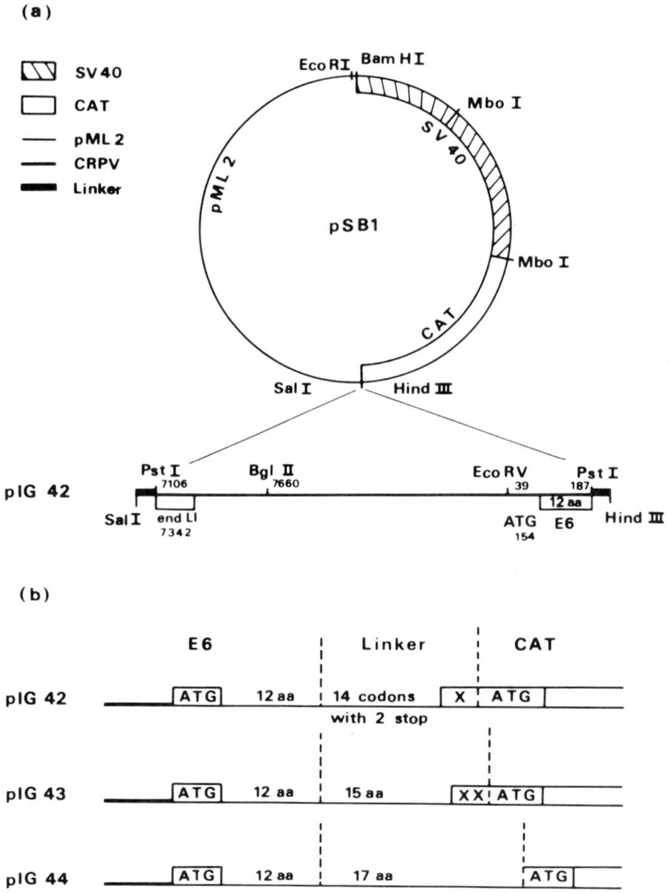


FIGURE 4. a) Expression vector used to test the promoter potential of CRPV non coding region : The Pst1 fragment (949 bp long) of CRPV was first inserted at the Pst1 site of a polylinker in pUC 18 excised by digestion with SalI and Hind III recloned between the Sal1 and Hind III sites of pSB1 (pIG42). Black boxes correspond to linker sequences coming from pUC18. The Hind III site was removed using Klenow polymerase to obtain plasmid pIG43. A HindIII linker inserted to produce the plasmid pIG44 which contains the first E6 ATG and the CAT ATG in the same reading frame.

b) Relative positions of E6 and CAT ATG initiator codons in pIG42, 43 and 44 : X are nucleotides disrupting the reading frame between the two ATG.

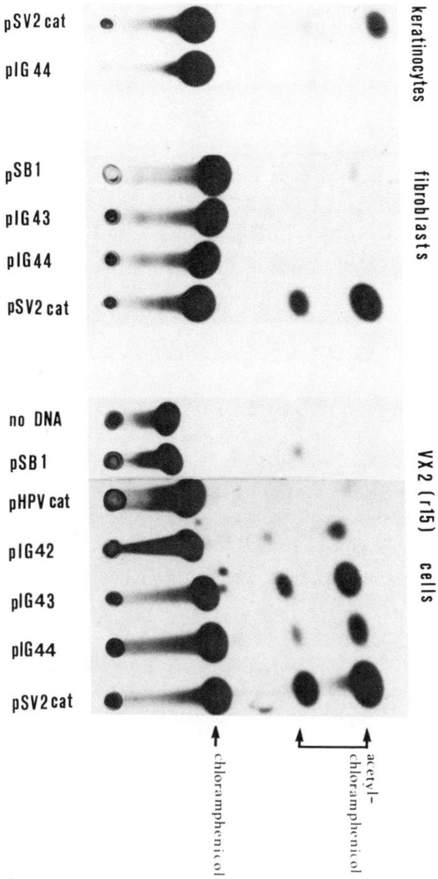


FIGURE 5. Assay of CAT activity in cells transfected with CRPV plasmids.

The day before transfection, cells were seeded at a density of $4.10^6$ VX2 cells or keratinocytes and $10^6$ fibroblasts per 10 cm dish. Cells were transfected with 10 ug of each plasmid DNA coprecipitated with calcium phosphate, according to standard procedures, and harvested 46 hours later. The enzyme activity was measured with 40 ul of cell extract (1/4 dish) after an incubation of 3 hours. The native chloramphenicol was separated from its acetylated derivatives by chomatography on a silica gel thin-layer plate. After autoradiography overnight, the spots were cut out and counted to quantitate the amount of chloramphenicol converted into its acetyl forms. Results are given in table 1.

shown). A similar CAT construction with the HPV1 non coding region also leads to negative results. We also transfected rabbit fibroblasts with the CRPV constructions without detecting significant CAT activity (figure 5, table I). We are currenlty investigating if the low activity of the CRPV promoter observed in normal rabbit keratinocytes (DRSK line -E. Georges et al., unpublished) is significant. We finally examined the promoter activity of the CRPV constructs in two cell lines established from the VX2 transplantable carcinoma(7). These cell lines both contain actively expressed CRPV genomes in an integrated state. The VX2T (clone 6) line retains the undifferenciated phenotype of the original tumor cells, whereas the VX2R (clone 15) shows the characteristics of a differenciated keratinocyte. The results of the CAT assay in the VX2 R (clone 15) cell line are shown in figure 5 and table I. CAT activity was reproducibly observed when these cells were transfected with plasmids pIG42, pIG43 and pIG44. Significant CAT activity was also detected in the extracts of transfected VX2T cells (not shown). Yet, the activity in VX2T was 2 to 5 times lower than in VX2R. The plasmid containing the HPV1 non coding region failed to yield any CAT activity in either type of cells. Compared to the activity of pSV2CAT in these cells, the CRPV fragments behaves as a relatively strong promoter in VX2R.

TABLE I

| Cell type | DNA transfected | Percentage of chloramphenicol acetylated | Percentage of SV40 activity |
|---|---|---|---|
| V x 2 (R15) | - | < 0.1 | 0 |
| | pSB1 | 0.3 | 1 |
| | pHPV1 CAT | 0.1 | 0.3 |
| | pIG 42 | 1 | 3.3 |
| | pIG 43 | 7.4 | 24.7 |
| | pIG 44 | 3 | 10 |
| | pSV2CAT | 30 | 100 |
| Rabbit fibroblasts | pSB1 | 0.3 | 2.5 |
| | pIG 43 | 0.1 | 0.8 |
| | pIG 44 | 0.1 | 0.8 |
| | pSV2CAT | 12 | 100 |
| Rabbit keratinocytes | pIG 44 | 0.1 | 3.3 |
| | pSV2CAT | 3 | 100 |

## CONCLUSIONS

We have identified a promoter fragment in the non coding region of the CRPV genome. Its activity is specifically detected in cells which already contain a transcribed CRPV genome, suggesting that viral early proteins may activate in trans the viral promoter. If such factors are present in the VX2 cells, they are unable to activate a promoter in the non coding region of HPV1. The higher activity of the CRPV promoter in the VX2R, compared to the VX2T imply that some cellular factors present in a differenciated keratinocyte increase the activity of the viral promoter. Both types of factors, cellular or viral, are not mutually exclusive, although keratinocytes factors alone does not seem to be sufficient, as shown by the lack of strong promoter activity in cultured rabbit keratinocytes. Identification of these factors could now be approached by characterizing proteins that bind specifically to the non coding segment of the CRPV genome, in extracts from VX2 R and T cells or from rabbit keratinocytes.

## ACKNOWLEDGEMENTS

We thank Gilles Thomas for help in the construction and analysis of plasmids and Jacqueline ARS for the preparation of the manuscript. This work was supported by grants from the CNRS (LA 270), from the Ministry of Industry and Research (82V1388), INSERM (PRC 134030 and 135018), from the ARC and from the Fondation pour la Recherche Medicale Française.

## REFERENCES

1. Danos O, Giri I, Thierry F, Yaniv M (1984). Papillomavirus genomes : sequences and consequences. J Invest Dermatol 83:7s.
2. Sarver N, Rabson MS, Yang YC, Howley PM (1984) Localization and analysis of the bovine papillomavirus transforming functions. J. Virol 52:377.
3. Yang YC, Okayama H, Howley PM (1985). Bovine papillomavirus contains multiple transforming genes. Proc Natl Acad Sci USA 82:1030.

4. Lusky M, Botchan MR (1985). Genetic analysis of Bovine Papillomavirus type 1 trans-acting replication factors. J Virol 53:955.
5. Syverton, JT (1952). The pathogenesis of the rabbit papilloma to carcinoma sequence. Ann NY Acad Sci 54:1126.
6. Nasseri M, Wettstein FO, Stevens SG (1982). Two colinear and spliced viral transcripts are present in non virus producing benign and malignant neoplasms induced by the shope (rabbit) papillomavirus. J Virol 44:263.
7. Georges E, Breitburd F, Jibard N, Orth G (1985). Two shope papilloma virus-associated VX2 carcinoma cell lines with different levels of keratinocyte differenciation and transplantability. J Virol (in press).
8. Giri I, Danos O, Yaniv M (1985). Structure of the genome of the cottontail rabbit (shope) papillomavirus. Proc Natl Acad Sci (USA) 82:
9. Danos O, Engel LW, Chen EY, Yaniv M, Howley PM (1983). A comparative analysis of the human type Ia and bovine type 1 papillomavirus genomes. J Virol 46:557.
10. Georges E, Croissant O, Bonneaud N, Orth G (1984). Physical state and transcription of the genome of the cottontail rabbit papillomavirus in domestic rabbit papillomas and in the transplantable VX2 and VX7 carcinomas. J Virol 51:530.
11. Danos O, Georges E, Orth G and Yaniv M (1985). Fine structure of the cottontail rabbit papillomavirus mRNAs expressed in the transplantable VX2 carcinoma. J Virol 53:735.
12. Nasseri M, Wettstein FO (1984). Viral transcipts in cottontail rabbit papilloma virus induced tumors : differences exists in benign and malignant as well as between non virus producing and virus-producing tumors. J Virol 51:706.
13. Kozak M (1983). Comparison of initiation of protein synthesis in procaryotes, eucaryotes and organelles. Microbiol Rev 47:1.
14. Gorman CM, Moffat LF, Howard BH (1982). Recombinant genomes which express chloramphenicol acetyl transferase in mammalian cells. Mol Cell Biol 2:1044.
15. Herbomel P, Bourachot B, Yaniv M (1984). Two distinct enhancers with different cell specificities coexist in the regulatory regions of polyoma. Cell 39:653.

**Papillomaviruses: Molecular and Clinical Aspects, pages 391–396**


# HUMAN PAPILLOMAVIRUS TYPE 16 DNA: EXPRESSION OF OPEN READING FRAMES IN E.COLI

Klaus Seedorf, Günter Krämmer and Walter G. Röwekamp

German Cancer Research Center
Institute of Cell and Tumor Biology
Im Neuenheimer Feld 280
D - 6900 Heidelberg, F.R.G.

ABSTRACT Sequence analysis of the DNA of HPV16 has revealed an arrangement of open reading frames similar to that found in BPV1, HPV1a, HPV6b, CRPV. A striking difference could be demonstrated in the open reading frame (ORF) coding for the suspected $E_1$ protein, showing splitting of the polypeptide sequence on two viral open reading frames. Almost the entire $E_6$ and the carboxyterminal part of the $L_1$ open reading frame have been expressed in E.coli.

## INTRODUCTION

The general structure of the papillomavirus DNA has been established recently (1, 2, 3, 4). Up to 6 open reading frames can be assigned to the early region of the viral genome. Additionally two open reading frames are found, named L2 and L1, which code for structural viral proteins. Transcriptional data have been obtained in different systems, suggesting a biological role of these gene products.

Results from BPV1 transfection experiments indicate the existance of two transforming genes in the early region. In cervical cancer cell lines and biopsies containing

HPV18 or HPV16 DNA respectively only a part of the early region is expressed (E6, E7 and most of E1), while E2 is either deleted or inactive (6). Nevertheless an intracellular protein analogue to T-antigens of the polyomavirus type has not yet been identified, though homologies between the large T of SV40 and polyomavirus and the E1 protein of papillomaviruses have been found (7).

To address this question we have initiated experiments to express several open reading frames of HPV16 in E.coli in order to raise antibodies against these polypeptides.

## RESULTS

The DNA of HPV16 originally cloned in bacteriophage λ from an invasive cervical carcinoma (8) was subcloned into the BamHI site of pUC8 in both orientations. Using the DNaseI/$Mn^{++}$ technique 5'- and 3'-end deletions were generated which increased progressively by about 200 bp (9). More than 95% of the genome were sequenced on each strand applying the dideoxy chain termination method of Sanger (10) on the pUC8 clones. Ambigous regions were additionally sequenced by partial chemical degradation according to Maxam and Gilbert (11). The HPV16 genome has a size of 7904 bp (4). Fig. 1 shows the distribution of the termination codons in the three possible reading frames. Homology comparisons between HPV16, HPV6b and BPV1 at the nucleotide level as well as at the amino acid level allowed us to designate the presumptive early ($E_6$, $E_7$, $E_1$, $E_2$, $E_4$, $E_5$) and late ($L_2$ and $L_1$) reading frames (Fig. 1). They are located on one DNA strand as has been shown for all other sequenced papillomaviruses. The general organization resembles that of the other viruses with three exceptions. In contrast to other papillomaviruses the $E_4$ and $E_5$ open reading frames do not possess a translation initiation codon. Additionally the suspected $E_1$ gene product is split into RF1 and RF3. Homology comparisons indicate that the frameshift occurs probably at base position 1137. Since a sequencing mistake (i.e. one missing nucleotide) between the stop codon in RF3 (pos. 1101) and the stop codon in RF1 (pos. 1168) could account for this result we verified the sequence in this region additionally by Maxam and Gilbert sequencing.

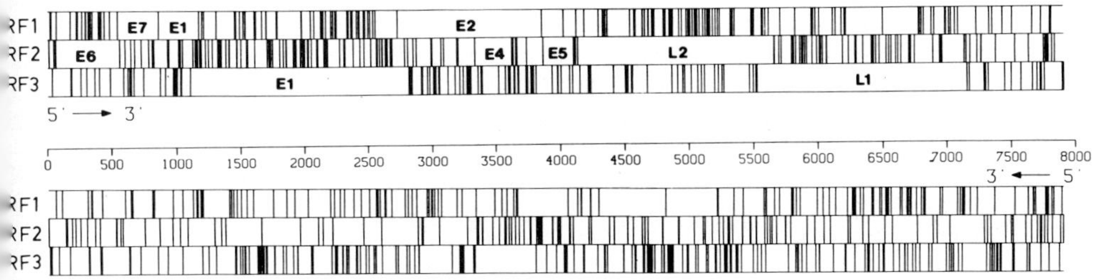


Figure 1. Distribution of translational termination codons of the HPV16 nucleotide sequence in all possible reading frames. Each vertical bar represents one termination codon. The open reading frames are designated in analogy to the organization of BPV1, HPV1a, HPV66 and CRPV DNA.

At the present time we do not know whether this interruption in the $E_1$ reading frame has any functional relevance. A possible involvement of $E_1$ in BPV plasmid maintenance (12, 13) as well as the conservation of structural features of the $E_1$ gene in BPV1, HPV1a, HPV6b and the large T-antigen of polyoma virus and SV40 (7) might suggest a general function of the $E_1$ protein in the control of DNA replication. Since HPV16 DNA occurs in benign tumours normally in an episomal state, whereas in malignant tumors it appears to be integrated in the host genome the interruption of the $E_1$ coding region might reflect a functional state of the HPV16 DNA. We have started to isolate HPV16 DNA from episomal and integrated origin in order to analyze this region in other isolates.

Expression of the open reading frame (ORF) $E_6$ and part of $L_1$ in E.coli.

In order to provide antibodies directed against polypeptides encoded by HPV16 DNA we have started to express several ORF's in E.coli. We have constructed a series of expression vectors based on the plasmid pPLc24 which contains the leftward promoter $P_L$ of phage λ and the first 98 amino acids of the replicase gene of the RNA phage $MS_2$ cloned downstream from the $P_L$ promoter (14). The pPLc24 vector allows insertion of an ORF only into a BamHI or into a HindIII site. Therefore we have introduced into this BamHI-HindIII site a polylinker sequence with cloning sites for EcoRI, BamHI, SalI, PstI, BglII, XbaI and HindIII. Additionally, we constructed three derivatives of this polylinker vector (pEx8, pEX1O, pEx12) allowing insertion in all three possible reading frames with respect to the $MS_2$ initiation AUG (unpublished results). A 3' fragment of the $L_1$ coding sequence starting from the EcoRI site (pos. 6818) and extending to a DdeI site (pos. 7761) with a stop codon at position 7152 was cloned into pEx12. Almost the entire ORF of $E_6$ starting from position 109 and extending to a PstI site at pos. 875 (translation initiation codon is at pos. 83, stop codon at pos. 557) was cloned into expression vector pEx12 as well.The synthesis of the $E_6$ and $L_1$ polypeptides in induced cultures of strain E.coli 537 (kindly supplied by H. Schaller) transfected with these expression vectors was monitored by the appearance of a new protein in the bacterial extracts (Fig. 2). In the induced cells a new major protein for $E_6$ (lane A') and for $L_1$ (3'-terminal third) was detected (lane B'). These proteins are absent in the induced cultures harbouring no plasmid (lane A + B). The observed molecular weights for the MS2-$L_1$ (21K) and the MS2-$E_6$ (25K) fusion proteins are consistent with the theoretical values of the calculated sizes of 21K and 23.5K respectively. We have started to purify these induced polypeptides in order to produce monoclonal antibodies.

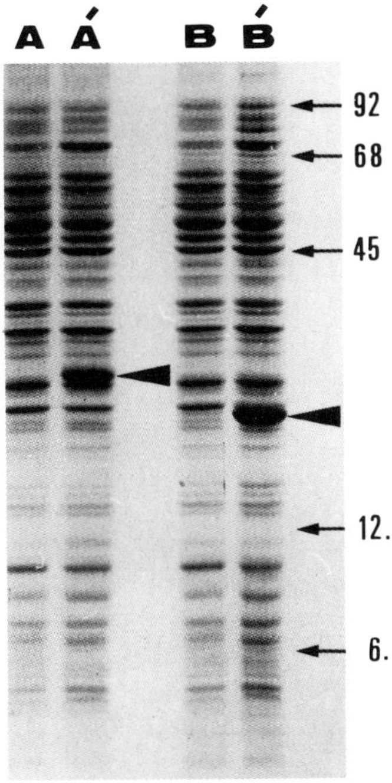


Legend to Figure 2. Expression of HPV16 $E_6$ and $L_1$ open reading frames in E.coli. Almost the entire $E_6$ and the carboxy terminal part of $L_1$ were cloned into appropriate expression vectors (see text for more details). The bacterial strains were grown to stationary phase at 28°C, diluted with 4 volumes of L broth, heated to 43°C and kept at this temperature for 3 hrs. Cells were spun down, lysed directly in Laemmli sample buffer and aliquots were applied to Laemmli gels. Lane A and B: Host bacteria containing no expression plasmid treated as indicated above. A': Expression of the $E_6$ open reading frame. B': Expression of part of the $L_1$ open reading frame. Small arrows indicate the positions of molecular weight standards, the large arrows show the positions of the newly expressed fusion peptides.

ACKNOWLEDGEMENTS

We thank Dr. H. zur Hausen, Dr. L. Gissman for helpful discussions, U. Schätzle for technical assistance, and M. Cole for typing the manuscript. Parts of this work were supported by a grant from the Deutsche Forschungsgemeinschaft to W.G.R. (RÖ 444/6-4).

REFERENCES

1. Chen EY, Howley PM, Levinson AD, Seeburg PH (1982). The primary structural and genetic organization of the bovine papillomavirus type 1 genome. Nature 299:529.
2. Danos O, Katinka M, Yaniv M (1982). Human papillomavirus 1a complete DNA sequence: A novel type of genome organization among papovaviridae. EMBO J 1:231.

3 Schwarz E, Dürst M, Demankowski C, Lattermann O, Zeck R, Wolfsperger E, Suhai S, Zur Hausen H (1983). DNA sequence and genome organization of genital human papillomavirus 6b. EMBO J 2:2341.
4. Seedorf K, Krämmer G, Dürst M, Suhai S, Röwekamp WG (1985). Human papillomavirus type 16 DNA sequence. Virology 114:in press.
5. Sarver N, Rabson MG, Yang YC, Byrne JC, Howley PM (1984). Localization and analysis of bovine papillomavirus type 1 transforming functions. J Virol 52:377.
6. Schwarz E, Freese UK, Gissmann L, Mayer W, Roggenbuck B, Stremlau A, Zur Hausen H (1985) Structure and transcription of human papillomavirus sequences in cervical carcinoma cells. Nature 314:111.
7. Clertant P, Seif J (1984). A common function for polyoma virus large-T and papillomavirus $E_1$ proteins? Nature 311:276.
8. Dürst M, Gissmann L, Ikenberg H, Zur Hausen H (1983). A papillomavirus DNA from a cervical carcinoma and its prelevance in cancer biopsy samples from different geographic regions. PNAS 80:3812.
9. Frischauf AM, Garoff H, Lehrach H (1980). A subcloning strategy for DNA sequence analysis. Nucl Acids Res 8:5541.
10. Sanger F, Nicklen S, Coulson AR (1977). DNA sequencing with chain-terminating inhibitors. PNAS 74:5463.
11. Maxam AM, Gilbert W (1980). In Grossmann L, Moldove K (eds): "Methods in Enzymology", New York: Academic Press, 65, p.499.
12. Nakabayashi Y, Chattopadhyay SK, Lowy DR (1983). The transforming function of bovine papillomavirus DNA. PNAS 80:5832.
13. Lusky M, Botchan MR (1984). Characterization of the bovine papillomavirus plasmid maintenance sequences. Cell 36:391.
14. Remaut E, Stanssens P, Fiers W (1981). Plasmid vectors for high-efficiency expression controlled by the $P_L$ promoter of coliphage lambda. Gene 15:81.

**Papillomaviruses: Molecular and Clinical Aspects, pages 397–406**


# *IN VITRO* REPLICATION OF DNA CONTAINING THE SV40 ORIGIN SEQUENCE

Frank Dean, C. Richard Wobbe, Lawrence Weissbach, Yasufumi Murakami and Jerard Hurwitz

Graduate Program in Molecular Biology and Virology
Sloan-Kettering Institute for Cancer Research
New York, New York 10021

High salt extracts of HeLa cells support replication of DNA containing the SV40 origin in the presence of SV40 large T antigen. The reaction leads to the accumulation of large molecular weight products that represent DNA containing one parental strand and one progeny strand as well as duplex molecules that contain both strands derived from the input deoxynucleoside triphosphates. The replication reaction is inhibited by aphidicolin and by camptothecin, two inhibitors known to inhibit eukaryotic DNA replication *in vivo*.

## INTRODUCTION

The replication of the papovavirus SV40 has been carried out *in vitro*. Reports from the laboratories of Ariga (1), Kelly (2) and Stillman and Gluzman (3) have shown that extracts isolated from a variety of different cells support SV40 DNA replication. They demonstrated that the bidirectional replication required the viral-encoded large T antigen and a functional SV40 origin sequence in the DNA. The reaction was sensitive to aphidicolin, suggesting that DNA polymerase α plays an important role in the replication process.

## RESULTS

We have confirmed and extended these findings. As shown in Table 1, extracts of HeLa cells supported DNA synthesis only in the presence of T antigen and duplex circular DNA containing the SV40 origin of replication.The products formed in the reaction (as a function of time) were analyzed by agarose gel electrophoresis (Fig 1). Replication products included RFI, RFII, intervening topoisomers, and discrete slower migrating species. High molecular weight DNA products were found only in the presence of both T antigen and DNA containing the SV40 origin.

**TABLE 1**

REQUIREMENTS FOR REPLICATION OF SV40 Ori$^+$ DNA

| Component Omitted | | DNA Synthesis (%) |
|---|---|---|
| None | | 100 |
| T antigen | | <2 |
| DNA | | <2 |
| DNA + ori$^-$ DNA | | <2 |
| DNA + topoisomerase I-treated ori$^+$ DNA | | 83 |
| DNA + *Pst* I RFIII of ori$^+$ DNA | | 3 |
| ATP | | 35 |
| Creatine phosphate and Creatine phosphokinase | | 9 |
| dATP, dGTP, dTTP and CTP, UTP, GTP | | 3 |
| dATP, dGTP, dTTP | | 3 |
| CTP, UTP, GTP | | 80 |
| + aphidicolin | 100 µM | <2 |
| | 400 µM | <2 |
| + camptothecin | 100 µM | 58 |
| | 500 µM | 42 |

Reaction mixtures (50 µl) containing 30mM Hepes buffer (pH7.5), 7mM $MgCl_2$, 0.5mM dithiothreitiol, 4mM ATP, 200 µM each of CTP, UTP, GTP, 100 µM each of dATP, dGTP and dTTP, 25 µM [α-$^{32}$P] dCTP, 40 mM creatine phosphate, 20 µg/ml of creatine phosphokinase, 0.3 µg of RFI plasmid (ori$^+$), 338 µg of HeLa extract and 0.6 µg of T antigen.Ori$^-$DNA consisted of a 2481-bp derivative of pBR322 lacking the 1881-bp EcoRV-Pvu II fragment. Ori$^+$ DNA consisted of the 311-bp origin-containing EcoRII fragment of SV40 cloned into the 2481-bp pBR322 derivative. Reactions were carried out for 120 min at 37$^o$C and the amount of acid-insoluble material formed was measured. The value 100% corresponded to the incorporation of 128 pmol of dCMP into an acid-insoluble form.

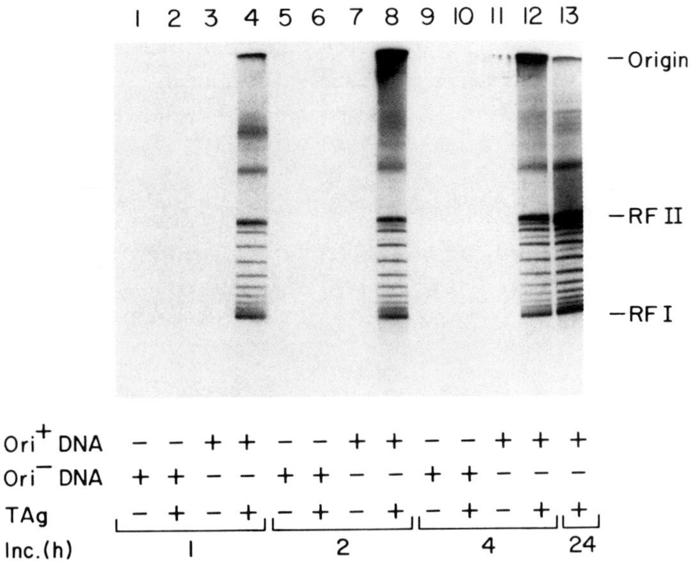


FIGURE 1. Time course of DNA synthesis and product distribution. Reactions were as described in Table I except that after the times indicated, they were terminated by the addition of 20 mM EDTA, 0.5% SDS, 20 μg tRNA as carrier and digested with 200 μg/ml proteinase K at 37$^{o}$C for 20 min. After phenol extraction and precipitation with ethanol, the products were subjected to agarose gel electrophoresis. The lanes contained ori$^{+}$ or ori$^{-}$ DNA, with or without the SV40 T antigen, as indicated.

Maximum DNA synthesis required, in addition to T antigen and the origin sequence, $Mg^{2+}$, ATP, creatine phosphate and creatine phosphokinase, dNTPs, circular duplex DNA (superhelical or relaxed) and rNTPs. The latter addition stimulated synthesis about 20%.

The reaction was sensitive to pancreatic DNase, RNase, aphidicolin and camptothecin. The high concentration of DNase (200 μg/ml) necessary to quantitatively reduce dNMP incorporation to background levels suggests that the DNA may be protected from nuclease attack in the presence of high levels of crude HeLa extract. The effect of RNase on the reaction remains to be clarified. The inhibition with aphidicolin is in keeping with the important role ascribed to DNA polymerase α in SV40 DNA replication (4). Removal of DNA polymerase α activity from crude cytosolic extracts with monoclonal antibodies that react with DNA polymerase α resulted in the quantitative loss of replication activity. The addition of purified DNA polymerase α-primase preparations to the depleted extracts did not restore ori$^{+}$/T antigen-dependent DNA synthesis; the addition of crude Hela nuclear extract (at levels that did not support DNA replication) partially restored replication activity (40-50%). These results suggest that other factors, possibly associated with DNA polymerase α, were either inactivated or lost during the depletion procedure. The nature of the stimulating activity is now under investigation.

The inhibition of DNA synthesis with camptothecin has been examined more carefully. Camptothecin is a known inhibitor of HeLa chromosomal DNA synthesis *in vivo* (5). *In vitro*, this compound, at a concentration of 10 μM, inhibited DNA synthesis 50% (as it does *in vivo*), but a high concentration of camptothecin (500 μM) inhibited replication maximally (60%).

As shown in Fig 2A and 2B, camptothecin inhibited the action of purified topoisomerase II and topoisomerase I. The former was measured by its ability to render kinetoplast DNA non-sedimentable in the presence of ATP while the latter was measured by its ability to relax supercoiled DNA. Studies with topoisomerase II indicated that the inhibitory effects were dependent on the enzyme concentration and not the concentration of DNA. Similar results were obtained with the epipodophyllotoxin derivatives (7) that specifically inhibit topoisomerase II (and not topoisomerase I). Camptothecin inhibited the synthesis of high molecular weight DNA more than the monomer-sized products which include RFI and RFII. These results suggest an important role for topoismerase I and/or topoisomerase II in the accumulation of these complex DNA replication forms. It is not clear which of the accumulated high molecular weight products represent *bona fide* intermediates or products accumulating due to nuclease or other artifacts catalyzed by the crude fractions. This problem will be resolved by further purification and isolation of the components essential for SV40 ori+/T antigen-dependent DNA synthesis.

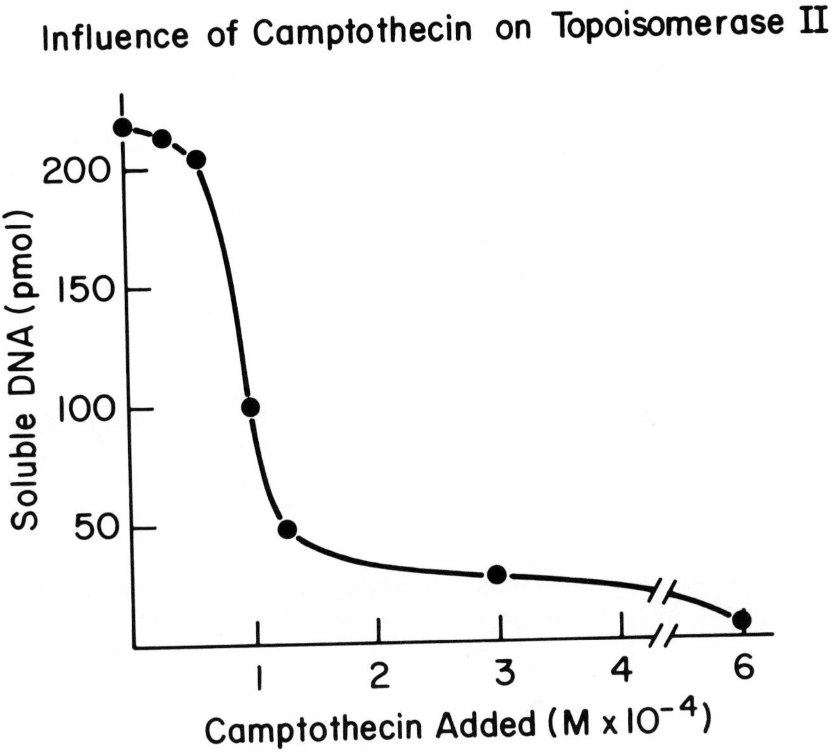


FIGURE 2A. Influence of camptothecin on topoisomerase II. Reaction mixtures (30 µl) contained 20 mM Tris buffer pH 8.0, 6 mM $MgCl_2$. 0.1 mM dithiothreitol, 20 µg/ml bovine serum albumin, 0.05 M NaCl, 1 mM ATP, 67.5 ng of $^3$H-labeled kinetoplast DNA (6), 8 ng of topoisomerase II and varying amounts of camptothecin (as indicated). After 15 min at 30$^o$C, reaction mixtures were centrifuged in an Eppendorf centrifuge for 15 min and an aliquot of the supernatant was counted. Reaction mixtures lacking ATP resulted in 16 pmol of soluble material. This value has been subtracted from those presented.

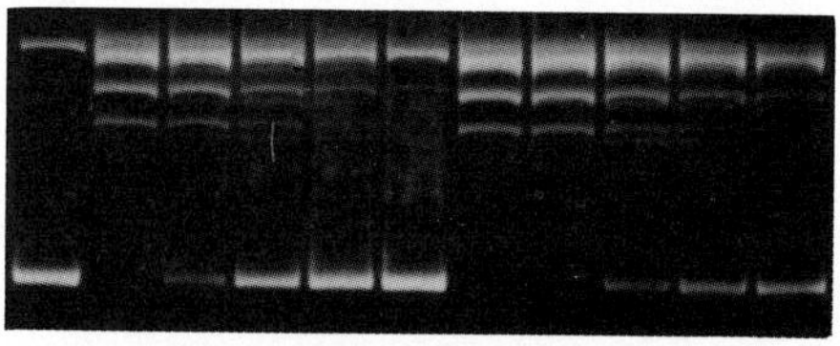


FIGURE 2B. Inhibition of topoisomerase I by camptothecin. Reactions were carried out in 20 μl containing 50 mM Tris·HCl, pH 7.9, 40 mM NaCl, 10 mM $MgCl_2$, 1 mM dithiothreitol, 0.5 mM EDTA, 30 μg/ml bovine serum albumin, and 0.3 μg supercoiled ori$^+$ plasmid DNA. After incubation for 30 min at 37$^0$ reactions were stopped with the addition of sodium dodecyl sulfate to 0.3% and EDTA to 10 mM, and electrophoresed in a 1.5% agarose gel. Calf thymus topoisomerase I was purchased from BRL, and varying amounts of both topoisomerase I and camptothecin were added, as indicated.

As shown by others (1-3), the replication of ori$^+$ DNA occurs by a semiconservative mechanism, initially leading to one strand derived from the added dNTPs and one strand from the parental DNA. This was established by utilizing of the restriction enzyme *Dpn* I. Since the plasmid DNAs were isolated from a *dam*$^+$ strain of *E. coli* (HB101), both strands were methylated. The restriction enzymes *Dpn* I and *Mbo* I cut DNA at their recognition sequence (GATC) only if the adenine residues on both strands are methylated or if neither adenine residue is methylated, respectively. Resistance to *Dpn* I cleavage indicates one round of semiconservative replication while hydrolysis by *Mbo* I indicates multiple rounds of replication. As shown in Fig 3, the amount of *Mbo* I sensitive DNA increased with incubation time. After 4 hr of incubation, approximately 20% of the incorporated label was detected in Mbo I sensitive DNA. Thus, some of the synthesis has resulted from two or more rounds of replication.

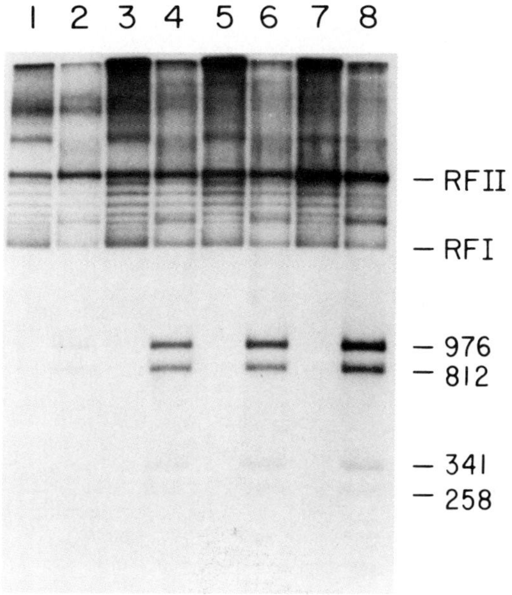


FIGURE 3. Mbo I digestion of replication products. $Ori^+$ DNA (0.3 μg) was incubated in reaction mixtures containing HeLa cell extract (350 μg of protein) and 0.6 μg T antigen for 1 (lanes 1 and 2), 2 (lanes 3 and 4), 4 (lanes 5 and 6) or 24 hr (lanes 7 and 8) followed by protease digestion, phenol extraction and ethanol precipitation as described in Fig 1. After dissolving the precipitate in buffer containing 50 mM Tris-HCl (pH 8.0), 10 mM $MgCl_2$, 1 mM dithiothreitol, 50 mM NaCl, 100 μg/ml bovine serum albumin, the DNA was incubated for one hr at $37^o$ without (lanes 1, 3, 5, 7) or with 5 units of MboI (lanes 2, 4, 6, 8) and electrophoresed in a 1.5% agarose gel. The positions of Mbo I bands, indicated at right, were determined from ethidium bromide stained, Dpn I digested $ori^+$ DNA simultaneously run with the above digests.

We have routinely observed four bands of high molecular weight products, in addition to supercoiled (RFI) and nicked (RFII) product monomers. We have shown that the high molecular weight products contain undetectable amounts of catenated DNA rings. We believe that these products contain substantially, but not completely, replicated DNA. The unreplicated DNA is located at random sites around the circle, its position determined either by the relative rates of movement of the two replication forks or by the random positioning of factors that prevent fork movement. If the latter were true, these factors are present at concentrations equal to or greater than the added DNA.

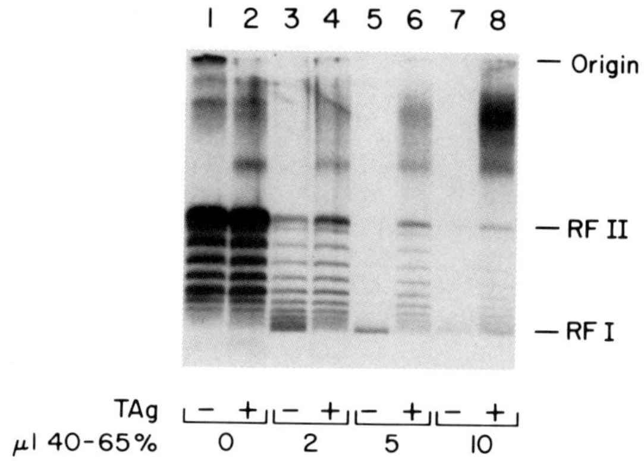


FIGURE 4. Influence of protein fractions on T antigen-dependent DNA synthesis. Crude extract was adjusted to 0.2 M NaCl and applied to a DEAE cellulose column equilibrated with buffer A (20 mM Hepes, pH 7.5, 1 mM dithiothreitol, 0.1 mM EDTA, 10% glycerol) containing 0.2 M NaCl. The flow through was adjusted to 40% saturation with ammonium sulfate and the precipitate removed by centrifugation. The supernatant was adjusted to 65% ammonium sulfate and recentrifuged. The pellets were dissolved with buffer A containing 50 mM

(Continued)

Fig. 4 (Continued)

NaCl and dialyzed extensively against the same buffer. Ten μl of the 40% ammonium sulfate fraction (28 mg/ml) was assayed under standard reaction conditions (Table I) in the presence of the indicated amounts of the 65% ammonium sulfate fraction (48 mg/ml). Products were prepared for electrophoresis as described in Fig 1.

Our initial attempts to isolate protein components have resolved the system into a number of fractions. As shown in Fig 4, the specificity of the reaction changed upon ammonium sulfate fractionation (or upon heparin-agarose chromatography). A 0-40% ammonium sulfate fraction alone showed T antigen-independent synthesis and virtually no response to T antigen. Upon combination with a 40-65% ammonium sulfate fraction (itself totally inactive in the presence or absence of T antigen), the T antigen-independent synthesis was completely inhibited and addition of T antigen resulted in the accumulation of high molecular weight products.

These observations are similar to those seen with replication carried out using the E coli ori C system (8) as well as those carried out with the adenovirus replication system. In the latter case, the protein factor that rendered origin⁻ DNA inactive was the adenovirus DNA binding protein (9). In the case of the ori C initiation reaction, dnaA site specific initiation was maintained by the addition of the HU protein, RNase H and topoisomerase I.

The availability of a system capable of replicating duplex circular DNA containing the SV40 origin in the presence of SV40 T antigen is a major step forward. Since the only viral protein essential for this DNA replication system is the T antigen, it will provide an important assay for the isolation and characterization of host proteins essential for bidirectional DNA replication.

## REFERENCES


(1) Ariga H, Sugano S (1983). Initiation of SV40 DNA replication in vitro. J Virol 48:481-491.

(2) Li JJ, Kelly TJ (2984). SV40 DNA replication in vitro. Proc Natl Acad Sci USA 81:6973-6977.

(3) Stillman B, Gluzman Y (1985). Replication and supercoiling of SV40 DNA in cell free extracts from human cells. In press.

(4) De Pamphilis ML, Wasserman PM (1980). Replication of eukaryotic chromosomes: A close-up of the replication fork. Ann Rev of Biochem 49:627-666.
(5) Horwitz SB, Chang CK, Grollman AP (1971). Studies on camptothecin: I effects on nucleic acid and protein synthesis. Mol Pharmacol 7:632-644.
(6) Englund PT (1978). DNA networks in crithidia fasciculata. Cell 14:157-163.
(7) Nelson EM, Tewey KM, Liu LF (1984). Intercalative antitumor drugs interfere with the breakage-reunion reaction of mammalian DNA topoisomerase II. Proc Natl Acad Sci USA 81:1361-1365.
(8) Kaguni JM, Kornberg A (1984). Replication *in vitro* at the origin (ori C) of the *E. coli* chromosome reconstitution with purified enzymes. Cell 38:183-190.
(9) Kaplan LM, Ariga H, Hurwitz J, Horwitz MS (1979). Complimentation of the temperature-sensitive defect in H5ts125 adenovirus DNA replication *in vitro*. Proc Natl Acad Sci USA 76:5534-5538.

# VII. EPITHELIAL CELL CULTURE

**Papillomaviruses: Molecular and Clinical Aspects, pages 409–411**


# WORKSHOP SUMMARY: EPITHELIAL CELL CULTURE

Lorne B. Taichman

Department of Oral Biology and Pathology
School of Dental Medicine
State University of New York at Stony Brook
Stony Brook, New York 11794

The workshop on "Epithelial Cell Culture" dealt with the biology of the keratinocyte and its interaction with papillomaviruses.

Dr. Lorne Taichman (SUNY Stony Brook) described his studies on the interaction of HPV1 and cultured human epidermal keratinocytes. Following infection with HPV1 particles, cultured keratinocytes exhibit no CPE, no transformation, and no evidence of late gene expression. However, HPV1 DNA is present as a multicopy monomeric episome which replicates primarily in the least differentiated cells. In addition, viral transcripts (5.9, 5.0 and 3.9 kb) were detected which hybridized with DNA of the E1 and E2 ORFs. When infected cells were subcultured, there was a diminution in the amount of viral DNA, and after several passes, no HPV1 DNA was detectable. A similar loss of HPV1 DNA was observed following infection and growth of malignant keratinocytes. By growing infected cells in BrdUrd and probing the density labeled DNA for HPV1 sequences, it was shown that the viral DNA replicated even though it was eventually lost from the culture. The conclusion Dr. Taichman drew from these results was that the loss of HPV1 from keratinocyte cultures could be due to a failure of viral DNA to segregate properly at the time of cell division.

What is the phenotype of the PV-transformed cell? To answer this question, Dr. Françoise Breitburd (Institut Pasteur) described studies done by the group of Gérard Orth on the properties of keratinocyte cultures derived from human and rabbit papillomas and carcinomas. Keratinocytes cultured from CRPV-induced papillomas underwent senescence after 4 passes and during growth, the CRPV DNA was lost in a manner similar to that observed in human keratinocytes infected with HPV1.

VX2 is a transplantable anplastic tumor derived initially from a CRPV-associated rabbit carcinoma. Two lines, VX2T and VX2R, contained multiple integrated copies of CRPV DNA and expressed similar transcripts (4.6, 2.0 and 1.2 kb). The state of viral DNA and the RNA composition in these two lines resembled that seen in the VX2 parent. The two lines did, however, differ in phenotype. The VX2T cells appeared much less differentiated. They contained few desmosomes, reduced levels and numbers of keratin proteins, and formed undifferentiated nonkeratinizing carcinomas in nude mice. The VX2R cells appeared more differentiated in that more keratin protein was present, a 65 kd keratin could be induced, desmosome-tonofilament complexes were abundant, and more differentiated, keratinizing tumors developed in nude mice.

Dr. Breitburd also described an interesting line of human keratinocytes (Skv-1) established from vulvar Bowenoid papules and which formed tumors with features of Bowenoid carcinoma in nude mice. The cells responded to growth in vitamin A-depleted medium by expressing a more differentiated phenotype. In addition, Skv-1 cells contained multiple integrated copies of HPV16 DNA while the original Bowenoid lesion contained primarily episomal HPV16 DNA and a minute amount of integrated viral DNA. This finding suggested that the culture conditions had selected for those cells that had integrated copies of HPV16 DNA.

A puzzling aspect of papillomavirus biology is the predeliction for certain PV types to infect specific epithelial sites. Dr. Tung-Tien Sun's (New York University) talk addressed this point by helping to define in biochemical terms how various epithelia actually differ. Using monoclonal antibodies to define the keratin content of a variety of keratinizing epithelia, Dr. Sun has discovered that the multiple keratin proteins are expressed according to very specific "rules". These rules may be summarized as follows: 1, Keratins are expressed in pairs, an acidic and a basic polypeptide which differ in molecular weight by 8 kd. 2, In basal keratinocytes, a 50 and 58 kd pair are synthesized. 3, Upon differentiation, keratinocytes in the epidermis synthesize a set of 56.5 and 65-67 kd keratins which are specific for this epithelium. 4, In culture and in hyperproliferative states (including PV-induced papillomas), the epidermal specific keratins are not made, and in their place a 48 and 56 kd pair of keratins are produced. 5, Other stratified squamous epithelia such as cornea and esophagus produce specific pairs of higher molecular weight keratins.

Simple epithelia such as mesothelial cells produce pairs of lower molecular weight keratins. Although keratin proteins are not known to play a direct role in papillomavirus expression, this regulated expression of keratin proteins helps to explain how various epithelial surfaces differ from one another.

The most constant feature of papillomavirus infection is transformation. How papillomaviruses induce tumors in keratinocytes is not known. Dr. Stuart Yuspa's work (National Cancer Institute) on chemical carcinogenesis in cultured keratinocytes from newborn mice was the starting point for a discussion of carcinogenic initiation. Dr. Yuspa has found that terminal differentiation of mouse keratinocytes is blocked when calcium levels in the culture medium are reduced to 0.02-0.09 mM. When calcium is restored to normal concentrations, the cells en masse undergo terminal differentiation. Treatment of mouse skin with carcinogens such as MMNG or DMBA results in the appearance of cell colonies that are resistant to this calcium-induced terminal differentiation. The number of colonies is directly dependent upon the dose and potency of the carcinogen used. A number of features of these resistant cells suggest that they are initiated cells. Cells in these foci are, at the outset, not tumorigenic in nude mice, but when induced to undergo multiple cycles of replication in culture, become tumorigenic. In addition, keratinocytes from the SENCAR strain of mice, which readily develop tumors following the application of promoter, give rise to calcium-resistant cells without prior application of an initiator. The resistance of these initiated cells to undergo calcium-induced terminal differentiation suggested that in the development of PV-induced lesions, there may be a similar block to the expression of the keratinocyte phenotype.

At the conclusion of the workshop, Dr. Clyde Dawe (Harvard University) described a curious polyomavirus which induces a variety of tumors including papillomatous growths of hair follicle keratinocytes. Vegetative viral replication is confined to the differentiating population of cells.

**Papillomaviruses: Molecular and Clinical Aspects, pages 413–426**


# EFFECTS OF ALPHA-INTERFERON ON CULTURED LARYNGEAL PAPILLOMA CELLS[1]

Bettie M. Steinberg,* Allan L. Abramson,* and Bernard Horowitz**

*Department of Otolaryngology, Long Island Jewish Medical Center and **Blood Derivatives Program, New York Blood Center

ABSTRACT We have investigated the effects of interferon on cultured cells derived from both normal laryngeal epithelium and laryngeal papillomas. Treatment with interferon at concentrations up to 1000 units/ml had no effect on outgrowth of primary cells from tissue explants. Autoradiography of primary cells labeled with tritiated thymidine showed a 76% reduction in labeled nuclei of both cell types when cultured in the presence of 100 units/ml interferon. Treatment of secondary papilloma cells with interferon resulted in a 70% reduction in incorporation of tritiated thymidine into TCA precipitable material, but there was no reduction of tritiated thymidine incorporation in normal cells treated with interferon. There was no significant reduction in the average number of copies of Human Papilloma Virus (HPV) DNA per cell after culture in the presence of interferon. This was in contrast to a drop in copy number in biopsy samples from two papilloma patients on interferon therapy.

## INTRODUCTION

Papillomas of the larynx are benign neoplasms located primarily but not exclusively on the vocal cords. They

1. This work was supported by National Institutes of Health Grant P01 NS19214

are characterized by frequent recurrences, sometimes persisting for the life of the patient and sometimes lasting for only a few months or years. Recurrences can be interrupted by extended periods of remission. It is not known what regulates either the remissions or the recurrences. We do know that the Human Papilloma Virus (HPV) DNA associated with the papillomas can also be found in the "normal" laryngeal tissues of a patient with either active disease or disease in remission (1). Presumably, it is this latent infection which is the source of recurrent lesions.

Laryngeal papillomatosis is most commonly managed by multiple surgical procedures. Recently, however, a number of clinical trials have suggested that interferon therapy can be of use in the management of this disease (2-5). It is not known what role interferon plays in this therapy. It could be acting as an antiviral agent, since Turek et al (6) showed that the copy number of Bovine Papilloma Virus (BPV) DNA was reduced when C127 cells were cultured in the presence of interferon for long periods of time. Conversely, it could be acting directly as an anti-tumor agent (7,8) or as a regulator of immune function (9). We have begun to investigate the effects of alpha-interferon on the growth of cultured epithelial cells derived from laryngeal papillomas to determine whether there is a direct antitumor-like or antiviral effect on these cells. The results of our studies are reported in this paper.

## METHODS AND MATERIALS

Primary and secondary cells were cultured as previously described (10) from biopsy fragments of normal and papillomatous tissues. Alpha-interferon (specific activity $2 \times 10^6$ units/mg protein) was prepared as described (11) and was provided by the New York Blood Center and used in culture at concentrations ranging from 10 to 1000 units per ml.

Effects on cell outgrowth were determined by measuring the increasing diameters of sheets of outgrowing primary cells from tissue fragments. The rate, in mm/day, was calculated from the slope of a plot of diameter against time in culture. After three weeks of culture in the presence of interferon, the primary cells were labeled for 24 hours with 10 μCi/ml [$^{3}$H]thymidine (New England Nuclear), and prepared for autoradiography (12). Results were normalized to the percentage of labeled nuclei in dishes without interferon.

Secondary cells were prepared by growing tissue explants for three weeks in the absence of interferon, releasing the cells from their collagen matrix with collagenase and trypsin, and suspending in liquid medium. They were plated at $10^5$ cells per 16 mm well in duplicate in media containing interferon ranging from 0 to 1000 units/ml. After four days, they were labeled with either 10μCi/ml [$^{3}$H]thymidine or [$^{3}$H]Amino Acid Hydrolysate (New England Nuclear) for 24 hours. Medium was removed, cells washed in PBS and scraped into Eppendorf tubes containing 5% TCA. After 60 minutes at 4°C, tubes were spun for 15 minutes, the pellets washed with 5% TCA and resuspended in 0.1 N NaOH. One aliquot was removed for Lowry protein determination (13), another aliquot added to scintillation fluid (Aquaflur, New England Nuclear). Results were calculated as cpm/μg protein and expressed as relative incorporation compared to control cultures without interferon. Values were normalized to reduce the variation seen between biopsy samples. The range of variation for each experiment is given in the figure legend or accompanying test. All incorporation studies are the averages of at least two experiments except where noted.

Keratin biosynthesis was detected by adding 20μCi/ml tritiated amino acids to secondary cultures for 48 hours after five days growth in the presence or absence of interferon. Keratins were then extracted, separated on 8.5% acrylamide gels as described (14) and detected by fluorography.

HPV DNA content was estimated by Southern blot analysis as previously described (1), comparing results to standard reconstructions of salmon sperm DNA plus cloned HPV-11 DNA. Cells were grown in the presence of interferon for seven weeks before extraction of DNA.

## RESULTS

Outgrowth of cells from a tissue sample is a combination of cell migration and cell division. We measured the effects of interferon on primary cell outgrowth. The results from a single experiment are

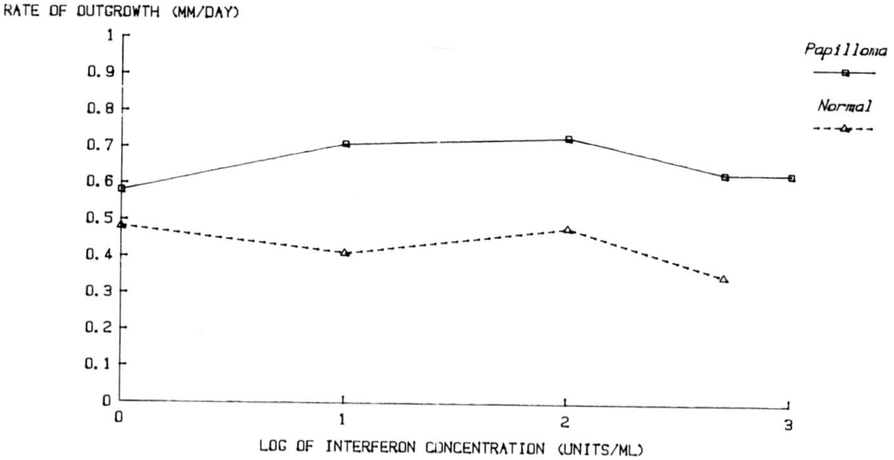


FIGURE 1. Effect of interferon on primary cell outgrowth. Biopsy tissues were minced and embedded in collagen gels supplemented with Hams F12, 15% fetal calf serum and 10 µg/ml hydrocortisone. Outgrowth of cells from the tissue explants was measured daily over a two week period, with continuous exposure to interferon. The "0" on the absissa indicates absence of interferon in this and subsequent figures.

shown in Figure 1. They are typical of the response seen. The rates of outgrowth varied from tissue to tissue, ranging from 0.3 mm/day to 0.85 mm/day in the absence of interferon (data not shown). This variation may reflect the condition of the biopsy fragment. It is not a function of the presence or absence of HPV infection. In no case was there any significant decrease in outgrowth with the addition of interferon. This would suggest that either there is no effect on cell division, migration or both.

We therefore determined the effect of interferon on thymidine incorporation by primary cells. Using our culture conditions, 10% to 16% of the nuclei in the untreated primary outgrowth were labeled during a 24 hour exposure to [$^3$H]thymidine, with some variation from tissue sample to tissue sample, but with no difference between normal and papilloma derived cells. If the primary cells were grown in the presence of interferon for three weeks, there was a marked effect

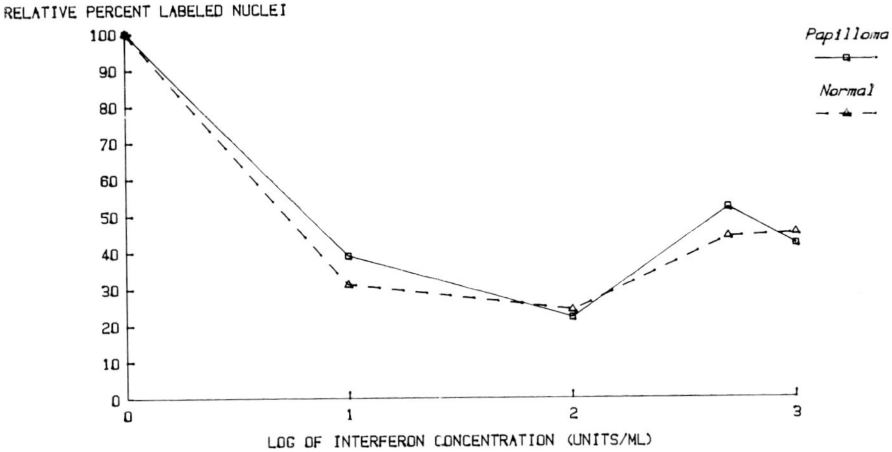


FIGURE 2. Effect of interferon on [$^3$H]thymidine incorporation into nuclei of primary cells. Cell explants were grown in the presence of interferon for three weeks, then labeled as described in Methods. Values are expressed relative to the percent labeled nuclei in the untreated dishes. Actual percentages of labeled nuclei ranged from a high of 16% to a low of 1.9% at 100 units/ml interferon.

on the number of labeled nuclei seen after autoradiography (Figure 2). Relative to the controls, there was a 76% reduction in labeling index with 100 units/ml interferon. Surprisingly, there was no difference in the response of the two types of cells. Both showed the same degree of inhibition. Moreover, both showed less inhibition when the dose of interferon was increased to 500 or 1000 units/ml. This was a consistent pattern, not the result of variability in the data.

We then investigated the effects of interferon on incorporation of precursors into macromolecules in secondary cells. Figure 3 shows the results of culturing cells in the presence of interferon for four days prior to labeling with [$^3$H]thymidine. In this experiment, the amount of labeled thymidine incorporated into acid insoluble material per μg cell protein was determined, rather than the number of labeled nuclei. Again, the papilloma cells showed a marked reduction in incorporation at 100 units/ml and less reduction at higher concentrations

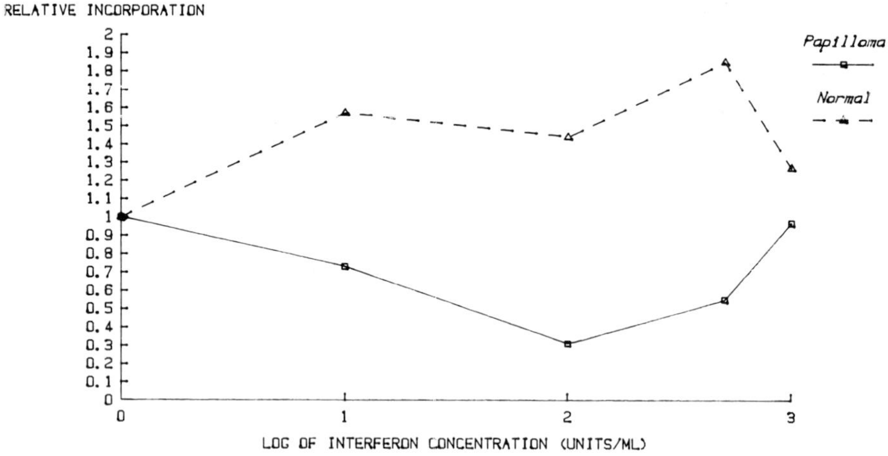


FIGURE 3. Effect of interferon on [$^3$H]thymidine incorporation by secondary cells. Cells were labeled for 24 hours after four days exposure to interferon as described in Methods. Data was calculated as cpm/µg cell protein, and expressed as relative incorporation compared to untreated cells. Actual cmp/µg protein for control papilloma cells ranged from 172 to 302. Normal cell controls ranged from 524 to 1539.

The value for 1000 units/ml is based on a single experiment, while the other values for papilloma cells are the average of two experiments, with a maximum standard deviation of 0.22. There was no inhibition of normal cells. The results shown in Figure 3 are the averages of three experiments with normal cells. Standard deviations for each set of data ranged from 0.29 to 0.64. Although rather large, there was no case where data for the two cell types overlapped except at 1000 units/ml. In every experiment, there was an enhanced incorporation of thymidine when the normal cells had been cultured in the presence of interferon. There is clearly a difference in the response of the two cell types.

Finally, we measured the effect of interferon on amino acid incorporation by the two types of secondary cells. The results are shown in Figure 4. There was a general decreased incorporation into TCA precipitable material with increasing concentration of interferon.

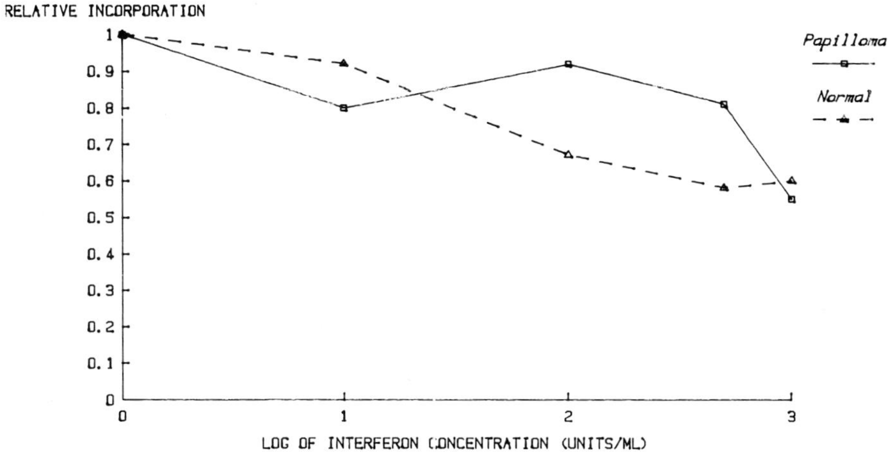


FIGURE 4. Effect of interferon on amino acid incorporation by secondary cells. Cells were grown in the presence of interferon for four days, then labeled with [$^3$H]amino acids as described in methods. Data was calculated as cpm/μg cell protein and expressed as relative incorporation compared to untreated cells. Actual cpm/μg protein in controls ranged from 1556 to 4752 for papilloma cells and 2577 to 5638 for normal cells.

There was no significant difference between the two cell types. The standard deviations for each interferon concentration ranged from 0.07 (10μ/ml) to 0.20 (500μ/ml) so that the difference seen can be attributed to experimental error.

There was no change in the specific keratins synthesized by either type of cell after growth in interferon (Figure 5). The molecular weights of keratins made in the presence of interferon were the same as those made by control cells. In no case did we detect the 51 kd and 59 kd keratins found in fully differentiated laryngeal epithelium. There was also no great difference in the amount of keratin synthesized, although it appears that there was a trend to increased amount with the presence of interferon. The nearly blank lane #4 for papillomas was an error in computing the amount of protein loaded in the well. Since the types of keratins synthesized are markers for the state of differentiation

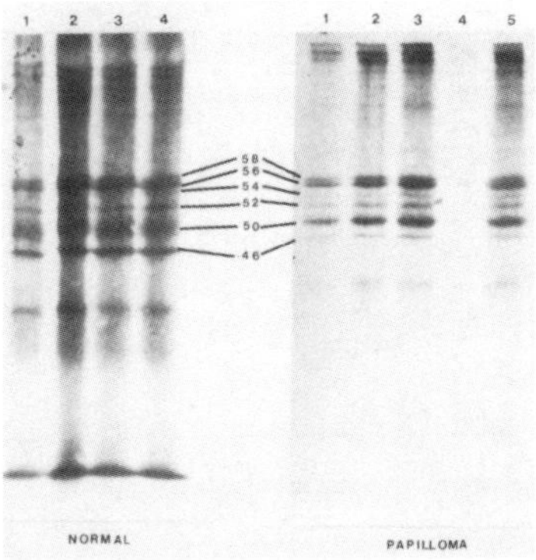


FIGURE 5. Effect of interferon on keratin synthesis. Keratins were labeled with $[H^3]$amino acids, extracted and analyzed as described in Methods. 30μg protein was loaded on each lane. Numbers between the two fluorograms show molecular weights of the keratin bands in kilodaltons. Lanes 1: no interferon, Lanes 2: 10 units/ml interferon, Lanes 3: 100 units/ml interferon, Lanes 4: 500 units/ml interferon, Lane 5: 1000 units/ml interferon. The absence of bands in Lane 4 of the papilloma is due to an error in calculating protein loaded in that lane.

of epithelial cells (14), it would suggest that interferon does not alter the degree of differentiation of these cultured cells.

We have begun to question the effect of interferon exposure on the amount of HPV DNA present in the cultured papilloma cells. Results are shown on Table 1. There was no rapid effect on the presence of HPV DNA since the copy number did not change in these cells. For comparison, we have included preliminary data from two patients on interferon therapy (Table 1). Patient 1 showed a significant drop in copy number within a two month period. Patient 2, just before interferon therapy began, was the source of the cultured cells used for this experiment. It may be significant that this patient did not show an appreciable and consistent drop in copy number with therapy (Table 1), even though there was a clinical reduction in symptoms (data not shown). Papilloma cells derived from other patients must be studied to learn whether a drop in copy number can occur in culture after exposure to interferon.

TABLE 1
EFFECTS OF INTERFERON TREATMENT ON HPV COPY NUMBER

| | Copy Number | | |
|---|---|---|---|
| Time of Treatment | Cells | Patient 1[a] | Patient 2[b] |
| 0 months | 5 | 15 | 3 |
| 2 months | 5 | 1 | 5 |
| 13 months | - | 1 | 10 |

a. Treated with $3 \times 10^6$ units interferon 3 X weekly for 2 months, increased to $6 \times 10^6$ units per injection for 8 months, then returned to initial dose after six months papilloma free.

b. Treated with $3 \times 10^6$ units interferon 3 X weekly for 3 months, gradually reduced to $1 \times 10^6$ units per injection at 6 months since nearly symptom free. Increased to $2 \times 10^6$ units per injection at 9 months of treatment as papillomas recurred.

## DISCUSSION

It is not possible to determine from these studies the actual mechanism whereby interferon therapy is able to induce a remission in laryngeal papillomatosis. The difference in thymidine incorporation of the secondary normal and papilloma cells would suggest that interferon has a direct anti-cellular effect on the proliferation of the papilloma cells (Figure 3). However, it must be remembered that those cells were only exposed to interferon for a total of five days. Primary cultures were treated with interferon for three weeks, and under those conditions both cell types showed similar inhibition of thymidine incorporation (Figure 2). This would suggest that there might not be a specific anti-proliferative effect on papilloma cells with continued treatment.

The variation in response might also reflect the difference between primary and secondary cells. When cells are trypsinized and replated, there is a selection for that subset of the original population which can reattach to a substrate and grow. This could yield a culture enriched in basal cells, for example, or distinguished by some other criteria. Such a selection might also be a factor in our observation that thymidine incorporation by normal primary cells was suppressed by interferon, while incorporation by normal secondary cells was not.

Thymidine incorporation might not be a valid indicator of cellular proliferation. In addition to trivial factors such as changes in thymidine uptake or pool sizes, there is another problem with thymidine incorporation studies. Davison et al (15) reported that thymidine incorporation did not correlate with direct cell counts or measurement of DNA content when studying proliferating epidermal keratinocytes in vitro. They suggest that under conditions of rapid growth the cells shift from a salvage pathway to de novo synthesis of pyrimidine nucleotides, and that these cells are unlike cultured fibroblasts in this respect. If thymidine incorporation were enhanced by preferential use of the salvage pathway when the papilloma cells were not growing rapidly, it might explain the increased relative thymidine incorporation with culture in the presence of 500 and 1000 units/ml interferon. At any rate, we have seen a change in thymidine incorporation with exposure of papilloma cells to interferon. Direct cell counts would be necessary to distinguish between inhibition of cell growth and an induced shift in pyrimidine biosynthesis pathways.

The questions regarding the meaning of the thymidine incorporation studies do not, however, conflict with our initial outgrowth studies (Figure 1). Clearly, the majority of the cells in the population are not rapidly dividing, since only 10 to 16% of the nuclei in control dishes were labeled during a 24 hour incubation with [$H^3$]thymidine. Even if the cells tend to use a de novo synthetic pathway, one would expect some [$H^3$]thymidine incorporation, resulting in nuclei with some number of grains after autoradiography. Therefore, the majority of cells in the population are either not replicating at all or replicating very slowly. We suggest that outgrowth is primarily the result of migration, which is not affected by interferon. In vivo, the number of cells is regulated in one of two diferent ways. Fibroblasts, which are the type of cell usually studied in culture, do not proliferate at all unless stimulated by mitogens like those found in the serum supplements used in tissue culture. Therefore, suppression of fibroblast growth is seen simply as a population of quiescent cells. The number of cells in a stratified squamous epithelium is regulated differently. In this case, there are a relatively small population of dividing stem cells which give rise to terminally differentiated nonreplicating cells, as well as replacing themselves. A shift in the percentage of differentiated cells produced, or the extent of their differentiation, can alter the balance between cell division and cell loss.

We have found that the increase in epithelial tissue mass in a laryngeal papilloma reflects a failure of the HPV infected cells to differentiate properly, rather than an increase in replication by the basal stem cells (R. Meade et al, manuscript in preparation). It was possible, therefore, that interferon therapy could have altered the differentiation of the papilloma cells.

One marker for differentiation is the synthesis of specific cytokeratins. All epithelial cells make a number of keratins with molecular weights ranging from 46 kd to 58 kd. There are additional keratins which are synthesized as the cells differentiate. In the larynx, these keratins have molecular weights of 51 kd and 59 kd (Romani and Steinberg, manuscript in preparation). We did not find any evidence for the induction of these specific keratins after interferon exposure in culture. Conversely, there was no reduction in the types of keratins, or amount of keratin, synthesized in the presence of interferon. This is consistent with our finding that interferon did not inhibit [$H^3$]amino acid incorporation (Figure 3) since approximately 30% of the total cellular protein synthesized by epithelial cells is keratin. We cannot state with certainty that interferon does not alter differentiation in vivo. Our cultured cells are grown in the presence of 15% serum. Fuchs and Green (16) have shown that the retinoids present in serum prevent the synthesis of differentiation-specific keratins in cultured epidermal cells. These experiments must be repeated with cells cultured in serum free medium in order to answer this question.

We have attempted to determine whether exposure to interferon during culture of papilloma cells reduces the amount of HPV DNA in the cells. While very preliminary, our data would suggest that unlike Turek's study (6) there was no decrease in viral copy number (Table 1). However, it may well be that there was a partial block to viral replication. In order to see a net loss, the cells would have to continue to divide, effectively "diluting out" the HPV. If there was a reduction in cell replication, it would reduce the likelihood of our detecting a decrease in copy number. Moreover, the cells used for this experiment were derived from a biopsy sample from a patient about to begin interferon therapy. We now know that even during periods of partial remission that this patient did not show a large drop in viral copy number. It may be that the failure of this patient to achieve complete remission for any length of time, even while on interferon, reflects these results.

There is, however, a problem with placing too much emphasis on HPV DNA copy number. We recently found that two tissue fragments from the same biopsy, when processed separately, contain significantly different copy numbers (data not shown). It has been known for some time that only small clusters of cells in a laryngeal papilloma synthesize viral particles, as evidenced by production of capsid antigen (17). If a tiny tissue fragment used for DNA extraction contained such a cluster, the average copy number would be much higher than if there were no productive cells in the fragment. Until in situ hybridization techniques are sensitive enough to detect the rather low numbers of HPV DNA present in these cells, it will not be possible to accurately determine the effects of interferon on viral presence. It may be possible, at our present levels of sensitivity, to determine whether interferon therapy reduces the likelihood of a productively infected cell. Serial sections through biopsies taken from patients on interferon therapy could be used for either capsid antigen detection or in situ hybridizations which do detect large numbers of HPV in a single cell. This could not be done with cultured cells, since they do not make capsid antigens and do not produce virus.

In order to determine the mode of action of interferon, additional studies are in progress. These include measurements of 2'5' oligoadenylate synthetase induction (18) and quantitation of actual cell numbers after prolonged culture. In addition, we shall attempt to measure levels of HPV specific mRNA in cells exposed to interferon. In this way, we may eventually begin to understand the mechanism of interferon therapy for laryngeal papillomatosis.

## REFERENCES


1. Steinberg BM, Topp WC, Schneider PS, Abramson A (1983). Laryngeal papilloma virus infection during clinical remission. New Eng Jour Med 308:1256-1264.
2. Haglund S, Lundquist PG, Cantell K, Strander H (1981). Interferon therapy in juvenile laryngeal papillomatosis. Arch Otolaryngol 107:327-332.
3. Goepfert H, Sessions RB, Gutterman JU, Cangir A, Dichtel WJ, Sulek J (1982). Leukocyte interferon in patients with juvenile laryngeal papillomatosis. Ann Otol Rhinol Laryngol 91:431-436.
4. McCabe B, Clark K (1983). Interferon and laryngeal papillomatosis: the Iowa experience. Ann Otol Rhin Laryngol 92:2-7.
5. Schouten TJ, Weiman W, Bos JH, Bos CE, Cremers CWR Jr, Schellenkens H (1982). Treatment of juvenile laryngeal papillomatosis with two types of interferon. Laryngoscope 92:686-688.
6. Turek LP, Burne JC, Lowy D, Dvoretzki I, Friedman RM, Howley PM (1982). Interferon inhibits bovine papilloma virus transformation of mouse cells and induces reversion of established transformants. UCLA Sym Mol Biol 25:181-191.
7. Borden EC, Hogan TF, Voelkel JG (1982). Comparative antiproliferative activity in vitro of natural interferons and for diploid and transformed human cells. Cancer Res 42:4948-4853.
8. Katoaka T, Oh-hashi F, Sakuai Y, Ida N (1982). Characteristics of in vitro antiproliferation activity of human interferon. Cancer Chemother Pharmacol 9:75-80.
9. Vilcek J, Gresser I, Merigan TC (ed.) (1980). Regulatory functions of interferons. Annals NY Acad Sci Vol 30.
10. Steinberg BM, Abramson AL, Meade RP (1982). Culture of human laryngeal papilloma cells in vitro. Otolaryngol Head-Neck Surg 90:728-735.
11. Horowitz B (1981). Human Interferon - properties, clinial application and production. Parenteral Sci and Tech, pp 223-226.

12. Rogers AW (1973). "Techniques of Autoradiography". New York: Elsevier Scientific Publication Co.
13. Lowry OH, Rosebrough NJ, Fair AL, Randall RJ (1951). Protein measurements with the Folin phenol reagent. Jour Biol Chem 193:265-275.
14. Fuchs E, Green H (1979). Changes in keratin gene expression during terminal differentiation of the keratinocyte. Cell 25:627-635.
15. Davison P, Liu S, Karasek M (1979). Limitations in the use of [$H^3$]thymidine incorporation into DNA as a marker of epidermal keratinocyte proliferation in vitro. Cell Tissue Kinet 12:605-614.
16. Fuchs E, Green H (1981). Regulation of terminal differentiation of cultured human keratinocytes by vitamin A. Cell 25:617-625.
17. Lack E, Jensen A, Smith H, Healy R, Pass F, Vauter G (1980). Immunoperoxidase localization of human papilloma virus in laryngeal papillomas. Intervirol 14:148-154.
18. Lodemann E, Kornhuber B, Gerein V, Ilberg CH (1984) (2'-5') Oligo (A) Synthetase as a monitor of interferon action in juvenile laryngeal papillomatosis. J Interferon Res 4:283-290.

**Papillomaviruses: Molecular and Clinical Aspects, pages 427–433**


# REPLICATION OF HPV 1 DNA IN MALIGNANT KERATINOCYTES IN CULTURE[1]

Sheila S. Reilly, Kathryn M. Albers, and Lorne B. Taichman

Department of Oral Biology and Pathology, School of Dental Medicine, State University of New York at Stony Brook, Stony Brook, New York 11794

ABSTRACT When malignant keratinocytes were infected with human papillomavirus type 1 (HPV 1) particles, viral DNA was observed as a multicopy monomeric episome. However, after several passages in culture, HPV 1 DNA was no longer detected. Similar results were obtained when normal keratinocytes were infected and passaged. Replication of HPV 1 DNA in malignant keratinocytes was demonstrated by the incorporation of bromodeoxyuridine (BrdUrd) into episomal DNA.

## INTRODUCTION

Papillomaviruses (PVs) are DNA viruses capable of inducing benign and occasionally malignant tumors of keratinocytes. Productive replication of papillomavirus, however, is seen only in benign lesions of keratinizing epithelia, specifically, in those cells that are in the process of terminal differentiation (9). The amount of progeny virus produced appears to be related to both PV type and site of infection (14). For example, some lesions such as HPV 1 induced plantar warts which occur in highly keratinized epithelium, are productive of large amounts of virus particles, while PV induced laryngeal warts and cervical carcinomas (HPV types 6,11,16, and 18) produce relatively small quantities of virus (3,10,14). Some animal papillo-

[1]This work was supported by a grant from the National Institute of Dental Research.

maviruses, such as bovine PV type 1, induce benign fibroblastic tumors, but vegetative viral replication does not occur in these cells.

In certain instances, such as in the genetic disorder epidermodysplasia verruciformis, and in Shope PV induced lesions of the cottontail rabbit, benign papillomatous growths develop into malignant carcinomas at a relatively high rate (5,8). When this transition occurs, the production of progeny particles formerly seen in the benign lesion is arrested (4,17). The reason why productive PV replication stops in the malignant cell is not known. To explore the PV replication in malignant keratincoytes, lines of keratinocytes established from naturally occurring squamous carcinomas (SCC lines) were infected with HPV 1 and persistence of the viral DNA was followed over several passages.

## METHODS

Normal newborn foreskin keratinocytes were cultured as described by Taichman and Prokop (16) in the medium described by Wu et al (18). The characteristics of SCC12B2, SCC25, SCC9, and SCL1 have been described previously (1,11). The carcinoma lines were cultured in fetal calf serum (10%), Dulbecco's modified Eagle's medium, 0.4μg/ml hydrocortisone, and penicillin/streptomycin. HPV 1 particles were isolated from plantar warts and cells were infected as described by LaPorta and Taichman (6). Total DNA from infected cells was extracted with phenol/chloroform and analyzed using a modified Southern technique (12). Cesium chloride density gradient analysis was performed as described by Taichman (13).

## RESULTS

Following infection of normal and malignant keratinocytes with HPV 1 particles, viral DNA was detected in cells as monomeric episomal DNA at 100-150 copies per cell (Figure 1). With repeated passage of the cells, the number of copies of HPV 1 DNA diminished until after 4-5 subcultures, no detectable viral DNA was observed (Figure 1). Different lots of fetal calf serum had no effect upon the loss of HPV 1 DNA nor did heat inactivating the serum. Two possible

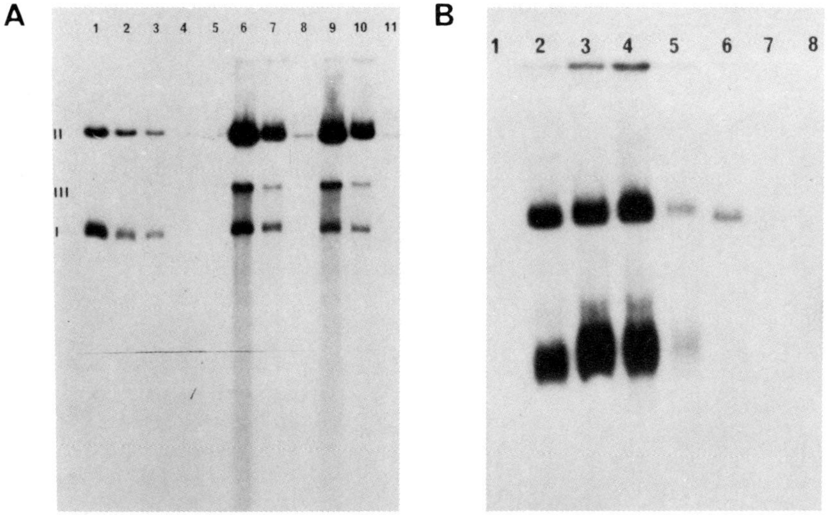


FIGURE 1. Lack of HPV 1 DNA persistence in infected normal and malignant (SCC25) keratinocytes. Total DNA was extracted from infected cells, digested with Sal I, (a no-cut enzyme for HPV 1), and probed for viral sequences by Southern hybridization. A) HPV 1 infected normal keratinocyte DNA: Lanes 1-4 are marker lanes and represent 50,20, 10, and 1 copy of HPV per diploid cell (the three bands correspond to forms I, II, and III DNA), lane 5 is an uninfected control, lanes 6-8 represent passes 1-3 in medium supplemented with untreated 10% fetal calf serum while lanes 9-11 represent passes 1-3 of cells grown in medium supplemented with 10% heat inactivated fetal calf serum (56°C for 20 min.). B) HPV 1 infected SCC25 DNA cut with Sal I: Lane 1 is an uninfected control, lanes 2 and 3 represent 24 and 48 hours postinfection, and lanes 4-8 represent passes 1-5.

explanations for the loss of HPV 1 DNA could be (1) a failure of the viral DNA to replicate in the infected keratinocytes or (2) production of interferon in the infected cultures. To test for the latter, medium was removed from keratinocyte cultures 24 and 48 hours postinfection and analyzed by Dr. Jan Vilcek (NYU Medical Center). No beta interferon was found.

To determine if HPV 1 DNA replicated in malignant keratinocytes, cultures of SCC cells were infected with HPV 1. Two days postinfection, BrdUrd (15μg/ml) was added to the medium for 16 hours. Total cellular DNA was extracted and centrifuged to equilibrium in CsCl density gradients to separate unsubstituted (LL) and BrdUrd (HL) DNA (Figure 2). DNA from these two fractions was dialyzed and spotted onto cellulose nitrate paper. HPV 1 specific DNA was detected by hybridization with 32P-labeled HPV 1 DNA (Figure 2). The presence of HPV 1 DNA in hybrid density DNA proves that HPV 1 replicated. As a control, HPV 1 virion DNA (20 copies per diploid cell) was added to DNA isolated from uninfected BrdUrd treated cells, and the mixture was centrifuged in CsCl. Viral DNA sequences were not detected at significant levels in the HL DNA fraction, proving that contamination of replicated HL DNA with unreplicated LL viral DNA did not occur. Therefore, a total absence of HPV 1 DNA replication cannot explain the lack of persistence in malignant keratinocytes. A partial block to HPV 1 replication has, however, not been excluded.

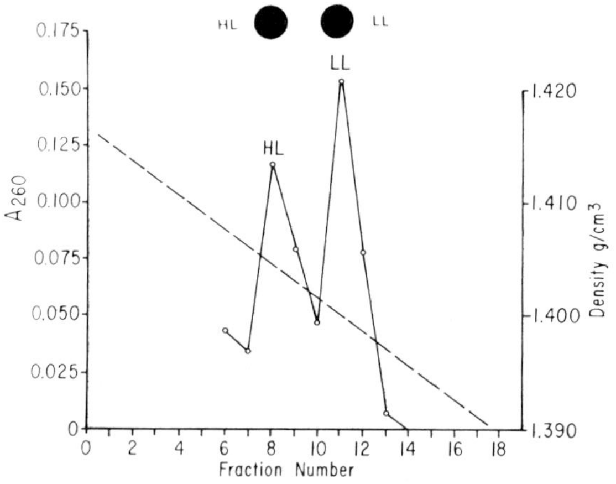


FIGURE 2. Detection of BrdUrd substituted DNA (HL) in CsCl gradients. HPV 1 infected SCC25 DNA was isolated from LL and HL peaks after centrifugation in CsCl, dotted onto nitrocellulose, and probed with 32P-labeled HPV 1 DNA. Hybridization indicates presence of HPV 1 sequences.

## DISCUSSION

Following infection of normal and malignant keratinocytes with HPV 1 particles, viral DNA was detected as monomeric episomal DNA at 100-150 copies per cell (Figure 1). With repeated passage, the number of copies of HPV 1 DNA diminished until after 4-5 subcultures, no viral DNA was detectable. Heat inactivating the fetal calf serum and the use of different serum lots were without effect.

To determine if HPV 1 DNA replicated, cultures of SCC cells were infected with HPV 1 virions and labeled in BrdUrd. The presence of BrdUrd substituted HPV 1 DNA proved that this episome was indeed replicating in the cells although the rate of replication has yet to be determined. Other explanations for the loss of viral sequences are possible. HPV 1 DNA could fail to partition properly at the time of cell replication, or infected keratinocytes could have a reduced plating efficiency and/or growth rate compared to their uninfected counterparts.

The loss of HPV 1 seen in this study was unexpected since previous results were positive (6), but other investigators have noted loss of HPV 1 DNA and Shope PV DNA following infection of normal keratinocytes with HPV 1 and Shope PV particles respectively (S. Burnett personal communication, 15). Keratinocytes cultured from human laryngeal papillomas however do maintain a constant copy number of HPV 6/11 DNA during 3 passes in culture (B. Steinberg, personal communication).

The conditions necessary for stable maintenance of the PV genome in keratinocytes are unclear. In bovine papillomavirus type 1 (BPV 1) transformed C127 cells, the viral DNA maintains stable plasmid replication in part through the action of two trans-acting functions. One function "rep" maps to two separate segments of the BPV genome and is responsible for episomal viral DNA maintenance. The other function "cop" is responsible for maintaining BPV 1 at high copy numbers (7). In HPV 1 infected cultured keratinocytes copy number rapidly diminishes although the viral DNA always remains episomal. Thus, if analogous sequences to "rep" and "cop" are present in the HPV 1 genome, they may not be fully functional.

The failure of HPV 1 to be maintained in normal keratinocytes makes it difficult to interpret the similar loss of HPV 1 in lines of squamous carcinoma cells. Malignancy involves a loss of the normal sequence of differentiative events in keratinizing epithelium. If these malignant changes disrupt those aspects of the differentiation program utilized by the papillomavirus in vivo, then cessation of vegetative replication that accompanies malignant transformation can be explained. Growth of normal keratinocytes in culture also leads to a disruption of the program for terminal differentiation (2). Hence, failure of HPV 1 to persist in either cell type in vitro and to replicate vegetatively in malignant carcinoma cells may stem from phenotypic alterations that occur in these keratinocytes.

## REFERENCES

1. Boukamp P, Tilgen W, Dzarlieva RT, Breitkreutz D, Haag D, Riehl RK, Bohnert A, Fusenig NE (1982). Phenotypic and genotypic characteristics of a cell line from a squamous carcinoma of the human skin. JCNI 68(3):415-427.
2. Eichner R, Bonitz P, and Sun T-T (1984). Classification of epidermal keratins according to their immunoreactivity, isoelectric point, and mode of expression. J Cell Biol 98:1388-1396.
3. Grussendorf-Conen EI, Gissman L, Hollers J (1983). Correlation between content of viral DNA and evidence of mature virus particles in HPV-1, HPV-4, and HPV-6 induced acanthomata. J Invest Dermatol 81:511-513.
4. Jablonska S, Dabrowski J, Jakubowicz K (1972). Epidermodysplasia verruciformis as a model in studies on the role of papova viruses in oncogenisis. Cancer Res 32:583-589.
5. Kreider JW, Bartlet GL (1981). The Shope papilloma-carcinoma complex of rabbits: a model system of neoplastic progression and spontaneous regression. Adv Cancer Res 35:81-108.
6. LaPorta RF, Taichman LB (1982). Human papillomavirus DNA replicates as a stable episome in cultured human epidermal keratinocytes. Proc Natl Acad Sci USA 79:3393-3397.
7. Lusky M, Botchan MR (1985). Genetic analysis of bovine papillomavirus type 1 trans-acting replication factors. J Virol 53:955-965.
8. Lutzner MA, Blanchet-Bardon C, Orth G (1984). Clinical observations, virologic studies, and treatment trials in patients with epidermodysplasia verruciformis, a disease induced by specific human papillomaviruses. J Invest Dermatol 83:18s-25s.

9. Orth G, Breitburd F, Favre M, Croissant O (1977). Papillomaviruses: possible role in human cancer. Hiatt HH, Watson JD, Winston JA (eds). In "Origins of Human Cancer", Cold Spring Harbor Laboratory. Cold Spring Harbor, NY pp1043-1068.
10. Pfister H, Gissman L, zurHausen H (1980). Characteristics of human and bovine papilloma viruses and of the humoral immune response to papilloma virus infection. Essex M, Todaro G, zurHausen H (eds). In "Viruses in Naturally Occurring Cancers", Cold Spring Harbor Laboratory. Cold Spring Harbor, NY pp 249-258.
11. Rheinwald JG, Beckett MA (1981). Tumorigenic keratinocyte lines requiring anchorage and fibroblast support cultured from human squamous cell carcinomas. Cancer Res 41:1657-1663.
12. Southern EM (1975). Detection of specific sequences among DNA fragments separated by gel electrophoresis. J Mol Biol 98:503-517.
13. Taichman LB (1979). The use of ultraviolet light in the fractionation of chromatin containing unsubstituted and bromodeoxyuridine substituted DNA. Nucleic Acids Res 6:2029-2030.
14. Taichman LB, LaPorta RF (1985). The expression of papillomaviruses in epithelial cells. Howley PM, Saltzman NP (eds). In "The Viruses", Plenum Press (in press).
15. Taichman LB, Breitburd F, Croissant O, Orth G (1984). The search for a culture system for papillomavirus. J Invest Dermatol 83:2s-6s.
16. Taichman LB, Prokop CA (1982). Synthesis of keratin protein during maturation of cultured human keratinocytes. J Invest Dermatol 78:464-467.
17. Watts SL, Ostrow RS, Phelps WC, Prince JT, Faras AJ (1983). Free cottontail rabbit papillomavirus DNA persists in warts and carcinomas of infected rabbits and in cells in culture transformed with virus of viral DNA. Virol 125:127-138.
18. Wu Y-J, Parker LN, Binder NE, Beckett MA, Sinaid JH, Griffiths CT, Rheinwald JG (1982). The mesothelial cells and nonkeratinizing epithelia. Cell 31:693-703.

# VIII. PAPILLOMAVIRUS TRANSFORMATION

**Papillomaviruses: Molecular and Clinical Aspects, pages 437–456**


# GENETIC ANALYSIS OF CELL TRANSFORMATION BY BOVINE PAPILLOMAVIRUS[1]

Daniel DiMaio, James Metherall, Kathryn Neary, and Donna Guralski

Department of Human Genetics
Yale University School of Medicine
New Haven, Connecticut 06510

ABSTRACT We have undertaken a statistical and mutational analysis of the genome of bovine papillomavirus, type 1. An analysis of codon usage within the viral genome suggests that most of the large open reading frames (ORFs) are expressed at the protein level, as is at least one of the small ORFs entirely overlapping with ORF E2. Constructed mutations located exclusively in ORF E2 or E5 interfere with efficient focus formation in mouse C127 cells. In cell lines containing the E2 mutants, the viral DNA appears integrated.

## INTRODUCTION

The conversion of a normal cell into a neoplastic one is a complex series of events that is still poorly understood, but it is clear that the papillomaviruses initiate or contribute to this process in a number of natural and experimental settings. These viruses cause predominantly benign tumors of epithelial cells, and in some cases these lesions progress to carcinomas (1). Although the study of tumor induction and progression in animals presents formidible experimental difficulties, bovine papillomavirus type I (BPV) and DNA of this virus can induce oncogenic transformation of rodent fibroblasts growing in culture (2,3). Thus, BPV provides an experimentally favor-

[1] This work was supported by grants from the National Cancer Institute, the Swebelius Cancer Research Fund, and the Anna Fuller Fund.

able system for studying the mechanism by which the action of a limited number of viral genes contributes to tumorigenesis.

The genome of BPV is a 7945 base pair circular double-stranded DNA molecule which can be divided into two functional segments (4). About two thirds of the genome is sufficient for in vitro oncogenic transformation of mouse fibroblasts and for extrachromosomal viral DNA replication in the nuclei of the transformed cells; the other third is expressed only in productively infected papillomas and encodes the virion structural proteins (5-10). Sequence analysis of BPV DNA revealed that the transforming segment contains eight long nucleotide stretches devoid of translation termination codons, and these open reading frames (ORFs) have been designated E1 through E8 (4). They are presumed to code for viral proteins involved in oncogenic transformation and plasmid replication, but no viral proteins have yet been identified in transformed cells. Each of these ORFs, all of which are located on the same strand of viral DNA, overlap entirely or in part with at least one other. The structure of spliced viral RNA found in the cytoplasm of transformed cells indicates that some of these ORFs are included in more than one mRNA species and could thus encode portions of more than a single protein (11,12). Moreover, some of the putative proteins are encoded by spliced mRNAs that originate from more than a single OFR. DNA sequences with regulatory capacity have also been localized to the transforming segment of the viral genome. These include a promoter region, a transcriptional enhancer, and sequences apparently involved in the maintenance of the viral DNA as a plasmid (13-18).

In an attempt to assign transforming functions to various portions of the viral genome, several groups have assayed the biological activity of cloned deletion and insertion mutants of BPV and of subgenomic DNA fragments and viral cDNAs under the control of regulatory signals derived from other viruses. These studies suggest that two independent segments of BPV DNA contain transforming activity, a 5' segment including E6 and E7, and a 3' region including E2, E3, E4, E5, and the 3' end of E1 (12,15-17,19). The assignment of transforming functions to specific viral genes is complicated by the compact organization of the genome and by the complex structures of the viral mRNA. Most subgenomic DNA fragments and cDNA segments contain more than a single ORF which could be expressed. Many of the mutations already studied lie within more than one ORF. Even a mutation within only a single ORF could affect expression of a separate coding region. This could occur, for example, if the mutation lies within a regulatory signal, modifies patterns of RNA processing, or influences the stability of an RNA expressing a different ORF.

To circumvent some of these problems, we are constructing mutations at predetermined sites in the viral genome to generate a collection of BPV mutants each containing a lesion in a single ORF. Moreover, where possible we are designing the mutations so that we can experimentally confirm their proposed modes of action. Before describing the mutants we have constructed, we present briefly an analysis of codon usage within the BPV genome. This analysis was undertaken in an attempt to identify which of the ORFs are most likely to be bona fide protein-coding regions.

## METHODS

### Codon Usage Analysis

We have developed a computer program that compares the codon usage within an ORF or a set of ORFs to the pattern characteristic of a specified set of reference genes. Two criteria must be met in order to conclude that codon usage of an ORF is similar to the usage pattern of the reference set. First, the usage pattern of the test and reference ORFs must differ from random usage, ie. not all codons encoding the same amino acid are used with equal frequency; this requirement is necessary to demonstrate that factors actually do influence the choice of synonymous codons. Second, the codon usage pattern of the test ORF must deviate away from random toward that of the reference set. Both of these requirements can be tested simultaneously by using a statistical F-test.

The variance between the observed usage and that of the reference set is compared to the variance between the observed and random usage. This calculation is shown below:

$$F= \frac{\sum_i (f_i^{obs}-f_i^{ran})^2}{\sum_i (f_i^{obs}-f_i^{ref})^2} \quad ; \quad df= \sum_j (n_j-1)$$

where $f_i$ is the frequency of use of codon i, $f^{obs}$ is the observed frequency within the test ORF, $f^{ref}$ is the codon usage frequency within the reference set and $f^{ran}$ is the usage frequency expected if all codons in a synonymous set are used with equal frequency (no correction for base composition is included in this calculation). The variances are summed over all amino acid-encoding codons, and their ratio is expressed as an F-value. The number of degrees of freedom (df) in this system is equal to the sum of n-1 for each amino acid, where $n_j$ is the number of codons specifying amino acid j. This sum is equal to 40.

As shown in figure 1, this analysis was extended to look at the codon usage pattern of different regions within an ORF to determine whether ORFs in other frames influence the pattern within the region of overlap. Here, F-values are calculated for regions of a specified length (50 codons), and these values are plotted as a function of position within the ORF.

The published nucleotide sequences of BPV and HPV 1a, as modified, were used to assemble the reference sets for the papillomavirus genomes (4, 20-23). Each viral reference set is comprised of the codons in ORFs E1-E8, L1, and L2 (extending in each case from the first codon downstream of the termination codon at the 5' end of the ORF to the codon immediately preceeding the next in phase termination codon). For comparison of individual ORFs to the aggregate viral usage, all codons of the test ORF (and portions of ORFs that overlap the test ORF in other reading phases) were first subtracted from the reference set. Codon usage reference sets for human genes, bovine genes, and human plus bovine keratin genes were constructed from sequences present in the GENBANK data base.

Cell Maintenance

Mouse C127 cells are grown on plastic in DME medium containing 10% fetal calf serum, penicillin, and streptomycin at 37° in a humidified atmosphere with 5% $CO_2$. The cells are passaged 1:15 two times a week. About twelve passages after thawing, untransformed C127 cells are discarded and a fresh vial of frozen cells is thawed. Normal and transformed cells can be frozen in medium containing 8% DMSO.

## Transformation Assay

Two to three days before transformation, approximately $10^5$ cells are distributed in 10cm petri plates. Cells should cover about 70% of the surface of the plate at the time of transformation. Three to six hours prior to the addition of DNA, the medium on the cells is replaced with 10ml fresh medium.

Viral DNA is digested to completion with Bam HI (it is not necessary to remove the enzyme following digestion). 50ng of the mixture of DNA fragments and 12 ug of carrier calf thymus DNA is added to 0.5ml of 2X HEBS at room temperature and an equal volume of 0.25M $CaCl_2$ is added dropwise while bubbling air through the sample (24). The solution is mixed vigorously for 5 seconds. After 20 minutes at room temperature, the solution is added dropwise into the medium in the plates. A granular precipitate which becomes more obvious with time should be visible by phase contrast microscopy. Cells are placed at 37°.

A 20% (v/v) solution of DMSO (spectroscopy grade) in medium is prepared and allowed to equilibrate to room temperature. 8 to 13 hours after the addition of DNA, medium containing the precipitate is removed from the cells and 2 ml of the DMSO mixture is added to each plate and dispersed by tilting. The cells in DMSO are kept for 3 minutes at room temperature with occasional tilting. 5 ml of room temperature PBS is then gently added and removed. After an additional rinse with 5 ml of PBS, 10 ml of room temperature medium containing 5 mM Na butyrate (Sigma) is added and the cells are incubated at 37° for 10 to 14 hours (25). The cells are then split 1:3 and incubated at 37° with twice weekly medium changes (without butyrate). Foci of transformed cells should start to become visible by 10 days, and they can be picked using cloning cylinders and expanded into cell lines.

## Construction and Analysis of Mutants

Standard in vitro mutagenesis procedures were used to construct deletion and insertion mutations (26). The base substitution mutation in ORF E2 was constructed by oligonucleotide-directed mutagenesis of a segment of BPV DNA cloned in M13mp8 (27). The structures of the mutations were determined by restriction analysis of small-scale plasmid DNA preparations (28). In most cases the exact nature of the mutation was determined by nucleotide sequencing (29).

Total DNA was purified from transformed cell lines, and viral DNA was detected by Southern blotting using $^{32}$P-labelled BPV DNA as a hybridization probe (30).

## RESULTS

### Codon Usage of the BPV Open Reading Frames

Most amino acids are encoded by any one of several codons, and many cellular and viral genes preferentially use specific members of each set of synonymous codons. It is not clear what factors influence the preferential use of one synonymous codon over another because these choices do not result in alterations in protein structure. Investigators have proposed a number of explanations to account for the patterns that are observed. These explanations include the sequence characteristics of the gene itself and selection for the level gene expression (31,32). Ikemura has demonstrated a good correlation between preferentially used codons and high levels of specific isoaccepting tRNAs in *E. coli* (32). Whatever the source of codon usage patterns, it is frequently found that there is a consistent pattern of codon usage preference among the protein-coding regions in a particular organism or virus (31).

The algorithm used for the pairwise comparison of codon usage in two sets of ORFs is described in the Methods section. When analyzed in this manner, it is apparent that BPV and HPV 1a exhibit very similar codon usage patterns, and that the usage patterns of both deviate substantially from the pattern of their natural hosts. BPV and HPV 1a codon usage also deviates from the pattern of sequenced human and bovine keratin genes which are actively expressed in epidermal tissue where these viruses undergo their lytic cycle (1).

Table 1 shows the extent to which the codon usage of individual papillomavirus ORFs conform to the usage characteristic for each virus type: the observed usage for ORFs E1, E6, L1 and L2 conform well to the aggregate usage, but E2 usage does not. E3, E4, and E8 (of BPV) all deviate substantially from the aggregate pattern (these three ORFs are each entirely contained within a larger ORF in a different reading frame). The pattern of E2 was somewhat unexpected because it is one of the largest ORFs in the viral genomes and is found in all papillomavirus genomes that have been sequenced. To analyse codon usage in this

TABLE 1
CODON USAGE ANALYSIS: COMPARISON
OF INDIVIDUAL OPEN READING FRAMES TO OVERALL USAGE

| ORF | BPV 1 | HPV 1a |
|---|---|---|
| E1 | 1.95 | 2.65 |
| E2 | 1.08 | 1.17 |
| E3 | 0.83 | -- |
| E4 | 0.73 | 0.51 |
| E5 | 1.37 | 0.76 |
| E6 | 1.52 | 1.71 |
| E7 | 1.20 | 0.63 |
| E8 | 1.00 | 1.23 |
| L1 | 1.48 | 2.44 |
| L2 | 1.72 | 2.65 |

Codon usage of individual ORFs of BPV and HPV 1a were compared to the aggregate pattern of each virus. Values greater than 1 indicate that the usage of the test ORF is more similar to the reference usage than it is to random; values less than 1 indicate that it is more similar to random. Levels of statistical significance: 1.50 equivalent to $p < 0.10$, 1.69 equivalent to $p < 0.05$, 2.11 equivalent to $p < 0.01$.

TABLE 2
TRANSFORMING ACTIVITY OF BPV DNA

| DNA | Foci/ ug BPV DNA |
|---|---|
| pBPV-142-6 | 1328 |
| pBPV-142-6 (digested) | 2282 |
| pBPV-β1 | 5000 |
| pBPV-BV1 | 1617 |

DNA transfer was performed as described in the methods section with Bam HI-cut pBPV-142-6 or with super-coiled plasmid DNA. Foci were counted 18 days after DNA transfer and normalized to the mass of the 69% transforming fragment of BPV DNA added for each plasmid.

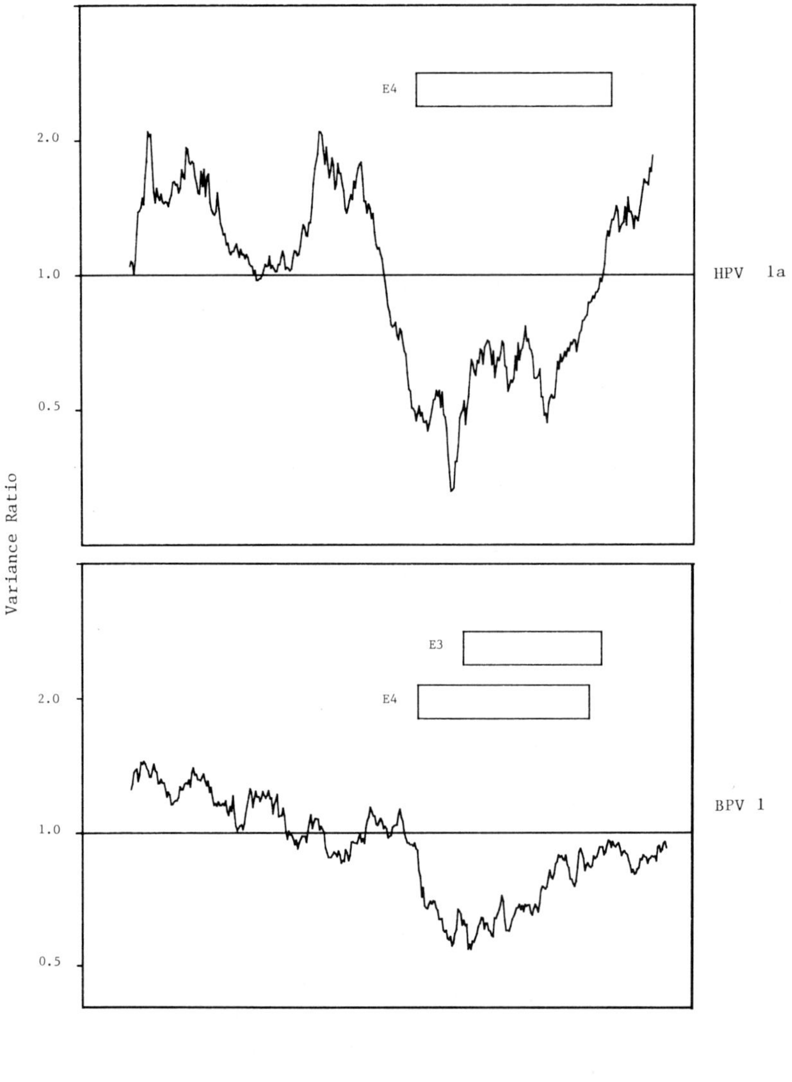


FIGURE 1. Codon usage pattern of E2. The conformity of the codon usage of a moving 50 codon segment of BPV and HPV 1a ORF E2 is plotted as a function of position of the segment on the map of the viral genomes. The relative positions of ORFs E3 and E4 are also shown.

ORF in more detail, we determined how codon usage varied in different portions of E2. In figure 1, the codon usage patterns of ORFs E1 and E2 are compared to the aggregate usage; the data are plotted as a function of position on the physical map of the viral genome. For both viruses, codon usage of E2 is more similar to the aggregate usage than to random usage over most of its extent, except for the region of overlap with ORF E3 and E4. Within this interval, the conformity of E2 is considerably lower and similar to that seen for the smaller ORFs. The decrease in this region is particularly dramatic for HPV. In contrast, although BPV ORF E8 does not conform well to the aggregate usage, the conformity of E1 is not significantly lower in the E8 overlap region.

Our interpretation of these data is based on the assumption that the appearance of a preferred pattern of codon usage indicates that the coding regions displaying this pattern are actually translated. Given this assumption, these results suggest the following: 1) E1 and E2 have been subjected to selective pressure at the level of codon usage, and thus are likely to encode proteins. 2) Selection for codon usage has also been exerted on E3, E4, or both, resulting in the sharp discontinuity of the E2 conformity at the boundaries of the overlap with these small ORFs. Thus, E3 and/or E4 are also likely to encode proteins. (The low conformity of all three ORFs in this region is probably an inevitable consequence of the amino acid sequence requirements of 2 (or 3) proteins encoded by overlapping ORFs). 3) E8 codon usage does not bear the imprint of the selective pressure that molded the other BPV ORFs, but because the E1 usage conformity is not sharply lower in the E8 region, this cannot be simply explained by simultaneous selection on 2 overlapping coding regions. This raises the possibility that E8 does not encode a protein.

Such inferences from sequence analysis must of course be corroborated by biological experiments. In the rest of this report we describe the in vitro transformation assay we are using to test the effects of mutations in specific ORFs and we summarize our results to date.

## Focus Forming Assay for BPV DNA

To test the biological activity of BPV DNA we are using a focus-forming assay on mouse fibroblasts (3). Because the properties of BPV mutants depend on the precise protocol of

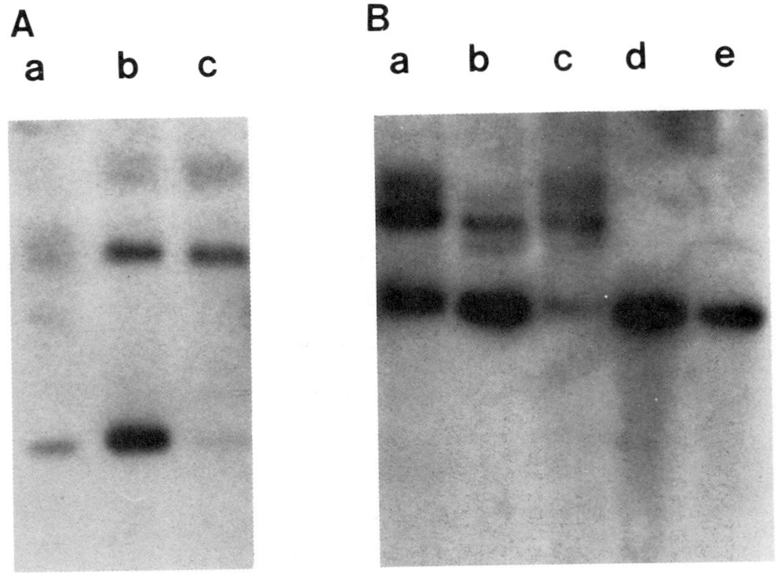


FIGURE 2. Viral DNA in secondary transformants. Transformed foci of C127 cells were generated with wild type viral DNA, and cellular DNA was purified from cell lines derived from these foci. Fresh C127 cells were transformed with 10 ug of transformed-cell DNA, and cell lines were (designated ST 1, 2, 3) established from individual transformed foci. DNA was isolated from these secondary transformants and analysed by Southern blotting using the gel- purified 69% subgenomic transforming fragment of BPV DNA as a hybridization probe. A) Undigested DNA; B) DNA digested with Hind III (a,b,and c) or Bam HI (d,e). Cellular DNA: a) ST1, b) ST2, c) ST3. pBPV-142-6 DNA: d) 500 ng, e) 100 ng.

the transformation assay (see below), we have presented a detailed protocol of our standard transformation assay in the Methods section. To determine the preferred form of the input viral DNA for this assay, we compared the efficiency of focus formation of BPV DNA excised from bacterial plasmid sequences to that of viral DNA contained in a variety of intact recombinant plasmids. These plasmids include the full length viral DNA joined at its Bam HI sites to pML2d (p142-6; ref. 33) and the 69% subgenomic transforming segment joined to a bacterial plasmid and either a full-length or a shortened stimulatory segment of cellular DNA (pBPV-B1 and pBPV-BV1, respectively, ref. 34,35).

The results of a representative transformation experiment are shown in table 2. The recombinant plasmid with the full length stimulatory segment displays the most potent transforming ability, but we decided not to use this plasmid as the parent for the BPV mutations because the nature of the stimulatory effect has not been elucidated. Instead, we have constructed mutations in pBPV-142-6, and prior to transfer the DNA is digested with Bam HI to separate the viral DNA from bacterial plasmid sequences which consistently exert an inhibitory effect on focus formation. Cell lines derived from foci generated in this manner with wild type BPV DNA contain the transferred viral genome as a plasmid. If total DNA is purified from these foci and used in another cycle of C127 cell transformation, secondary foci are readily generated, and they also contain unintegrated viral DNA (figure 2).

## Involvement of E2 ORF in Focus Formation

We have assembled a collection of constructed mutants with mutations that lie exclusively in the E2 ORF (see figure 3). We have constructed a deletion mutation that removes nucleotides number 2878 to 3089, an insertion mutation at nucleotide #3023 that results in a frameshift, and a single base substitution mutation at nucleotide #3081 that generates a chain termination codon (amber). In addition, J. Schiller and D. Lowy have sent us viral DNAs containing insertion/deletion mutations located (approximately) at nucleotide #2875, 3678, and 3360 (the latter mutation lies within the region of overlap between the E2, E3, and E4 ORFs). The ability of these cloned mutant DNAs to transform cells was assayed by the focus forming assay described above, and each forms foci at about 2% the efficiency of wild type DNA. In addition, the few

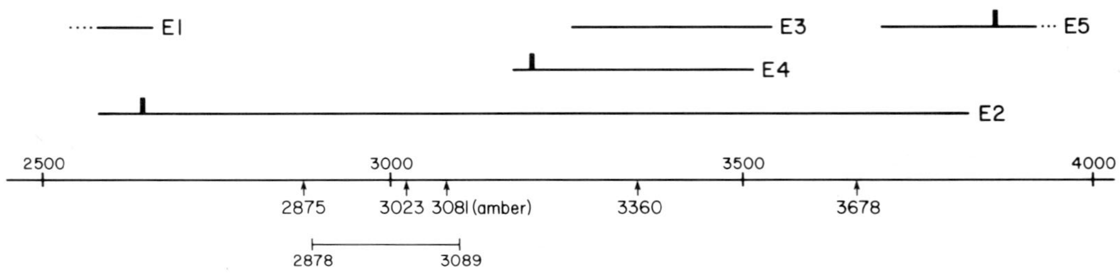


FIGURE 3. Positions of mutations in ORF E2. The horizontal line extending across the figure represents the physical map of the BPV genome with the nucleotide positions numbered. Above the line, the BPV ORFs in the region of the E2 ORF are shown. Translation of all OFRs proceeds left to right, and the vertical bars represent the most 5' methionine codon in each ORF. The positions of mutations are indicated below the line.

foci that formed following transfer of the mutant DNA appeared later and seemed to grow more slowly than did foci generated with wild type DNA. Interestingly, mutant 3678, in which the mutation is located the furthest towards the 3' end of the E2 ORF, seemed slightly less defective than did the other mutants. For the frameshift mutation at 3023 and the amber mutation, the transforming activity of genomes constructed from purified restriction fragments proved that the sequence alterations responsible for the transformation defect were located within the 211 base pair Nco I fragment exclusively encoding E2. Mutant viral DNA was maintained in the cell lines derived from the rare foci generated with the DNA containing the amber mutation, but the DNA was associated with the high molecular weight cellular DNA.

The transformation defect caused by several, independently-derived mutations located at different positions within the E2 ORF suggests that this region of DNA is translated into a protein which plays a role in cellular transformation. To prove this, we are attempting to suppress the transformation defect of the E2 amber mutant by introducing the appropriate suppressor tRNA into cells with the mutant viral DNA (36). We have not yet been able to suppress the focus-forming defect by co-transformation with the suppressor tRNA gene and the amber mutant, or by cloning the suppressor tRNA gene into a BPV vector containing the E2 amber mutation. We believe that this inability to suppress the defect is due to toxicity of high levels of suppressor tRNA to mammalian cells over the two week course of the focus-forming assay. Thus, although we have not yet proved that the amber mutation exerts its effects by causing premature termination of translation of the E2 ORF, this remains our working hypothesis.

## Involvement of ORF E5 in Transformation

We decided to test the transforming ability of E5 mutants in our standard assay because it has been found that some E5 mutants display a focus-forming defect in a transformation assay that does not register any effect of mutations in E2 (J. Schiller and D. Lowy, personal communication). The scheme shown in figure 4 was devised to determine whether any transformation defect of the E5 mutants is due to the absence of the putative protein translated from the E5 ORF. If the production of the E5 protein is important for focus formation, none of the transformation competent mutants with small deletions in the

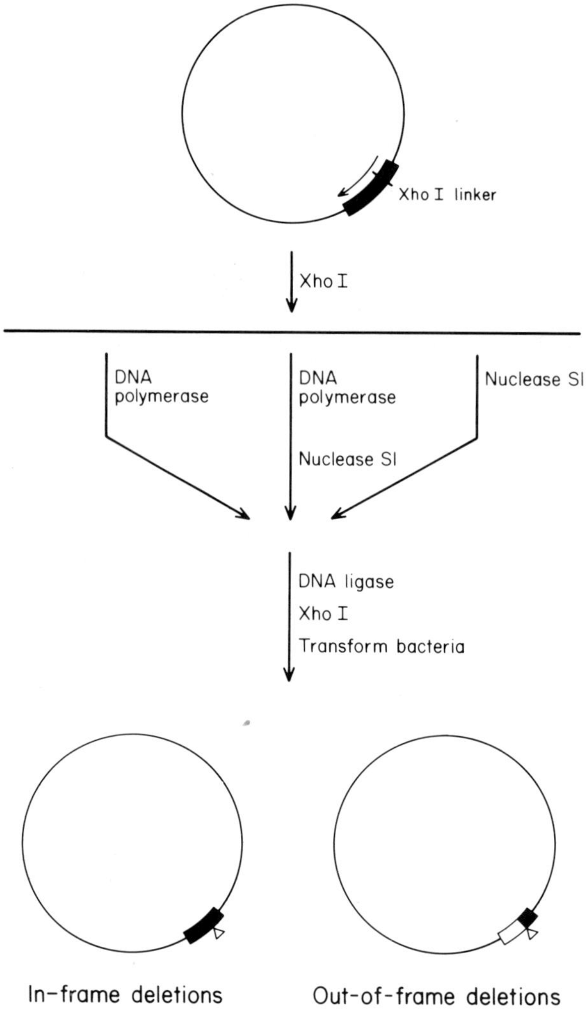


FIGURE 4. Generation of frameshift mutations. For purposes of illustration, a Xho I site is shown as the site of linearization; in practice any restriction endonuclease with a unique cleavage site could be used. After modification of the ends of the DNA and recircularization, Xho I digestion is used to enrich for molecules that have lost the Xho I site. Individual plasmids are isolated from bacteria and tested for transforming ability and the maintenance of an in-frame ORF.

N terminal portion of the E5 ORF should have suffered a frameshift at the site of the deletion.

To gain access to this portion of the E5 ORF, we exploited the existence of a unique Bst XI restriction endonuclease cleavage site four base pairs 3' to the sole (and presumably the initiator) methionine codon in E5. Recombinant viral DNA was linearized at this site by digestion with Bst XI or Xho I (the latter enzyme was used on BPV DNA containing Xho I linkers inserted at the Bst XI site and provided by J. Schiller and D. Lowy). As outlined in figure 4 for DNA containing the Xho site, the ends of the linear DNA molecules were enzymatically modified to generate a set of mutants with small insertions or deletions in E5. A variety of enzymatic treatments were performed on both starting plasmids in an attempt to maximize the number of mutants with relatively minor sequence changes in this region. So far, we have generated at least seven different deletion/insertion mutations at this position in E5. The wild type DNA and two mutants transform efficiently, and sequence analysis documented that in these cases ORF E5 is retained in frame. Other mutants, including at least three with a frameshift mutation in E5, are defective for focus formation. More mutants are being constructed and tested. An exact correspondence between transformation competence and in-frame deletions would strongly suggest that the E5 ORF is translated into a protein product required for efficient focus-formation on C127 cells.

## DISCUSSION

We are constructing mutations in each of the ORFs of BPV DNA and determining their effect in a focus forming assay in mouse fibroblasts. These experiments are designed to identify viral genetic functions required for efficient cellular transformation and to determine whether these functions are expressed via proteins encoded by the viral genes.

The codon usage analysis suggests that most of the major BPV ORFs are translated. E8 may be an exception; in fact, other sequenced papillomavirus genomes do not contain an ORF at the location of BPV E8 (E8 of HPV 1a is located in a different portion of the viral genome and is apparently unrelated to BPV E8) (20-23). One or both of the small reading frames entirely overlapping with E2 is likely to be expressed. The dramatic drop in E2 usage conformity for HPV 1a, which contains E4 but not E3, indicates that E3 is not required to generate this pattern. Because E3 is not present in other papillomaviruses and because BPV E3 contains no methionine codon nor obvious splice acceptor sequence, it seems less likely than E4 to encode a protein.

The mutational analysis of BPV ORFs E2 and E5 suggests that these two ORFs are translated into proteins playing a role in transformation. For ORF E2, several independently derived mutations at different locations within this ORF cause a dramatic decrease in focus forming ability in our standard transformation assay. Among these mutations is the substitution of a single base which prevents the synthesis of an intact E2 protein. Because we have not yet suppressed this chain termination mutation, the conclusion that E2 encodes an essential protein is still tentative. Similar results have been reported for a series of deletion mutations in the E2 region (17). The data are still preliminary for ORF E5, but a correlation between the ability of viral DNA to transform efficiently and the integrity of the reading phase of E5 seems to be emerging. The putative E5 protein can apparently tolerate limited amino acid changes at the position of these mutations. A similar frameshift analysis of E2 is underway, as is a complementation analysis of the E2 and E5 mutants.

Several observations indicate that there is not an absolute requirement for ORF E2 in transformation. 1) The mutants described above are not totally defective in our standard focus forming assay. 2) Transformed cell lines containing a mutant E2 gene are able to form colonies in soft agarose. 3) If the amber mutant is transferred into cells together with the G418 resistance gene from Tn-5 (37,38), most drug resistant colonies contain at least some cells that appear morphologically transformed. 4) Several of the E2 mutants that are defective in our standard transformation assay have been found to be able to efficiently form foci using a different transformation assay in mouse fibroblasts (J. Schiller and D. Lowy, personal communication). We are attempting to determine the critical differences between the two assays.

The observation that viral DNA containing an E2 mutation is associated with high molecular weight DNA in transformed cells also suggests a role of the E2 gene product in the maintenance of the viral DNA as a plasmid, and similar observations have been made by others (17). At face value, these results are not consistent with the report of Lusky and Botchan that plasmid maintenance can proceed in the absence of substantial segments of the E2 ORF; however, the various laboratories have studied DNA molecules with numerous structural differences which could influence their behavior (15, 17, 39). Nevertheless, the published data clearly demonstrate that under some conditions the E2 gene product is not required for plasmid maintenance.

Although our experiments indicate that the E2 gene product plays a role in cellular transformation and viral DNA replication, others have developed assays where the E2 gene is dispensible. One interpretation of these results is that the E2 protein plays an indirect role in these activities, perhaps by stimulating the expression of other viral genes that are directly required for replication and transformation. The E1 and E7 ORFs seem likely candidates for encoding this proposed replication function (39), and the E5 ORF may be an important transforming gene.

## ACKNOWLEDGEMENTS

The authors wish to thank Dr. Edward Benz for use of his IBM PC/XT computer. We also thank Drs. John Schiller and Douglas Lowy for sending us cloned BPV mutants. In addition, the support of the Edward Mallinckrodt, Jr. Foundation is gratefully acknowledged.

## REFERENCES

1. Pfister H (1984). The Biology and Biochemistry of Papillomaviruses Rev Physiol Biochem Pharm 99: 111-181.
2. Borion M, Levy JP, Thomas M ,Freidman JC, Bernard J (1964). Some properties of bovine papillomavirus. Nature 201:423-424.
3. Dvoretzky I, Shober R, Chattopadhy SK, and Lowy DR (1980). A quantitative in vitro focus forming assay for bovine papillomavirus. Virology 103:369-375.
4. Chen CY, Howley PM, Levinson AD, Seeburg PH (1982). The primary structure and the genetic organization of bovine papilloma virus type 1 genome. Nature 299:530-535.
5. Lowy DR, Dvoretzky I, Shober R, Law M-F, Engel L, Howley PM, (1980). In vitro tumorigenic transformation by a defined sub-genomic fragment of bovine papilloma virus DNA. Nature 297:72-74.
6. Lancaster WD, (1981). Apparent lack of integration of bovine papillomavirus DNA in virus-induced equine and bovine tumor cells and virus-transformed mouse cells. Virology 104:251-255.

7. Law M-F, Lowy DR, Dvoretzky I, Howley PM (1981). Mouse cells transformed by bovine papillomavirus contain only extrachromosomal viral DNA sequences. Proc Natl Acad Sci USA 78:2727-2731.
8. Amtmann E, and Sauer G (1982). Bovine papillomavirus transcription: polyadenylated RNA species and assessment of the direction of transcription. J Virol 43:59-66.
9. Engel LW, Heilman CA, Howley PM (1983). Transcriptional organization of Bovine Papillomavirus Type I. J Virol 47:516-528.
10. Heilman CA, Engel L, Lowy DR, Howley PM, (1982). Virus-specific transcription in bovine papillomavirus transformed mouse cells. Virol 119:22-34.
11. Stenlund A, Zabielski J, Ahola H, Moreno-Lopez J, Pettersson U (1985). The messenger RNAs from the transforming region of bovine papilloma virus type 1. J. Mol. Biol. In press.
12. Yang Y-C, Okayama H, Howley PM, (1985). Bovine papillomavirus contains multiple transforming genes. Proc Natl Acad Sci USA 82:1030-1034.
13. Campo MS, Spandidos DA, Lang J, Wilkie N (1983). Transcriptional control signals in the genome of bovine papillomavirus type 1. Nature 303:77-80.
14. Lusky M, Berg L, Weiher H, Botchan M (1983). Bovine papillomavirus contains an activator of gene expression at the distal end of the early transcription unit. Molec and Cell Biol 3:1108-1122.
15. Lusky M, Botchan M (1984). Characterization of the bovine papillomavirus plasmid maintenance sequences. Cell 36:391-401.
16. Nakabayashi Y, Chattopadhyay SK, Lowy, DR (1983). The transforming function of bovine papillomavirus DNA. Proc Natl Acad Sci USA 80:5832-5836.
17. Sarver N, Rabson M, Yang Y-C, Byrne JC, Howley PM (1984). Localization and analysis of bovine papillomavirus type 1 transforming functions. J Virol 52:377-388.
18. Waldeck W, Rosl F, Zentgraf H (1984) Origin of replication in episomal bovine papilloma virus type 1 DNA isolated from transformed cells. EMBO J 3:2173-2178.
19. Schiller J, Vass WC, Lowy DR (1984). Identification of a second transforming region of bovine papillomavirus. Proc Natl Acad Sci USA 81:7880-7884.

20. Clad A, Gissman L, Meier B, Freese UK, Schwartz E (1982). Molecular cloning and partial nucleotide sequence of human papillomavirus type 1 DNA. Virol 118:254-259.
21. Danos O, Katinka, Yaniv M, (1982). Human papillomavirus 1a complete DNA sequence: a novel type of genome organization amoung Papovaviriae. EMBO J 1:231-236.
22. Danos O, Engel L, Chen EY, Yaniv M, Howley PM (1983). Comparative analysis of human type 1a and bovine type 1 papillomavirus genomes. J Virol 46:557-566.
23. Schwartz E, Durst M, Demankowski C, Lattermann O, Zech R, Wolfsperger E, Suhai S, zur Hausen H (1983). DNA sequence and genome organization of human genital papillomavirus type 6b. EMBO J 2:2341-2348.
24. van der Eb AJ, Graham FL (1980). Assay of transforming activity of tumor virus DNA. Meth Enzymol 65:826-839.
25. Gorman CM, Howard B (1983). Expression of recombinant plasmids in mammalian cells is enhanced by sodium butyrate. Nucl Acids Res 11:7631-7648.
26. Shortle DS, DiMaio D, Nathans D (1981). Directed mutagenesis. Ann Rev Genetics 15:265-294.
27. Zoller M, Smith M, (1983) Oligonucleotide directed mutagenesis. Meth Enzymol 100:468-500.
28. Holmes D, Quigley M (1981). A rapid boiling method for the preparation of bacterial plasmids. Anal. Biochem. 114:193-197.
29. Maxam AM, Gilbert W (1980). Sequencing end-labelled DNA with base specific chemical cleavages. Meth Enzymol 65:499-560.
30. Southern E (1979) Gel electrophoresis of restriction fragments. Meth Enzymol 68:152-176.
31. Grantham R, Gautier C, Govy M, Jacobzone M, Mercire R, (1981). Codon catalogue usage is a genome strategy modulated for gene expressivity. Nucl Acids Res 9:r43-74.
32. Ikemura T (1985) Codon usage and tRNA content in unicellular and multicellular organisms. Molec Biol Evol 2:13-34.
33. Sarver N, Byrne JC, Howley PM (1982). Transformation and replication in mouse cells of a bovine papillomavirus-pML2 plasmid vector that can be rescued in bacteria. Proc Natl Acad Sci USA 79:7147-7151.
34. DiMaio D, Treisman RH, Maniatis T (1982). Bovine papilloma virus vector that propagates as a plasmid in both mouse and bacterial cells. Proc Natl Acad Sci USA 79. 4030-4034.

35. Zinn K, DiMaio D, Maniatis T (1983). Identification of two distinct regulatory regions adjacent to the human B interferon gene. Cell 34:865-879.
36. Laski FA, Ramamoorthy B, RajBhandary UL, Sharp, PA (1982). An amber suppressor tRNA gene derived by site-specific mutagenesis: cloning and function in mammalian cells. Proc Natl Acad Sci USA 79:5813-5817.
37. Colbere-Garapin F, Horodniceanu F, Kourilsky P, Garapin, A-C (1981). A new dominant hybrid selective marker for higher eucaryotic cells. J Molec Biol 150:1-14.
38. Southern PJ, Berg P, (1982). Transformation of mammalian cells to antibiotic resistance with a bacterial gene under control of the SV40 early region promoter. J Molec and Appl Genet 1:327-341.
39. Lusky M, Botchan M, (1985). Genetic analysis of the bovine papilloma virus type 1 trans-acting replication factors. J Virol 53:955-965.

**Papillomaviruses: Molecular and Clinical Aspects, pages 457–472**


# The Bovine Papillomavirus E6 Gene: Identification of its Transforming Function and Protein Product

John T. Schiller[1], Elliot J. Androphy, William C. Vass, and Douglas R. Lowy

Laboratory of Cellular Oncology
National Cancer Institute
Bethesda, MD 20205
(301) 496-9513

ABSTRACT We have genetically analyzed the transforming activity of the Bovine papillomavirus type 1 genome and determined that it contains at least two genes that can independently transform mouse C127 cells. One of these genes is encoded by the E6 open reading frame. This reading frame was cloned into a bacterial expression vector that directed the synthesis of large amounts of an E6 fusion protein which was used to generate antibodies to E6 in rabbits. These antibodies specifically immunoprecipitated a 15.5 kilodalton protein from C127 cells transformed by the E6 gene. Analysis of the E6 protein in transformed cells indicated that it exists as a monomer and is distributed equally between the nucleus and the non-nuclear membranes.

## INTRODUCTION

Papillomaviruses (PV) induce benign tumors (warts or papillomas) of the cutaneous and mucosal epithelia. In some instances, a subset of these papillomas appear to undergo malignant degeneration (1,2). A close association

---

[1]This work was supported in part by PHS grant 5-F32-CA-07327 awarded to J.T.S. by the National Cancer Institute, DHHS.

between human (H) PV infection and certain epithelial malignancies has given added significance to elucidation of PV genetics and biology (3,4). Bovine papillomavirus type 1 (BPV-1), which induces fibropapillomas in its natural host, is the PV whose genetics has been studied in greatest detail. Since DNA sequence analysis suggests that all PV genomes share a similar genetic organization (5,6), it is probable that understanding of BPV genetics will have direct relevance to other PVs, including HPVs.

Infection with BPV or its viral DNA genome can induce morphologic transformation of certain established cell lines in vitro, such as NIH 3T3 and C127 mouse cells (7,8). Cells transformed by BPV display a fully transformed phenotype: they form foci of proliferating cells in monolayer culture, colonies in agar, and tumors in nude mice. In these cells the viral DNA genome replicates as an unintegrated multi-copy episome (9). This extrachromosomal replication of the viral DNA is not required for morphologic transformation; following DNA mediated gene transfer, some mutant viral genomes transformed the cells even though the viral genetic information became integrated into the host chromosomal DNA (10,11). Cultured cells which contain the PV genome do not release progeny virus particles, since the genes that encode structural viral proteins are not transcribed in these cells (12).

Genetic analysis of BPV has begun to assign specific functions to defined regions within the viral DNA genome. The transforming and extrachromosomal maintenance functions have been mapped to a 5.4 kb segment of the 8 kb viral genome (this segment is called 69T because it represents 69% of the viral genome (8); see Fig. 1). Since 69T lacks the open reading frames (ORFs, potential protein coding segments) that encode the structural virion proteins (ORFs L1 and L2), it is clear that ORFs L1 and L2 are dispensible for these functions. As shown in Fig. 1, DNA sequence analysis of BPV indicates the presence of at least 8 ORFs (E1-E8) within this 5.4 kb transforming segment (13). Sequences from these ORFs are expressed as RNA in transformed cells (and in warts) (12,14,15). However, no protein product encoded by any of these putative non-structural genes has been identified for any PV, presumably because of the low level of expression of these genes in infected cells. In this report, we summarize our data indicating that BPV encodes at least two transforming genes, one of which corresponds to the E6

ORF (16), and that an E6 encoded protein can be identified in C127 cells transformed by this gene (17).

## METHODS

Random XhoI linker insertion mutations were introduced into the full-length BPV genome cloned in pML2d (18) by the method of Heffron et al. (19). Deletion mutants were generated by elimination of the sequences between pairs of XhoI linker inserts. pMX800 was constructed by the ligation of the 0.9 kb LTR containing EcoRI to BalI fragment of Moloney murine sarcoma virus (20) to the HpaI to EcoRI fragment of pMX633 (Fig. 1). XhoI linker insertions were introduced into pMX800 by replacing its HpaI to XmaI fragment with the corresponding fragment from full-length BPV insertion mutants.

In the transfection assays, 0.5 ug of undigested DNA was precipitated with calcium chloride (21) and 0.2 ml was added to a 35 mm seeded on the previous day with $2.5 \times 10^5$ C127 or NIH 3T3 cells. The cells were treated as described previously (22), except that dimethyl sulfoxide was not used.

The prokaryotic expression vector, which is identical to a previously published vector (23), was constructed by inserting a 736 bp fragment of pOG7 (which contains the phage lamda $P_L$ promotor, ribosome binding site, and N-terminus of the phage CII protein) into the ClaI site of pBR322. A 589 bp HpaII fragment of BPV was inserted; in-frame translation predicted a fusion of the N-terminal 13 amino acids of CII to 140 amino acids of the E6 ORF. This DNA was introduced into bacteria N6405, a $N^+$ E. coli which contains a lysogenic temperature-sensitive repressor (cI857ts) of $P_L$. Synthesis of the fusion protein was induced at 42°C and extracted from the bacteria (23). Rabbits were immunized with acrylamide gel slices containing this fusion protein.

Immunoprecipitations were performed using the rabbit antisera and protein-A bound to Sepharose beads (Pharmacia) in RIPA buffer (50mM Tris pH 7.4, 1mM EDTA, 150 mM NaCl, 1% deoxycholate, 0.1% sodium dodecyl sulfate [SDS], 1% aprotinin), and run on 15% polyacrylamide gels. For blocking experiments, non-radiolabeled bacterial lysates were pre-incubated with antisera, washed and then incubated with pXH800 lysate. Subcellular fractionations were performed using minor modifications of two different procedures (24,25).

## RESULTS

### BPV Contains More than One Transforming Gene.

To establish which gene(s) might be required for BPV transformation, we have generated a series of single site mutants of this genome by randomly inserting an 8 bp XhoI linker into the full-length BPV-1 genome. Forty single site insertions were analyzed and, although every major ORF was interrupted by at least one of the linker insertion mutations, each mutant retained at least some capacity to transform mouse C127 cells. Since the majority of the linker insertions should have resulted in a frame-shift mutation within the interrupted ORF, these results suggested that BPV-1 contained more than one transforming segment. The right-hand 2.3 kb of the 5.4 kb transforming segment had previoulsy been identified as containing a transforming gene (pHLB1, fig.1) (10). We therefore sought to determine if an ORF outside of 2.3 T might contain a transforming gene.

### The E6 ORF is a Transforming Gene.

In order to test this possibility, a clone was constructed (pXH633) from which the ORFs in 2.3 T had been deleted (although it retained the polyadenylation signal and enhancer element present at the extreme right-hand end of 2.3T; Fig. 1). This clone, which contained an intact E6 and E7 ORF, was still capable of transforming the C127 cells, although with a lower efficiency than that of the full lenth genome. An interesting feature of pXH633 and other clones (see below) that contained only E6 and E7 was that, although they induced a fully transformed phenotype in C127 cells, they did not induce the morphologic transformation of NIH 3T3 cells This result is in contrast to those obtained with 2.3T (clone pHLB1, Fig.1) or with the full-length viral genome, which transforms both C127 and NIH 3T3 cells. Deletion of putative regulatory elements from the BPV genome (clone pXH635) totally abolished this transforming activity. However, in clone pXH800, the activity was restored by addition of a retroviral regulatory element (the long terminal repeat [LTR], which contains sequences for enhancement, promotion, and initiation of RNA synthesis) to the otherwise non-transforming clone pXH635. Finally, deletion of the remaining non-coding sequences of 2.3 T

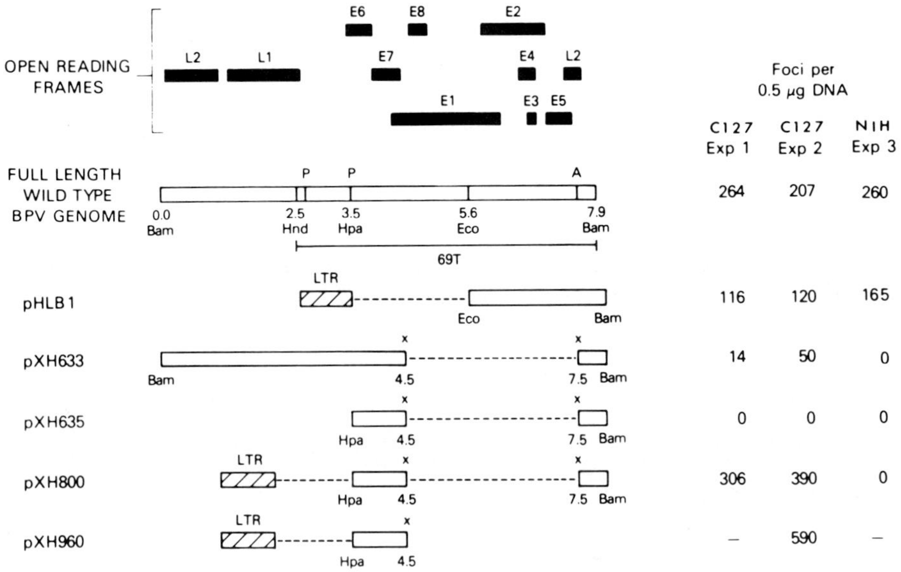


FIGURE 1. Transformation by BPV subgenomic clones. The genome of BPV-1 linearized at the unique BamHI site in which it was cloned into the pBR322 derivative pML2d is shown. The numbers below the BPV genome indicate the distance in kb from the BamHI site at 0.0. The locations of putative promoters and polyadenylation signal are designated "P" and "A" respectively. Open bars represent BPV seqences included in the clones, and dashed lines indicate deleted sequences. Sites of XhoI linker insertions are denoted by "X". Bam, BamHI; Hnd, HindIII; Hpa, HpaI; and Eco, EcoRI recognition sites.

did not abolish the transforming activity (clone pXH960). These results suggested that sequences within E6 and/or E7 encoded a gene that could transform C127 cells, but not NIH 3T3 cells.

Further mutational analysis of the 1 kb segment in clone pXH800, which contained the E6 and E7 ORFs, strongly suggested that the E6 ORF represented the transforming gene (Fig. 2). For example, deletion of the majority of the E7 ORF (clone pXH997) did not significantly impair the transforming activity of this segment. Conversely, a mutant that introduced a frame shift in the E6 ORF did abolish the transforming activity of this clone (pXH875). One mutant with a linker insertion in the 5' end of the E6 ORF (pXH831) retained the transforming activity of pXH800, but DNA sequence analysis indicated that it was an in-frame substitution rather than a frame-shift mutation. Elimination of the XhoI restriction site in the linker of pXH831 by a fill-in reaction, which should have introduced a change in reading frame, abolished the transforming activity of the mutant (data not shown).

Expression of E6 in Bacteria and Production of E6 Antibodies.

Having demonstrated that E6 was a transforming gene, we then sought to identify in transformed cells the E6 protein that presumably mediates this function. We used a prokaryotic expression vector in order to produce large quantities of an E6 polypeptide for generating antibodies specific to E6. The E6 ORF was inserted into the vector so that the plasmid would encode a fusion protein containing the N-terminal 13 amino acids of the phage lamda CII protein and 140 amino acids of the E6 ORF. The E6 sequences in the vector began three codons upstream from the first (translation initiation) AUG of E6 and extended down past the termination codon of the ORF. When placed in E. coli, this vector directed the synthesis of the predicted 17.5 kilodalton (kd) E6 fusion protein (data not shown). This band was excised from SDS-polyacrylamide gels and rabbits were immunized with this protein preparation. The immunization protocol resulted in rabbit sera that reacted with the fusion protein under reducing and non-reducing conditions by immunoprecipitation (Fig. 3) and by immunoblotting (not shown).

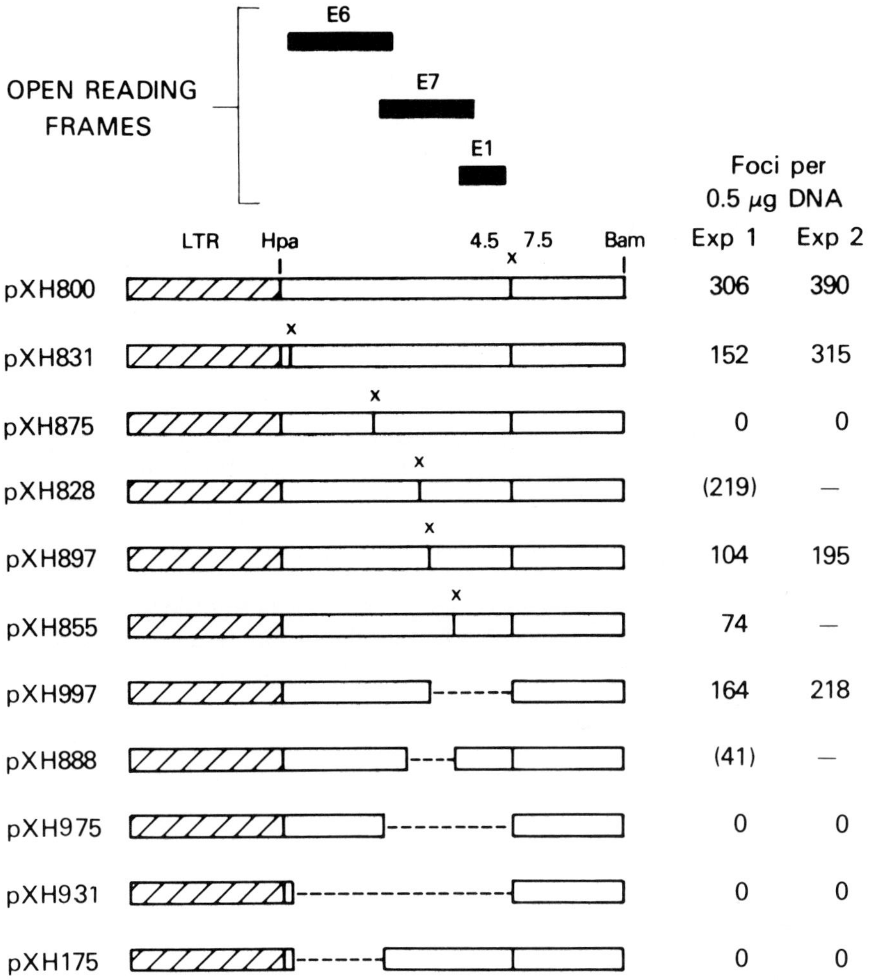


FIGURE 2. Mutational analysis of the 5' transforming region. Designations are the same as in Fig. 1. Only the $NH_2$ terminus of E1 is present in the 1-kb HpaI-to-XhoI fragment of pXH800. DNAs were transfected onto C127 cells in both experiments. Numbers in parentheses refer to a third experiment in which pXH800 induced 149 foci per 0.5 ug of DNA.

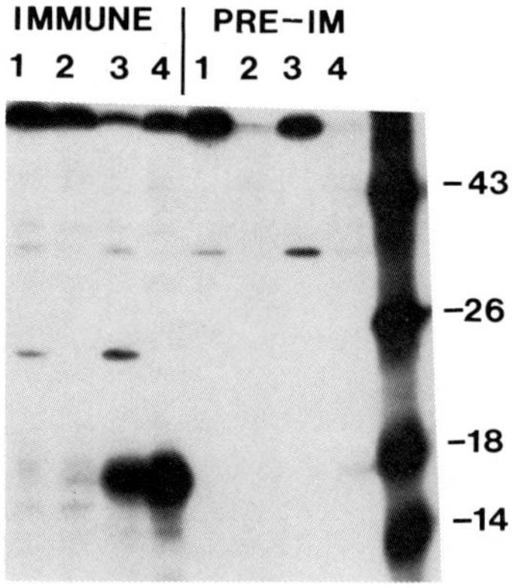


FIGURE 3. Immunoprecipitation of the bacterially made E6 fusion protein. #'s 1 and 2 are SDS extracts from non-E6 containing bacteria, and #'s 3 and 4 are SDS extracts from E6 containing bacteria. #'s 2 and 4 were boiled in 100 mM dithiothreitol prior to immunoprecipitation. Immune rabbit sera used in first four lanes, pre-immune sera for right four lanes.

Identification of the E6 Protein.

The above experiments confirmed the presence of the E6 ORF, as predicted from DNA sequence analysis (13). However, they did not indicate that this ORF actually encoded a polypeptide in mammalian cells morphologically transformed by E6. In principle, it should be easier to detect a putative E6 protein in cells that expressed the gene at high levels. We therefore sought to identify the protein in C127 cells transformed by the LTR activated clones pXH800 and pXH997 (Fig. 2), since E6 RNA levels were found to be at least 10 times greater in cells transformed by these constructions than in cells transformed by the full-length BPV genome.

When cells transformed by either of these LTR activated clones were metabolically labeled with (35)S-cysteine, the sera from the rabbit that possessed antibodies to the bacterial fusion protein specifically immunoprecipitated a 15.5 kd protein (Fig. 4). This size corresponds to the molecular weight predicted from DNA sequence analysis for the E6 protein, if the protein is initiated from the first AUG within the ORF and is not subjected to post-translational modification. Since much of E7 is deleted from clone pXH997, these results strongly suggest that the protein is encoded entirely by E6. Finding this protein in pXH997 indicates that the 15.5 kd molecule does not represent an E6/E7 fusion protein predicted from mRNA analysis of BPV transformed cells; sequence analysis of the spliced E6/E7 RNA suggests that this putative protein would be 20.5 kd. The 15.5 kd band was also the only specific band observed when the immunoprecipitates were run under non-reducing conditions. This suggests that the protein is not in disulfide linkage with other E6 molecules or with other proteins. When NIH 3T3 and C127 cells transformed by the full-length BPV genome were analyzed, they also synthesized the 15.5 kd protein, but at levels approximately 10-fold lower than those found in cells transformed by the LTR driven E6 ORF (not shown).

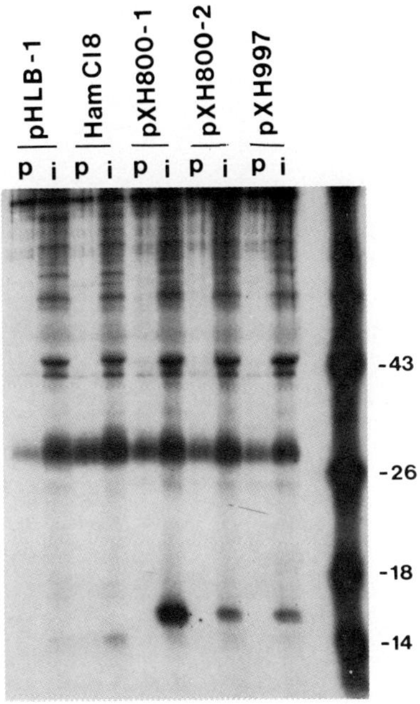


FIGURE 4. Immunoprecipitation of E6 from transformed cell lines. p=pre-immune sera, i=immune sera. 25 x $10^6$ CPM of (35)S-cysteine were used per lane. Cell lines are as in text and in Fig. 2. Ham Cl 8 is a Ha-ras transformed C127 cell line. 13 day autoradiogram exposure.

Immunoprecipitation inhibition experiments confirmed that the protein found in the transformed mouse cells was encoded by E6 (Fig. 5). Immunoprecipitation of the 15.5 kd band was specifically blocked only by a non-radiolabeled bacterial extract containing the E6 fusion protein. An extract from bacteria which did not contain E6 failed to block the immunoprecipitation of the 15.5 kd band.

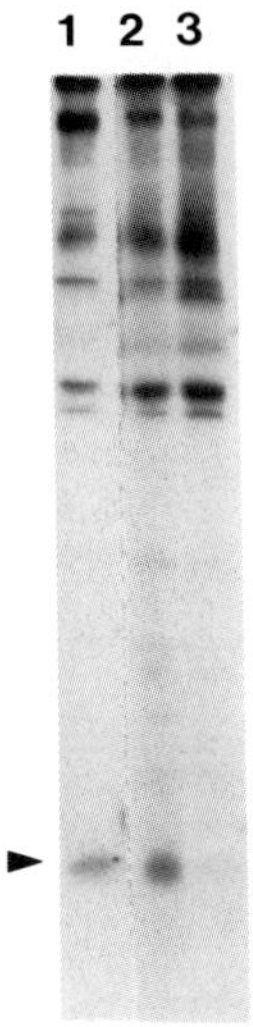


FIGURE 5. Immunoprecipitation inhibition experiment. Identical (35)S-cysteine labeled lysates from pXH800 cells were immunoprecipitated using rabbit antisera. Lane 1: no pre-incubation with bacterial lysate. Lanes 2 and 3: antisera added to non-radiolabeled extract from non-E6 containing bacteria , lane 2, and E6-containing bacteria, lane 3, prior to incubation with the pXH800 lysate.

The E6 Protein is in Nuclear and Membrane Fractions.

After determining that the 15.5 kd protein is the product of E6, we sought to localize the protein in transformed cells by sub-cellular fractionation. Cells transformed by pXH800 were metabolically labeled with cysteine and separated into nuclei, cytoplasm, and membranes (Fig. 6) (24) . Approximately equal quantities of the E6 protein were found in the nuclear and membrane fractions by two different methods of fractionation (24,25). As controls, C127 cells transformed by the unrelated ras oncogene (Ham Cl 8) did not contain the 15.5 kd band when fractionated by these methods. The completeness of the frationation was confirmed by identification of c-ras, which is found in membranes, and c-myc, which is found in nuclei, in the appropriate fractions of the pXH800 lysate, as well as by the use of other markers.

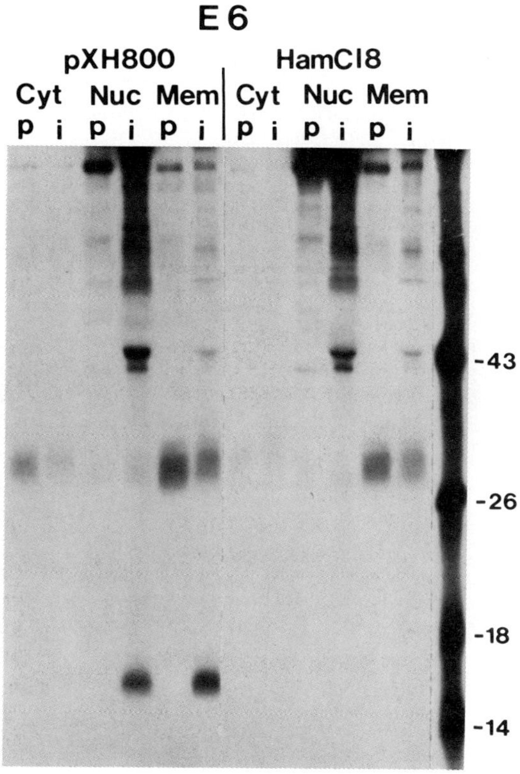


FIGURE 6. Immunoprecipitation of BPV E6 from sub-cellular fractions of transformed cells. pXH800 cells were fractionated using a Dounce homogenizer with cells suspended in 0.25 M sucrose in the prescence of $MgCl_2$ using a modification of the procedure of Hann (24). Ham Cl 8 is a Ha-ras transformed C127 cell line. p = pre-immune sera, i = immune sera, Nuc = nuclei, cyt = cytoplasm, mem = membranes.

## DISCUSSION

These data indicate that BPV contains at least two transforming genes; we have localized one of these genes to the E6 ORF and identified its protein product. The 15.5 kd E6 protein appears to be initiated at the first AUG of the ORF and encoded entirely by the BPV E6 ORF. Our results suggest further that the protein is not in disulfide linkage to other E6 molecules or to other proteins. In other studies not discussed here, we have localized another transforming gene to the E5 ORF in 2.3T (26).

Recent data suggest that E6 may be functionally significant in malignant tumors. Carcinomas induced by the cottontail rabbit PV as well as human cervical carcinomas which contain HPV DNA appear to selectively retain and express sequences from the E6 ORF (27,28). Each PV genome that has been subjected to DNA sequence analysis has been found to have an ORF that is analogous to the BPV E6 ORF (5,6). There is some homology at the amino acid level among these different E6 ORFs (Fig. 7). All of these polypeptides are relatively rich in cysteines. Many of the cysteine residues are arranged in repeats of cysteine-x-x-cysteine, which has been suggested to be a characteristic feature of nucleic acid binding proteins (NBPs) (29). These E6 polypeptides are also relatively rich in basic amino acids, which is another feature of NBPs. Since some of E6 is found in the nucleus, it may be a NBP.

SV40 large-T antigen has a nucleotide binding region and, like E6, is found in the nucleus and plasma membrane (30). However, only small amounts of large-T antigen are found on the plasma membrane, whereas the BPV E6 protein is distributed relatively equally between the nucleus and the non-nuclear membranes (the membrane fraction that contains E6 has not been identified). Furthermore, large-T antigen can be extracted from the nucleoplasm (30), while the E6 protein is not present in this fraction (unpublished observation).

The approach we have used to identify the BPV E6 protein should be applicable to the analogous E6 ORF of other PVs, as well as to other PV gene products. Since most PV-associated dysplasias and carcinomas do not synthesize detectable levels of structural viral antigens, identification of non-structural gene products such as E6 may prove useful diagnostically. The identification of the E6 protein should permit analysis of the biochemical properties of the molecule, as has been carried out for other transforming proteins, and facilitate the study of the pathogenesis of warts and PV-associated malignancies.

COMPARISON OF E6 PROTEINS

```
                              *              *  *
BPV 1: MDLKPF..ARTNPFSG.....LDC.LWCR.......EPLTEVDAFR.CMVK.DF.HVVIREGCRY..
HPV 1: MAT.PIRTVRQLSES......L.C.IPY...I.DVLLPCNFCNYFLSNAEKLLFDHFDLHLVWRDNL
HPV 6: MESANASTSATTID......QL.CKT.FNLSMHTLQINCVFCKNALTTAE........IYSYA.YKH
HPV16: MHQKRTAMFQDPQERPRKLPQL.C.TELQTTIHDIILECVYCKQQLLRREVYDFAFRDLCIV..YRD
          ++  + ++  ++     +X X +     +++  X+XX+X+ +X  +X+ +X + +X  + +X+

             *    *                                                 *  *
     ..GACTI.CLGN.CLATERRLWQGVPV..........TGEEAELLHGK..TLDRLC....IRCCYCG
     VFG.....CCQG.CARTVSLLEF.VLYYQES......Y.EVPEIE....GILDRPLLQIELRCVTCI
     LKVLFRGGYPYAACAC....LEFHGKINQYRHFDYAGYATTVEEET.KQDILD.VL....IRCYLCH
     ..GNPYAVC.DN CLKF......YSKISEYRHYCYSLYGTTLEQQYNK.PLCD.LL....IRCINCQ
       X     X  + X+ +   X++ ++X ++++  +  X +++X +  X  XXX+X+    XXX+ X

                                                  *  *   *
     ....GKLTKN.GKHRHVLFN.EPFCKTRAN..IIR....GRCYDC...CRHGSRSKY....P
     K....KLSVA.EKLEVVS.NGERVHRVR.N......RLKAKCSL....CRLYA.......I
     KPLCHKPLCEVEKVKHIL....T..KAR..FIKLNCTWKGRCLHCWTTCMEDM.......LP
     KPLC..PE.EKQKQRHLD....K..KQR..FHNIRGRWTGRCMSC...CRS.SRTRRETQL
     X+++ X+  + +X++XX+ + +   X X ++  ++ +++XXX  X  XX  ++      ++

     * = conserved cysteine        X = 3/4 or 4/4       + = 2/4
```

Figure 7. Comparison of E6 proteins. The amino acid sequence of BPV-1 and HPVs 1, 6, and 16 , based on their DNA sequences, have been aligned for comparison of their homologous peptides. (5,6,31)

ACKNOWLEDGEMENTS

We thank Max Gottesman for plasmid pOG7 and E.coli strain N6405, Robert Eisenman for antibody to c-myc, and Alex Papageorge and Nancy Hubbert for helpful discussions and technical assistance.

## REFERENCES

1. Orth G, Favre M, Breitburd F, Croissant O, Jablonska S, Obalek S, Jarzabek-Chorzelska M, Rzesa G (1980). Epidermodysplasia verruciformis: a model for the role of papillomaviruses in human cancer. In Essex M, Todaro G, zur Hausen H (eds): "Viruses in Natural Occuring Cancers," New York: Cold Spring Harbor Laboratory, p.259.
2. Ostrow RS, Bender M, Niimura M, Seki T, Kawashima M, Pass F, Faras AJ (1982). Human papillomavirus DNA in cutaneous primary and metastasized squamous cell carcinomas from patients with epidermodysplasia verruciformis. Proc Natl Acad Sci USA 79:1634.
3. Durst M, Gissmann L, Ikenberg H, zur Hausen H (1983). A papillomavirus DNA from a cervical carcinoma and its prevalence in cancer biopsy samples from different geographic regions. Proc Natl Acad Sci USA 80:3812.
4. Boshart M, Gissmann L, Ikenberg H, Kleinheinz A, Scheurlen W, zur Hausen H (1984). A new tupe of papillomavirus DNA, its presence in genital cancer biopsies and in cell lines derived from cervical cancer. EMBO J 3:1151.
5. Danos O, Engel LW, Chen EY, Yaniv M, Howley PM (1983). Comparative analysis of the human type 1a and bovine type 1 papillomavirus genomes. J Virol 46:557.
6. Schwarz E, Durst M, Demankowski C, Lattermann O, Zech R, Woldsperger E, Suhai S, zur Hausen H (1983). DNA sequence and genome organization of genital human papillomavirus type 6b. EMBO J 2:2341.
7. Dvoretzky I, Shober R, Lowy D (1980). Focus assay in mouse cells for bovine papillomavirus. Virology 103:369.
8. Lowy DR, Dvoretsky I, Shober R, Law M-F, Engel L, Howley PM (1980). In vitro transformation by a defined subgenomic fragment of bovine papillomavirus DNA. Nature (London) 287:72.
9. Law M-F, Lowy DR, Dvoretzky I, Howley PM (1981). Mouse cells transformed by bovine papillomavirus contain only extrachromosomal viral DNA sequences. Proc Natl Acad Sci USA 78:2727.
10. Nakabayashi Y, Chattopadhyay SK, Lowy, DR (1983). The transforming function of bovine papillomavirus DNA. Proc Natl Acad Sci USA 80:5832.

11. Lusky M, Botchan MR (1985). Genetic analysis of bovine papillomavirus type 1 trans-acting replication factors. J Virol 53:955.
12. Engel LW, Heilaman CA, Howley PM (1983). Transcriptional organization of bovine papillomavirus type I. J Virol 47:516.
13. Chen CY, Howley PM, Levinson AD, Seeburg PH (1982). The primary structure and the genetic organization of bovine papilloma virus type 1 genome. Nature 299:530.
14. Amtmann E, Sauer G (1982). Bovine papillomavirus transcription: polyadenylated RNA species and assessment of the direction of transcription. J Virol 43:59.
15. Heilman CA, Engel L, Lowy DR, Howley PM (1982). Virus-specific transcription in bovine papillomavirus transformed mouse cells. Virol 119:22.
16. Schiller JT, Vass WC, Lowy, DR (1984). Identification of a second transforming region in bovine papillomavirus DNA. Proc Natl Acad Sci USA 81:7880.
17. Androphy EJ, Schiller JT, Lowy DR. Manuscript submitted for publication.
18. Sarver N, Byrne JC, Howley PM (1982). Transformation and replication in mouse cells of a bovine papillomavirus-pML2 plasmid vector that can be rescued in bacteria. Proc Natl Acad Sci USA 79:7147.
19. Heffron F, So M, McCarthy BJ (1978). In vitro mutagenesis of a circular DNA molecule by using synthetic restriction sites. Proc Natl Acad Sci 75:6012.
20. Dhar R, McClements WL, Enquist LW, Vande Woude GF (1980). Nucleotide sequences of integrated Moloney sarcoma provirus long terminal repeats and their host and viral junctions. Proc Natl Acad Sci 77:3937.
21. Graham FL, van der Eb AJ (1973). A new technique for the assay of infectivity of human adenovirus 5 DNA. Virology 52:456.
22. Lowy DR, Rands E, Scolnick EM (1978). Helper-independent transformation by unintegrated Harvey sarcoma virus DNA. J Virol 26:291.
23. Lautenberger JA, Court D, Papas TS (1983). High-level expression in Escherichia coli of the carboxy-terminal sequences of the avian myelocytomatosis virus (MC29) v-myc protein. Gene 23:75.
24. Hann SR, Eisenman RN (1984). Proteins encoded by the human c-myc oncogene: differential expression in neoplastic cells. Mol Cell Biol 4:2486

25. Cooper JA, Hunter T (1982). Discrete primary locations of a tyrosine protein kinase and of three proteins that contain phosphotyrosine in virally transformed chick fibroblasts. J Cell Biol 94:287.
26. Schiller JT, Vass WC, Lowy DR. Manuscript submitted for publication.
27. Danos O, Georges E, Orth G, and Yaniv M (1985). Fine structure of the cottontail rabbit papillomavirus mRNAs expressed in the transplantable VX2 carcinoma. J Virol 53:735.
28. Schwarz E, Freese UK, Gissmann L, Mayer W, Roggenbuck B, Stremlau A, zur Hausen H (1985). Structure and transcription of human papillomavirus sequences in cervical carcinoma cells. Nature 314:111.
29. Wain-Hobson S, Sonigo P, Danos O, Cole S, Alizon M (1985). Nucleotide sequence of the AIDS virus, LAV. Cell 40:9.
30. Staufenbiel M, Deppert W (1983). Differential structural systems of the nucleus are targets for SV40 large T antigen. Cell 33:173.
31. Rowekamp, W, Seedorf, K, personal communication.

**Papillomaviruses: Molecular and Clinical Aspects, pages 473–486**


# STEPWISE TUMORAL PROGRESSION IN RODENT FIBROBLASTS TRANSFORMED WITH BOVINE PAPILLOMA VIRUS TYPE 1 (BPV1) DNA[1]

François Cuzin*, Guerrino Meneguzzi*, Bernard Binétruy*, Christa Cerni[+], Gisèle Connan*, Milaine Grisoni* and Odile de Lapeyrière[§]

*INSERM U273 and CNRS LP7300, Centre de Biochimie, Université de Nice, 06034, Nice, France,
[+]Institute for Tumor Biology, Cancer Research Center, University of Vienna, A-1090 Vienna, Austria and
[§]INSERM U119, 27 bd Leï Roure, 13009 Marseille, France

ABSTRACT Four distinct stages were tentatively defined in the oncogenic transformation process induced by BPV1 in rat FR3T3 and mouse C127 cells. Stage 1 lines, selected in G418 medium after transfer of a BPV1-*neo* plasmid, expressed normal cell morphology and growth control, maintained autonomous non-rearranged copies of plasmid DNA and produced transformed derivatives at a low frequency which increased after treatment with a tumour promoter (TPA). Stage 2 lines were derived either by focus selection after transfer of viral DNA or by spontaneous transformation of Stage 1 cells; their phenotype *in vitro* was intermediate between that of normal cells and that of "highly transformed" lines (polyoma virus or *ras* transformants); unlike cells transformed by polyomaviruses, however, they produce highly invasive tumours in the animal. Stage 3 cell lines, established back in culture from these tumours, exhibited increased plating efficiencies in suspension and tumorigenicity, but maintained an organized cyto-skeleton and remained dependent on serum factors for growth in culture. Stage 4 lines were also selected by

[1] This work was supported by grants from the Centre National de la Recherche Scientifique, Ministère de la Recherche and Association pour la Recherche sur le Cancer (France).

tumour formation in the animal, but directly from Stage 1 cells; they were characterized by the disappearance of actin cables and by a further increase in tumorigenicity; at this stage, the proviral genomes were either highly rearranged or, in one case, was entirely lost.

## INTRODUCTION

Infection with BPV1 virus (1), or transfection with cloned fragments of viral DNA (2), induce oncogenic transformation of rodent fibroblast cells in culture. As in other papillomavirus-induced tumours, proviral genomes are maintained as non-integrated circular molecules (3,4). Transformation requires only part of the genome of BPV1 (69 % BamHI-HindIII fragment) (2). When this fragment was linked to a bacterial vector, we observed that the transformed cells maintained in a plasmidial state both viral and vector DNA, but in most instances, with extensive deletions in the non-selected bacterial sequences (5). This was not the case after selection for expression of a drug-resistance gene included in the bacterial sequences, most of the resistant clones maintaining non-rearranged copies of the plasmid DNA (6).

We analyzed growth properties and other transformation-related characters in a series of cell lines which had been selected either by growth in G418-containing medium, or by focus formation in normal medium, or by growth as tumours in the animal. One series were rat FR3T3 derivatives, for which comparisons can be made with a large number of available lines, transformed by other viral or cellular oncogenes (see ref. 7 for review) and by complete BPV1 DNA (8). Another group of lines were derived from mouse C127 cells, extensively used in other laboratories for studies on BPV1 transformation (2,3). Depending on the selection applied, distinct transformation phenotypes were observed, both in the rat and in the mouse cells. They were reproducible enough to be, not too arbitrarily, described as four transformation stages. Unlike that observed with polyomavirus, adenovirus and cellular oncogenes (see ref. 7 for review), this progression does not start from the most normal rodent embryo fibroblasts, but only from previously immortalized pseudo-normal cell lines: no transformed focus or drug-resistant colony was produced in our hands by transfection of BPV1 DNA in cells of primary cultures, suggesting that the virus does not exert an immortalization function. This was confirmed using colony formation at low cell input as an assay for immortalization, as previously done for the polyoma _plt_ gene and for rearranged _myc_ genes (9) (Table 1). Lack of immortalization potential may be related with the fact that papillomas develop _in vivo_ from continuously dividing basal epidermal cells.

TABLE 1
IMMORTALIZATION ASSAY AFTER TRANSFER OF BPV1 DNA

| Plasmid DNA | Inserted genes | Plating efficiency[a] |
|---|---|---|
| pBR322 | none | 1 |
| pPY1 | polyoma early genes (9) | 15 |
| pBPV9 | complete BPV1 genome (10) | 1 |
| pV69 | BPV1 transforming region (6) | 0 |

[a]colonies after plating 3,000 cells per plate (9)

STAGE 1: NORMAL GROWTH CONTROL, PLASMIDIAL MAINTENANCE OF VIRAL SEQUENCES, HIGH FREQUENCY OF SPONTANEOUS TRANSFORMATION, TPA REACTIVITY.

Transfer into rat FR3T3 and mouse C127 cells of a BPV1(BamHI-HindIII)-_neo_ construct (pV69) yielded resistant colonies in the presence of the drug G418 with a frequency ten to twenty fold higher than that of focus formation in normal medium (6). G418-resistant cell lines established in this way, either from FR3T3 cells or from C127 cells, could not be distinguished from the original normal cells by their growth properties. In 10% serum, they only grew up to a low saturation density, they did not grow in suspension in agarose medium and could not survive in the presence of only 0.5% serum. They maintained the extended, flat morphology of normal cells and immunofluorescence staining of myosin revealed organized cytoskeletal structures (figure 1).

Cells grown in selective medium maintained autonomous copies of pV69 DNA, without any rearrangement detectable at the level of Southern blot analysis (6, see figure 3). In

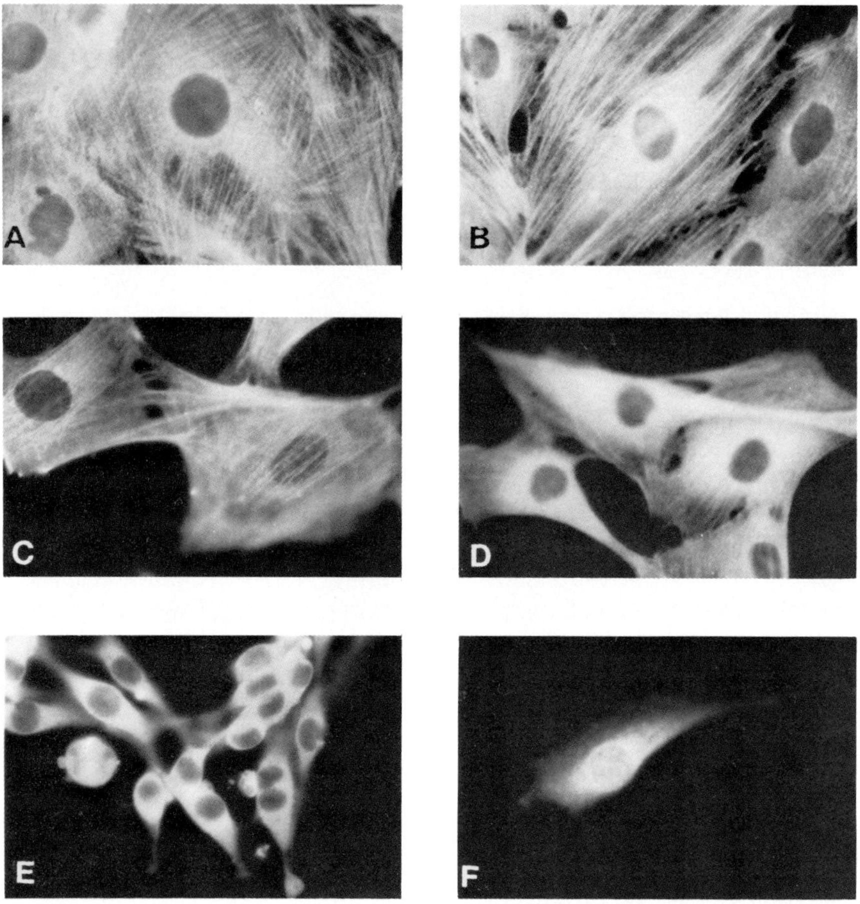


FIGURE 1. Indirect immunofluorescence staining of myosin in Fischer rat cells representative of the various transformation phenotypes: (A) untransformed FR3T3 cells; (B) RV691 line (Stage 1); (C) RVLC12 line (Stage 2); (D) RVLC14-TD2 (Stage 3); (E) RV694-TD1 (Stage 4); (F) polyoma virus-transformed PYT21 cells (9). See ref. 8 for experimental procedure.

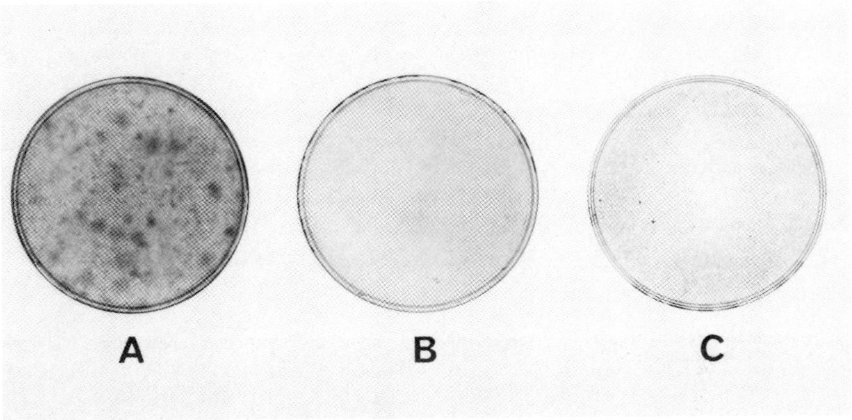


FIGURE 2. Effect of TPA on Stage 1 pV69 transformants. A. RV697 cells were treated with TPA for 12 days as indicated in the Text and subsequently maintained in normal growth medium; Giemsa staining after 4 weeks.
B. RV697 culture treated in parallel without TPA.
C. FR3T3 cells treated with TPA as in A.

the absence of selective pressure, these lines progressively loose resistance to G418. Reversion to the sensitive phenotype corresponded to the loss of the autonomous DNA and occured with variable frequencies from one line to another; sensitive cells represented between 10 and 50% of the culture after 3 generations and at least 95% after 15 generations.

These apparently normal lines exhibited an unusually high rate of spontaneous oncogenic transformation, as determined by monitoring the appearance of dense foci upon serial subcultures (6). Similar observations had been made on cells which received oncogenes such as polyoma virus plt gene or rearranged myc genes and, in these two cases, phenotypic transformation could be induced by exposure to a tumour promotor (TPA), which had no effect on the original normal cells (11). TPA treatment was applied on RV697 rat cells, a line which presents a low rate of spontaneous transformation. Cells were maintained for 12 days in Dulbecco-Eagle medium (DMEM) containing TPA ($2x10^{-5}$ M in 0.01% DMSO) and thereafter retruned to normal DMEM. Dense foci appeared within 4 weeks (figure 2), demonstrating a clear effect of TPA, possibly related to that previously described by Amtmann and Sauer (12) of a synergistic effect of papillomaviruses and TPA in cell transformation. As previously noted for cells which express the polyoma virus plt or rearranged myc genes (7,11), the apparent normal state of Stage 1 cell lines appears as a "high risk state", where the cells become responsive to environmental stimuli which do not induce transformation of normal cells.

## STAGE 2: AGRESSIVE TUMORIGENIC PROPERTIES CONTRASTING WITH A LIMITED DEVIATION FROM NORMAL GROWTH CONTROL IN CULTURE AND WITH NORMAL CELL STRUCTURE AND MORPHOLOGY

Stage 2 transformants were obtained either by direct selection for foci after transfection of pV69 or BPV1 DNA or, as indicated above, by spontaneous transformation of Stage 1 cell lines (TPA-induced transformants derived at Stage 1 exhibited somewhat different properties and have not yet been extensively studied).

Their phenotype, similar to that previously described for FR3T3 cells transformed with complete BPV1 DNA (8), corresponds to a low transformation level. Most noticeably, these cells retained the flat morphology and the organized cytoskeleton of the normal fibroblast (figure 1) and they grew only in the presence of high serum concentrations. They exhibited a broad range of saturation densities and plating efficiencies in agarose medium. High numbers of extrachromosomal copies of pV69 DNA were observed in all cases (see figure 3), as previously documented for the equivalent BPV1 transformants (8).

In spite of their apparent low level of transformation, FR3T3 cells transformed with BPV1 DNA were highly tumorigenic when injected in syngeneic rats (8), and the same result was obtained with the comparable Stage 2 cell lines transformed with pV69 DNA (table 2). Unlike tumours induced by polyoma- and SV40-transformed cells, primary tumours induced by BPV1 (or pV69) transformants did not remain localized at the site of injection, but quickly invaded inner organs and lung and liver metastasis were observed.

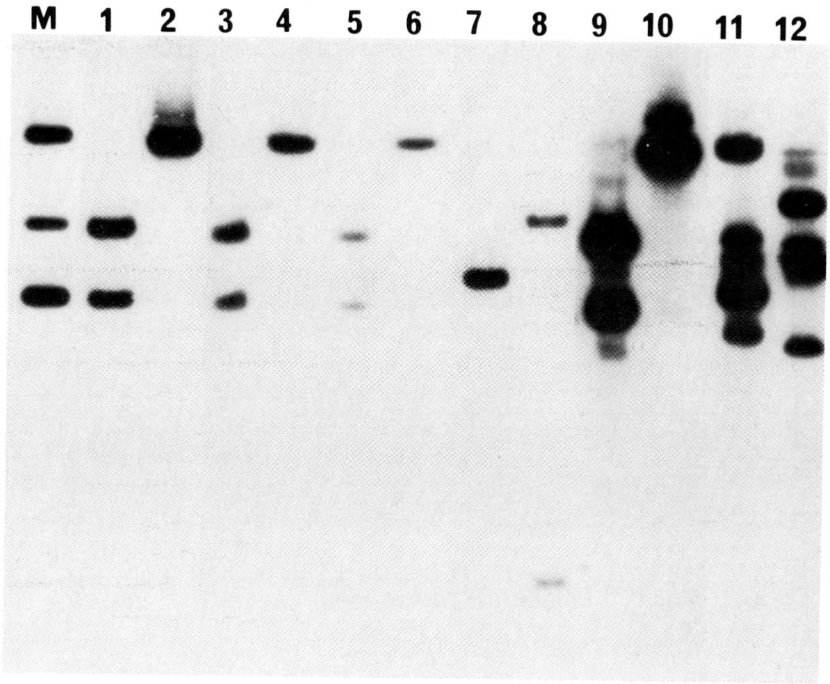


FIGURE 3. Blot-hybridization patterns of a radioactive pV69 DNA probe with restriction-cleaved total cellular DNA of representative cell lines. M: markers: from top to bottom: linearized pV69 DNA (8 KB), BamHI-HindIII BPV1 fragment (5.5 KB), pVV2 DNA (4 KB) (see ref. 6 for detailed structure of the DNAs); lanes 1 & 2: RV691 (Stage 1), 3 & 4: RVLC12 (Stage 2), 5 & 6: RV1-TD1 (Stage 3), 7 to 12: RV691-TD2, RV691-TD3, RV695-TD1 (Stage 4). Lanes 1, 3, 5, 7, 9, 11: cleavage with BamHI (2 cuts in pV69 DNA); lanes 2, 4, 6, 8, 10, 12: cleavage with HindIII (1 cut).

TABLE 2
TUMORIGENICITY IN FISCHER RATS
OF REPRESENTATIVE CELL LINES[a]

| Stage | Cell line | Latency (weeks) | Tumor incidence (animals with tumours after twelve months) | Macroscopic lung metastasis |
|---|---|---|---|---|
| 1 | RV691 | 24 | 8/19 | 3/4 |
| 2 | RVLC14 | 6 | 31/31 | 2/10 |
| 3 | BPV1-TD3 | 4 | 10/10 | 10/10 |
| 4 | RV691-TD2 | 0.5 | 9/9 | 9/9 |

[a]subcutaneous injection of $4 \times 10^6$ cells in 3 week-old Fischer rats.

## THE TRANSFORMED PHENOTYPE OF CELL LINES SELECTED BY TUMORAL GROWTH IN THE ANIMAL (STAGES 3 AND 4)

### Stage 3 Lines: Increased Level of Transformation in Culture, High Tumorigenicity and Invasiveness and a Flat Morphology.

We previously reported that cell lines initially transformed with BPV1 DNA and established in culture after tumoral growth in the animal, exhibited, as one would expect, some of the properties that were previously associated with tumorigenicity (efficient growth in suspension, high level of plasminogen activator production). It was striking, however, to observe that these tumour-derived cells still maintained organized cytoskeletal structures and needed high serum concentrations for growth in culture (8). These results were confirmed, with only minor variations, for cell lines established back in culture from tumours induced by Stage 2 pV69 transformants. These lines

(Stage 3) maintained a flat morphology (figure 1) and a complete dependence on high serum concentrations, but they produced very large colonies in agarose medium and exhibited increased tumorigenicity (table 2) in terms of latency (a few weeks), invasiveness of primary tumours and metastatic potential.

Stage 4: Cell Lines Selected Directly from Stage 1 by Tumoral Growth: Elevated Tumorigenic Potential, Altered Morphology, Highly Rearranged Viral Genomes.

In order to determine whether Stage 1 cells, which appear in culture as rather normal, are able to induce tumours in syngeneic immunocompetent hosts, series of Fischer rats were injected subcutaneously with FR3T3 derived Stage 1 cells. Results are summarized in table 2.

No tumour could be detected by palpation in these animals for the first 3-4 months after injection. At this stage, however, several animals died without having developed any obvious symptom. In two such cases, autopsy revealed the presence of internal sarcomas, in the diaphragm and in the intestinal lymph nodes, respectively. Henceforth, most animals developed tumours at the site of injection, with latency periods extending up to several additional months.

All lines derived from these long latency tumours exhibited the same high plating efficiencies in gelified medium and the same high levels of plasminogen activator production as Stage 3 cell lines. Their tumorigenicity was even higher, since injection in young Fischer rats produced detectable tumours within three days. By contrast with the other three groups of transformants, these cells had undergone important morphological changes and exhibited completely disrupted cytoskeletal structures (figure 1). This change in cell structure, consistently observed in Stage 4 lines derived from these long latency tumours, was occasionally also observed in rare cell lines derived from the short latency tumours (Stage 3). Rather than unique situations, Stages 3 and 4 may thus represent extreme cases in a continuum of tumour progression stages. It must be, however, underlined that among a large series of cell lines studied, transformed either by viral DNA or by pV69 plasmid DNA, Stage 3 tumour cells without an organized cytoskeleton remained exceptional.

## STATE OF THE BPV1 DNA SEQUENCES IN TUMOURS AND TUMOUR-DERIVED CELL LINES

Blot analysis with pV69 probes produced in all cases identical patterns for the primary tumors, their metastasis or the derived cell cultures. Digestion of tumor DNA with endonucleases which either do not cleave, or cleave once pV69 DNA, and comparative study of total DNA and low molecular weight DNA extracted (Hirt) from TD cultures, indicated that in all samples examined the plasmidial DNA replicates as free, oligomeric molecules. Unlike what was observed in Stage 1 and Stage 2 cell lines, these plasmidial molecules had often undergone rearrangements. Representative results are shown in figure 3.

Rearrangements were in most instances limited in Stage 3 lines, a number of them producing in fact the same blot-hybridization profile as the original cell lines, as previously described for equivalent cell lines transformed with BPV1 DNA (8). By contrast, the more advanced Stage 4 cells exhibited in all cases highly rearranged patterns and a variable number of copies as compared with the original lines. In one Stage 4 tumour DNA, no fragment hybridizing with the pV69 probe could be evidenced.

## DISCUSSION

Transformation phenotypes induced in rat and mouse fibroblasts by complete BPV1 DNA (8) and by pV69 DNA (this report) appear different in several important respects from those previously observed in the same cells after transformation by other agents (Polyomaviruses, Retroviruses). The Papillomavirus transformants exhibited impressive tumorigenic potentials, with highly invasive primary tumours and frequent metastasis. In clear contrast, however, with observations made in other systems (13), cells could be established back in culture from these tumours (Stage 3) which maintained the flat morphology and organized cytoskeletal structures of a normal fibroblast. These observations underline how difficult it is to generalize correlations established in one given system between the properties of cells in culture and their malignant potential in the organism.

Since the early work of Rous and Beard (14), stepwise progression of viral papillomas towards malignancy was documented in animals systems and suggested for several human cancers (this Symposium). The proper *in vitro* models for the study of carcinoma evolution were, however, difficult to develop because of the problems inherent to the culture of epithelial cells and their transformation in culture (15). For this reason, experimental models which reproduce some aspects of this stepwise progression may be useful, including systems as artificial as the transfection in rodent fibroblasts of constructs made from a bovine virus DNA and an *Escherichia coli* plasmid DNA. In fact, pV69-transformed FR3T3 and C127 cells provide us with situations where a definite succession of transformation phenotypes can be analyzed *in vitro* and *in vivo*.

As in other cases, such as the multistep process induced by Polyomaviruses and by cellular oncogenes (see ref. 7 for review), it would be definitely too simplistic to consider tumoral progression as a straightforward transit through a linear succession of steps, dependent only on selection by environmental conditions. For instance, one of the selective medium for transformed growth that we used extensively is the young Fischer rat. Although in principle relatively constant, this particular environment will not always lead to the emergence of the same type of tumour cell: direct selection from Stage 1 cells will produce a Stage 4 progeny, after a long latency, suggestive of rare events and/or multiple intermediate stages, whereas if Stage 2 transformants are first established *in vitro* from the same Stage 1 cells, selection will eventually lead to the emergence in the rat of Stage 3 cells.

Upon transformation with pV69 DNA, a first stage was identified, in which the cell replicates the transforming DNA as an autonomous entity, but does not express a transformed phenotype on the basis of the usual criteria. For reasons which are not clear at the present time, using this particular construct appears to stabilize a transition state in rodent fibroblasts, which could be recognized also after transfection with other BPV1-based plasmid DNAs (16) but was less stable and could not be further characterized. It shares an important feature with the initial step previously identified (7,9) in the tumoral pathway induced in the same rat fibroblast cells by Polyomaviruses and cellular oncogenes: it involves either limited changes (Polyoma), or no apparent change (BPV1) in cellular growth control in culture, cell physiology or cell structure, but the cells differ from truly normal cells because they can now be transformed by various transforming agents, typically chemical promoters, to which the original cell did not react. These two groups of "high risk" cells, Stage 1 lines established after transfer of pV69 DNA and cell lines immortalized by the plt and myc oncogenes, are, however, different in several important respects. The phenotypes induced by the polyoma, or SV40, large T proteins, by rearranged myc genes and by adenovirus E1A genes are all very similar and include two characteristic properties that were never observed in BPV1 transformants, clonal immortality in culture and ability to grow at low serum concentrations ((7) and E. Mougneau, N. Glaichenhaus and F. Cuzin, unpublished data). It is therefore likely that the molecular mechanisms involved in the two systems will eventually appear as different.

Identification of the molecular events involved in BPV1 transformation will ultimately depend on progresses made in the analysis of their genetic structure and their protein products (this Symposium). One preliminary set of observations suggest that transition from Stage 1 to Stage 2 may be related with an increased level of BPV1 transcripts. In Stage 1 mouse cells, Northern analysis identified three polyadenylated mRNA species hybridizing with a pV69 probe (8.2, 5.8 and 2.1 KB respectively), which were 4 to 5-fold more abundant in cells of the corresponding Stage 2 lines. These differences in the amounts of viral transcripts could not be correlated with any detectable difference in the number of copies or in the degree of methylation of pV69 DNA in these cells.

Another feature common to Polyomavirus- and Papillomavirus-induced transformation is the fact that some of the tumour cells at the terminal stages have lost the viral genomes (17 and figure 3). This observation may suggest that the viral oncogene(s) might only act at one or several early stage(s) of progression and that one of the consequences of the "high risk state" they induce is an increased probability of activation of cellular oncogenes. As previously discussed, the observed maintenance of organized cytoskeletal structures make BPV1 tumour cells (up to Stage 3) different from Polyomavirus transformants or from the same rodent lines after transformation by an activated ras oncogene (our unpublished results). This consideration would suggest that oncogenes different from the previously identified "Group II" genes (see ref. 7 for review) are active in Stage 3 cells. We are currently performing transfection experiments using cellular DNA from Stage 2 to Stage 4 cells in order to test these hypotheses.

## ACKNOWLEDGMENTS

We thank Elen van Obberghen-Schilling for editorial help. We are indebted to Linda Carbone, Colette Godefroy, Françoise Tillier and Marie-Louise Varani for expert technical assistance.

## REFERENCES

1 Thomas, M, Boiron, M, Tanzer, J, Levy, JP, Bernard, J (1964). In vitro transformation of mice cells by bovine papilloma virus. Nature 202:709.

2 Lowy, DR, Dvoretsky, I, Shobert, R, Law, MF, Engel, L, Howley, PM (1980). In vitro tumorigenic transformation by a defined sub-genomic fragment of BPV DNA. Nature 287:72.

3 Lancaster, WD (1981). Apparent lack of integration of bovine papilloma virus DNA in virus-induced equine and bovine tumor cells and virus-transformed mouses cells. Virology 108:251.

4 Law, MF, Lowy, DR, Dvoretzky, I, Howley, PM (1981). Mouse cells transformed by bovine papilloma virus contain only extrachromosomal viral DNA sequences. Proc Natl Acad Sci USA 78:2727.

5 Binétruy, B, Meneguzzi, G, Breathnach, R, Cuzin, F (1982). Recombinant DNA molecules comprising bovine papilloma virus type 1 DNA linked to plasmid DNA are maintained in a plasmidial state both in rodent fibroblasts and in bacterial cells. The EMBO J 1:621.

6 Meneguzzi, G, Binétruy, B, Grisoni, M, Cuzin, F (1984). Plasmidial maintenance in rodent fibroblasts of a BPV1-pBR322 shuttle vector without immediately apparent oncogenic transformation of the recipient cells. The EMBO J 3:365.

7 Glaichenhaus, N, Mougneau, E, Rassoulzadegan, M, Cuzin, F (1985). Cooperation between viral and cellular oncogenes corresponding to definite steps in tumoral progression. Adv Cancer Res, in press.

8 Grisoni, M, Meneguzzi, G, de Lapeyrière, O, Binétruy, B, Rassoulzadegan, M, Cuzin, F (1984). The transformed phenotype in culture and tumorigenicity of Fischer rat fibroblast cells (FR3T3) transformed with Bovine Papilloma Virus Type 1. Virology 135:406.

9 Rassoulzadegan, M, Naghashfar, Z, Cowie, A, Carr, A, Grisoni, M, Kamen, R, Cuzin, F (1983). Expression of the large T protein of polyoma virus promotes the establishment in culture of "normal" rodent fibroblast cells. Proc Natl Acad Sci USA 80:4354.

10 Matthias, PD, Bernard, HU, Scott, A, Brady, G, Hashimoto-Goth, T, Schütz, G (1983). A bovine papilloma virus vector with a dominant resistance marker replicates extrachromosomally in mouse and E. coli cells. The EMBO J 2:1487.

11 Connan, G, Rassoulzadegan, M, Cuzin, F (1985). Focus formation in FR3T3 and embryonic rat fibroblasts exposed to a tumour promoter after transfer of polyoma plt and myc onocogenes. Nature, 314:277.

12 Amtmann, E, Sauer, G (1982). Activation of non-expressed bovine papilloma virus genomes by tumour promoters. Nature 296:675.

13 Verderame, M, Alcorta, D, Egnor, M, Smith, K, Pollack, R (1982). Cytoskeletal F-actin patterns quantitated with fluorescein isothiocyanate-phalloidin in normal and transformed cells. Proc Natl Acad Sci USA 77:6624.

14 Rous, P, Beard, JW (1935). The progression to carcinomas of virus-induced papillomas (Shope). J Exp Med 62:523.

15 La Porta, RF, Taichman, LB (1982). Human papilloma viral DNA replicates as a stable episome in cultured epidermal keratinocytes. Proc Natl Acad Sci USA 79:3393.

16 Law, MF, Byrne, JC, Howley, PM (1983). A stable bovine papillomavirus hybrid plasmid that expresses a dominant selective trait. Mol Cell Biol 3:2110.

17 de Lapeyrière, O, Hayot, B, Imbert, J, Courcoul, M, Arnaud, M, Birg, F (1984). Cell lines derived from tumors induced in syngeneic rats by FR 3T3 SV40 transformants no longer synthesize the early viral proteins. Virology 135:74.

Papillomaviruses: Molecular and Clinical Aspects, pages 487–500


# THE PAPILLOMA TO CARCINOMA PROGRESSION OF COTTONTAIL RABBIT (SHOPE) PAPILLOMA VIRUS INDUCED TUMORS: CHARACTERIZATION OF PAPILLOMA DERIVED CELL LINES[1]

Mohammed Nasseri[2] and Felix O. Wettstein

Department of Microbiology and Immunology
UCLA School of Medicine,
and Molecular Biology Institute
University of California
Los Angeles, California 90024

ABSTRACT A cell line derived from a cottontail rabbit papilloma has been characterized and contains the equivalent of 10-20 gene copies of CRPV-DNA maintained extrachromosomally. A major plasmid is 9.1 kb and a minor one has the size of CRPV-DNA, 7.8 kb. Viral RNA can not be detected by dot blot hybridization. After treatment with the tumor promotor 12-0-tetradecanoylphorbol-13-acetate (TPA) viral RNA was synthesized at detectable levels, however, the cells remain negative for viral antigens in immunofluorescent tests. TPA treatment results also in a change of the growth properties and reduces the number of plasmids per cell. This has permitted the isolation of CRPV-DNA positive and negative cell lines. The parent sflEp cell line, as well as single cell cloned lines isolated after TPA

---

[1]This work was supported by PHS Grant CA-18151 awarded by the National Cancer Institute, DHHS and by a grant from the Cancer Research Coordinating Committee of the University of California.

[2]Present address: Department of Biological Chemistry, University of Rochester Medical Center, Rochester, New York 14642.

treatment are nontumorigenic in nude mice and rabbits. Exposure of CRPV-DNA positive and negative cell lines to x-ray as a carcinogen did not result in the generation of tumorigenic cells or cells capable of growing in soft agar. Finally, co-transfection of viral DNA negative lines with cloned CRPV-DNA and the neomycin gene permitted the selection of G418 resistant colonies. When grown in the absence of G418 the resistance marker was lost and the cells were CRPV-DNA negative, suggesting that these cells had a low ability to integrate DNA introduced by transfection.

## INTRODUCTION

Cottontail rabbit (Shope) papilloma virus (CRPV) induces virus producing papillomas (warts) in its natural host the cottontail rabbit (1). Papillomas are also induced in domestic rabbits, however, these yield little or no virus (2). In both experimentally infected domestic and cottontail rabbits a similar percentage, about 10-20%, of the tumors regress spontaneously (3). In both hosts, a papilloma growth period of several weeks is followed by a more or less stationary phase. About nine months after infection of domestic rabbits and twelve months with cottontail rabbits carcinomas start to develop at the site of papillomas. This malignant progression is high in domestic rabbits affecting 65 to 75% of the animals and 20-30% in cottontail rabbits (3). Because of the more frequent progression in domestic rabbits and the greater ease of keeping these animals in captivity they have become the preferred species to study tumor progression.

Benign and malignant domestic rabbit tumors contain equivalent amounts of viral DNA ranging from ten to over one hundred viral gene copies per diploid cell DNA equivalent (4,5). In papillomas most viral DNA is present as unit sized circular form I or II DNA. In primary carcinomas and particularly in metastatic tumors large circular plasmids predominate and in some of these tumors part of the viral DNA (up to 25%) is integrated (6). In the transplantable carcinoma Vx2 which has been propagated for 45 years all viral DNA is integrated in tandem repeats in three different sites (7). Tumor progression is also paralleled by an increase in viral DNA methyla-

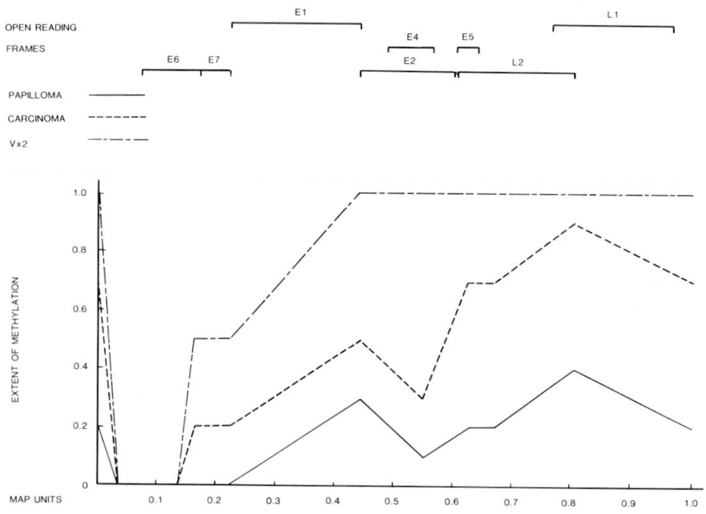


FIGURE 1. Methylation of CRPV-DNA in a domestic rabbit papilloma, a domestic rabbit carcinoma and the Vx2 transplantable carcinoma. The curves for the papilloma and the carcinoma are derived from numerical data of Wettstein and Stevens (8) and that for Vx2 from Nasseri and Wettstein (7).

tion (8,9). The DNA methylation is non-random and in the highly methylated Vx2 carcinoma, some sites remain unmethylated (8) (Fig. 1). The viral transcripts present in benign and malignant domestic rabbit tumors are very similar. The two major transcripts (2.0 and 1.3 kb) could code for a truncated E6 and a E7 protein (10,11) (see Fig. 2). Two minor transcripts at least twenty fold less abundant than the major ones could code for a full length E6 and a E2 protein. Transcription of these four RNA species involves at least three different cap sites, each preceded by a TATA box (Wettstein and Nasseri, submitted). A comparison of the relative abundance of these four species between benign and malignant tumors

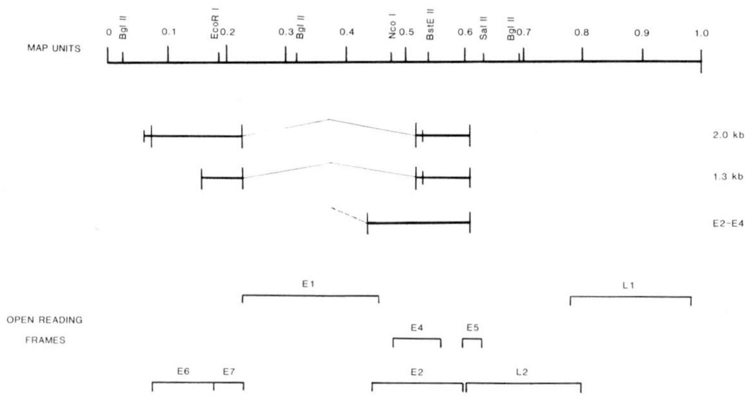


FIGURE 2. Map of the "early" transcripts present in domestic rabbit papillomas and carcinomas. The data are derived from Nasseri and Wettstein (10) and Wettstein and Nasseri (submitted). The open reading frame map is from Giri et al. (12). Large and small vertical bars represent major and minor exon ends respectively.

did not reveal significant differences except for the previously reported generally somewhat higher abundance of 1.3 to the 2.0 kb RNA in malignant tumors compared to benign ones (10). So far the increased methylation in malignant tumors can not be correlated with changes in the transcription.

## RESULTS

Studies on the benign to malignant progression in animals so far have been limited to the analysis of the beginning and end stages of the process. In order to develop an experimental approach for the study of the events leading to tumor progression we have initiated experiments to develop appropriate in vitro systems. Several homologous (rabbit epithelial cells) and heterologous (mouse fibroblast) lines were used in DNA transfection experiments (manuscript in preparation). However, since CRPV, like many other papilloma viruses, has a strict specificity for the host and the epithelial tissues, it is obvious that the experiments on epithelial cells from wild rabbits would provide biologically more relevant results. Fortuitously, an epithelial cell line derived from papillomatous tissue of a cottontail rabbit (sflEp) was available from the American Tissue Culture Collection (ATCC). This cell line had not been analyzed previously. Analysis by Southern blotting and hybridization under stringent conditions of undigested high molecular weight DNA from these cells revealed that the cells contained at least two species of extra chromosomal DNA of CRPV sequences. The results of a Southern blot filter hybridization of digested and undigested DNA from sflEp and Vx2 cells and of a cottontail rabbit papilloma are shown in Figure 3. Several bands are present in undigested DNA but little if any CRPV sequences comigrate with cellular DNA (Fig. 3, lane 4). A minor band has about the mobility of supercoiled CRPV DNA (Fig. 3, lane 1). After digestion with EcoRI, a single cut enzyme for CRPV-DNA, two major bands are present. One, comprising two thirds to three quarters of the viral DNA, has a size of 9.1 kb and the other has one of 7.8 kb. Digestion with BglII which cuts CRPV DNA into three fragments (Fig. 3, lanes 8, Vx2 DNA, and 9, CRPV DNA) results in a major band of 9.1 kb and two minor bands comigrating with the two smaller BglII CRPV-DNA fragments. The relative intensity of the bands suggests that the 9.1 kb plasmid has one BglII and one EcoRI site, while the 7.8 kb plasmid has one EcoRI and at least two BglII sites. The intensity of the CRPV-DNA in sfIEp cells (Fig. 3, lane 3) and in the Vx2 tumor (Fig. 3, lane 5) is about equal and this indicates that the equivalent of 10-20 viral genomes is present per sflEp cell.

The presence of the CRPV DNA in sflEp cells which were established from a papillomatous lesion of a cottontail rabbit suggests that this cell line is a papilloma (or benign) line. In order to verify this, the tumorigenicity of sflEp cells were tested using both rabbits and nude mice. First, 10 x $10^6$ cells were injected intrave-

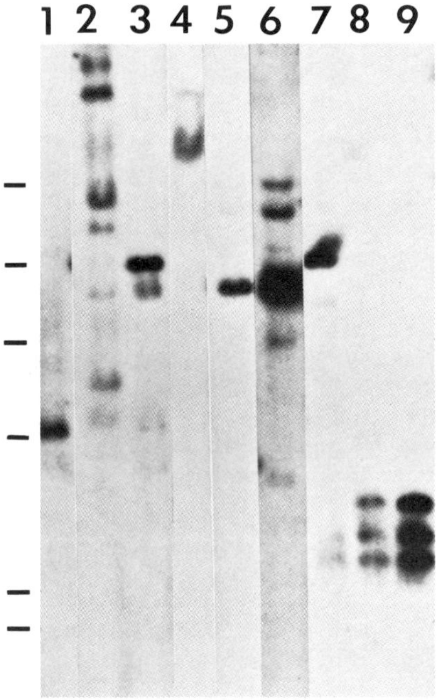


FIGURE 3. CRPV-DNA analysis of the cottontail rabbit papilloma derived cell line, sflEp. The sflEp cell line from the American Tissue Culture Collection was grown in Eagles medium supplemented with 10% fetal calf serum. Cell harvest, DNA extraction and Southern blotting was as described previously (6,7). Lane 1, cottontail rabbit papilloma DNA, undigested; lane 2, 2.5 ug undigested sflEp DNA; lane 3, 2.5 ug EcoRI digested sflEp DNA; lane 4, 2.5 ug undigested carcinoma DNA; lane 5, 2.5 ug EcoRI digested Vx2 DNA; lane 6, same as lane 5, long exposure; lane 7, 2.5 ug BglII digested sflEp DNA; lane 8, 2.5 ug BglII digested Vx2 DNA; lane 9, BglII digested cottontail rabbit papilloma DNA. The lines on the left indicate the position of molecular weight marker of lambda DNA HindIII digested with sizes of 23.1, 9.4, 6.5, 4.3, 2.3 and 2.0 kb.

nously into each of five domestic rabbits and second, 2 x $10^6$ cells were inoculated subcutaneously into each of five nude mice. None of the animals showed any tumors by four months. As control, rabbits were given intravenously Vx2 cells and nude mice were inoculated with CRPV DNA transformed NIH 3T3 cells. All the control animals showed tumors in about four weeks. Further, our studies on infected epithelium of cottontail and domestic rabbits using immunofluorescence and in situ molecular hybridization (4) indicated that no vegetative virus replication occurred in the basal layer which is the target epithelial cell layer for the infection with virus or viral DNA. The fact that sf1Ep cells carry viral DNA sequences together with the finding that the cells did not show any immunofluorescence when tested with antisera from tumor bearing animals (data not shown) thus indicates that they may represent a stage equivalent to the basal layer.

The maintenance of the viral DNA as plasmid suggest that same viral function(s) is expressed in these cells. However, Northern blot analysis of RNA extracted from these cells did not reveal virus specific sequences (data not shown) under conditions where viral RNA in non-virus producing domestic rabbit tumors could easily be detected.

TPA Treatment.

It has been shown with other virus-cell systems that in latently infected cells a very efficient induction of viral antigen expression could be achieved by treatment with a cocarcinogen, the tumor promoter 12-O-tetradecanoylphorbol-13-acetate (TPA) (13). When sf1Ep cells were treated with a single dose of 10 ng/ml of TPA for 3-6 days, rather striking changes occurred in all cultures. A large number of foci of morphologically altered cells developed within two weeks (Fig. 4) and ultimately the whole culture exhibited a new morphologic cell type which was stable in the absence of TPA. In addition, the growth properties of the cells changed drastically. The parent cell line doubled only once per week and the cells had a poor plating efficiency. After TPA treatment the doubling time was about one day and the plating efficiency was markedly increased. However, these cells remained negative in immunofluorescent tests (data not shown). The antisera employed here were positive at a 1:100 dilution in immunofluorescent tests on sections of cottontail rabbit papillomas. Since induction of the transcripts of bovine papilloma virus in transfected

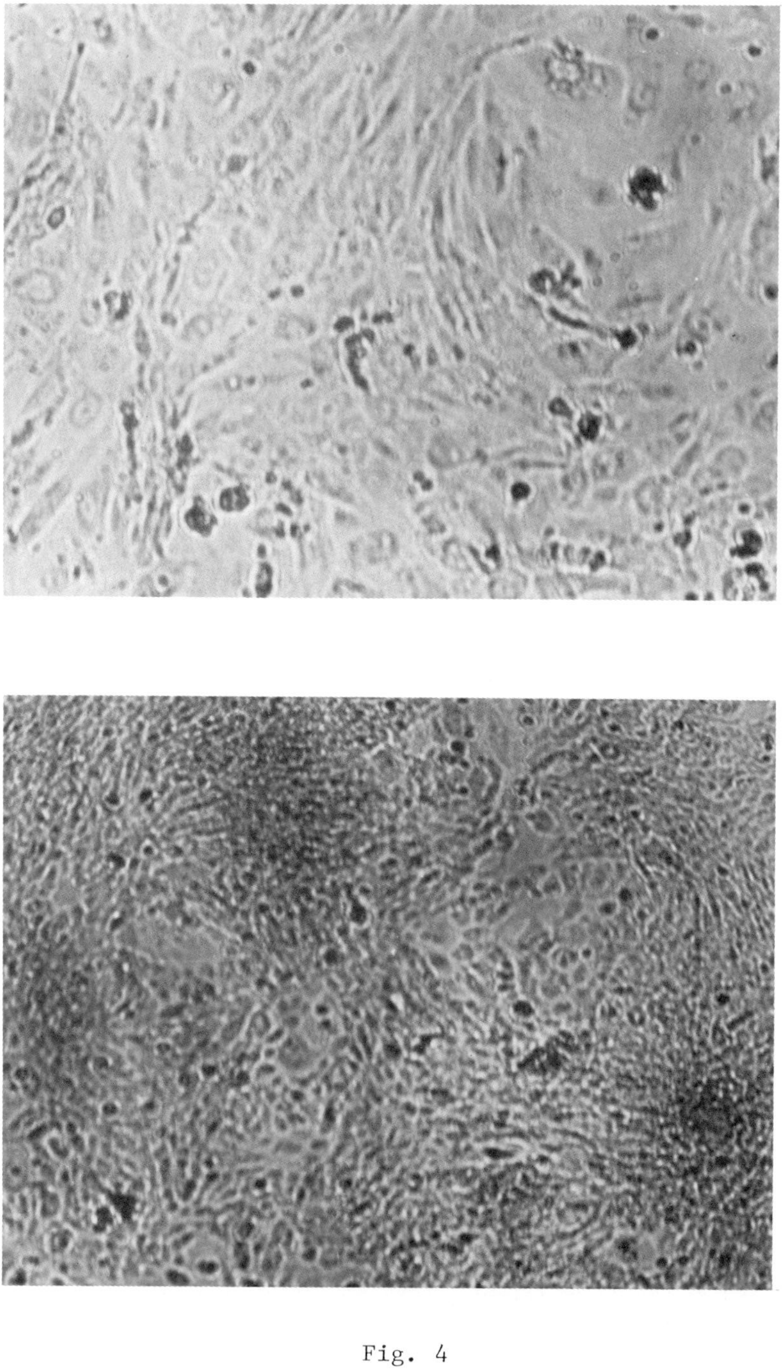

Fig. 4

FIGURE 4. Development of foci after TPA treatment of sflEp cells. A) Top: splEp cells untreated (450x). B) Bottom: splEp cells after 10 days exposure to TPA (400x). Three distinct foci are visible (left side, top, and right side) in some areas between the foci there are still some cels visible with the morphology of the parent sflEp cells.

mouse embryo fibroblast (MEF) tissue culture was achieved by others (14) using TPA we looked for possible poly A+ RNA expression in transformed cells. RNA was extracted from cells expanded from a tissue culture exposed for 3 days to TPA (sfT3). The presence of virus specific RNA sequences was tested by dot blot hybridization (Fig. 5). As can be seen in the figure the parent sflEp cells are negative while the sfT3 cells are positive for viral RNA. The amount of viral RNA was, however, 4 to 8 times lower than in a domestic rabbit papilloma included as a positive control.

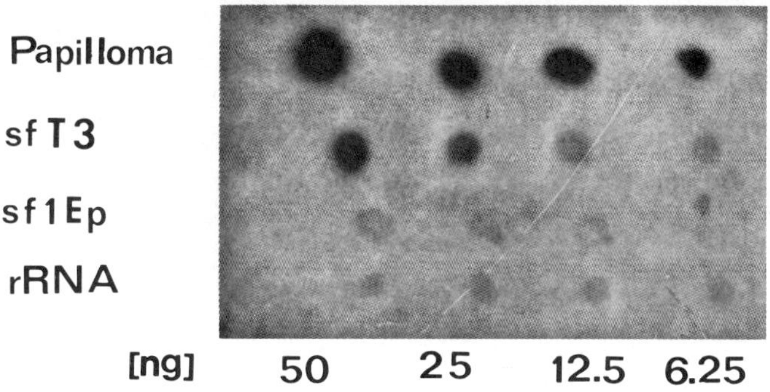


FIGURE 5. Spot-blot hybridization of RNA from untreated and TPA treated epithelial cells. Total RNA was isolated from a domestic rabbit papilloma sfT3 and sflEp cells, glyoxalated spotted on Gene Screen (New England Nuclear Corp.) and hybridized as previously described (10). Ribosomal RNA (rRNA) served as a negative control.

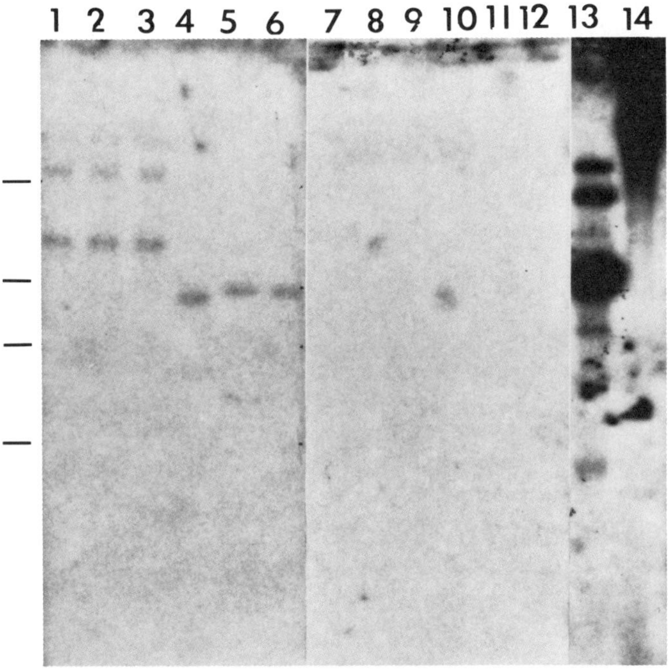


FIGURE 6. Southern blot analysis of DNA isolated from CRPV-DNA positive and negative cell lines. DNA was isolated, electrophoresed and hybridized as described previously (7). Lanes 1-6 CRPV-DNA positive cells; lanes 7-12 CRPV-DNA negative cells; lanes 13 and 14 Vx2-DNA. The DNA was analyzed undigested; lanes 1-3, 7-9 and 14 or after digestion with a single cut enzyme, lanes 4-6, 10-12 and 13. The molecular weight markers on the left are as indicated under Fig. 3. The sizes shown are 23.1, 9.4, 6.5 and 4.3 kb.

The TPA induced changes were further investigated by single cell cloning. Several single cell clones were derived from cultures exposed to TPA for 3, 4, 5 and 6 ($SFT_3$, $SFT_4$, $SFT_5$, $SFT_6$) days. Only lines, though not all, derived from single clones of 3 day TPA exposed cultures were CRPV-DNA positive (31, 32, 33); all others were negative (34, 41, 42, 43, 51, 52, 53, 54, 61). Even in the positive lines the viral DNA content was lower than in the parental sf1Ep line (Fig. 6). A comparison between the band intensity of CRPV DNA positive lines and the Vx2 transplantable carcinoma which contains 10-20 viral gene copies per cell (Fig. 6) suggests that not more than one viral DNA plasmid was present per cell.

X-Ray Irradiation of Cottontail Rabbit Epithelial Cells.

The ability to isolate after TPA treatment CRPV-DNA negative and positive cell lines provided the experimental basis to compare CRPV DNA positive and negative cells in their ability to undergo further changes toward a malignant state when exposed to x-ray as a carcinogenic agent. In the first step the sensitivity of the lines to x-ray was measured and it was found that at 150 rads there was minimal cell killing while at 350 rads approximately 50% of the cells were killed and complete killing was observed at 750-900 rads.

In these experiments a CRPV-DNA negative single cell clone (clone 51), a positive clone (clone 31) and the parent sflEp cells were exposed to x-ray at a rate of 120 rads per minute for a total exposure of 150, 200, 250, 300 and 350 rads. Two methods were chosen to select for the cells which had been transformed to a malignant state; colony formation in soft agar and tumor formation in nude mice. After x-ray irradiation the single cell clones were grown for 4-7 days and the much slower growing sflEp cells for one month prior to tests.

In all cases 2 x $10^6$ cells were injected into each of two nude mice for each level of irradiation and each cell type. Over a four month observation time no tumors were induced. As positive controls nude mice injected with cells derived from CRPV-DNA induced foci on NIH 3T3 developed tumors in 4-6 weeks (manuscript in preparation). Further, when colony formation in soft agar was used, no colonies were scored for any irradiated 31 or 51 clones or sflEp cells, however, control SV3T3 cells gave colonies within two weeks with an efficiency of greater than 90%.

Co-Transfection of Cottontail Rabbit Epithelial Cells.

A CRPV DNA negative line (cell line 51) was transfected with CRPV DNA inserted into the SalI site of the pLAII plasmid. Since the cell line could not be maintained as a monolayer for prolonged periods, it was not possible to select for foci and cotransfection was employed using as a selective marker, the neomycin resistance gene (15). Seven G418 resistant colonies were picked within 45 days (51-1 to 51-7) and the lines were expanded further in the absence of G418 for three weeks. When tested by spot hybridization all lines were negative with respect to CRPV-DNA and subsequent analyses showed that resistance to G418 was lost. Further, no neomycin resistance gene was detected in dot blot hybridization. This suggested that the cells when compared to NIH 3T3 cells had a much lower efficacy to integrated transfected DNA.

## DISUCSSION

Detailed analysis of transcripts present in benign and malignant CRPV induced tumors so far have not revealed any qualitative differences in spite of the rather significant increase in DNA methylation associated with tumor progression. In order to provide an experimental basis for the study of factors involved in the process of progression itself, at the cellular level, we have characterized a papilloma derived cell line. This cell line (sflEp) available from the American Tissue Culture Collection contains a low number (10-20) of viral gene copies per cell and is negative for the expression of viral antigen in immunofluorescent tests. These findings indciate that the cell line may be equivalent to cells of the basal layer known not to support vegetative replication of the virus. The cells did not contain detectable amounts of viral transcripts but as shown with another system (14) measurable levels of transcription could be obtained by treatment with TPA. In addition, exposure to TPA changed the growth properties of the cells. Since no comparable line without CRPV-DNA sequences was available it is not known if the TPA effect is mediated through increased viral transcription. The fact that viral DNA negative lines with altered growth properties could be isolated indicates that at least continued viral gene expression is not required.

The notion that the parent sflEp cell line and the TPA derivatized lines may represent a benign state is supported by their inability to form tumors in nude mice and in rabbits. Since it is known that carcinogens can shorten the lag period in the appearance of malignant tumors in animals (16), experiments were undertaken to see if treatment of these cells with a carcinogen could bring about transformation particularly of cells carrying CRPV-DNA. The experiments performed so far, employing x-ray as the carcinogen, did not yield cells which were anchorage independent for growth or could form tumors in nude mice. Other carcinogens may have to be tested to more fully explore the potential of these cells to serve as a tissue culture model for tumor progression.

The availability of CRPV-DNA negative epithelial cell lines is particularly important in order to study in culture the effect of different viral genes. Since papilloma viruses in general are restricted to epithelial cells, studies with epithelial cells may be more meaningful than those employing fibroblasts. A difficulty with the cell lines tested so far is that they exhibit a low efficacy to integrate transfected DNA.

ACKNOWLEDGEMENTS

We thank Drs. J.G. Stevens and M. Cook for helpful discussions and M. Poshmforoush for technical assistance.

REFERENCES

1. Shope RE, Hurst EW (1933). Infectious papillomatosis of rabbits. J Exp Med 58:607.
2. Shope RE (1935). Serial transmission of virus of infectious papillomatosis in domestic rabbits. Proc Soc Exp Biol Med 32:830.
3. Syverton JT (1952). The pathogenesis of the rabbit papilloma-to-carcinoma sequence. Ann NY Acad Sci 54:1126.
4. Stevens JG, Wettstein FO (1979). Multiple copies of Shope virus DNA are present in cells of benign and malignant non-virus-producing neoplasms. J Virol 30:891.
5. Watts SL, Ostrow RS, Phelps WC, Prince JT, Faras AJ (1983). Free cottontail rabbit papillomavirus DNA persists in warts and carcinomas of infected rabbits and in cells in culture transformed with virus or viral DNA. Virology 125:127.
6. Wettstein, FO, Stevens JG (1982). Variable-sized

free episomes of Shope papilloma virus DNA present in all non-virus-producing neoplasms and integrated episomes are detected in some. Proc Natl Acad Sci USA 79:790.
7. Nasseri M, Wettstein FO (1984). Cottontail rabbit papillomavirus-specific transcripts in transplantable tumors with integrated DNA. Virology 138:362.
8. Wettstein FO, Stevens JG (1983). Shope papilloma virus DNA is extensively methylated in non-virus-producing neoplasms. Virology 126:493.
9. Sugawara K, Fujinaga K, Uamashita T, Ito, Y (1983). Integration and mehtylation of Shope papilloma virus DNA in the transplantable Vx2 and Vx7 rabbit carcinomas. Virology 131:88.
10. Nasseri M, Wettstein FO (1984). Differences exist between viral transcipts in cottontail rabbit papillomavirus-induced benign and malignant tumors as well as non-virus-producing and virus-producing tumors. J Virol 51:706.
11. Danos O, Georges E, Orth G, Yaniv M (1985). Fine structure of the cottontail rabbit papilomavirus mRNAs expressed in the transplantable Vx2 carcinoma. J Virol 53:735.
12. Giri I, Danos O, Yaniv M (1985). Structure of the genome of the cottontail rabbit (Shope) papillomavirus. Proc Natl Acad Sci USA 82:1580.
13. zur Hausen H, O'Neill F, Freese UK, Hecker E (1978). Persisting oncogenic herpesvirus induced by the tumor promotor TPA. Nature 272:373.
14. Amtmann E, Sauer G (1982). Activation of non-expressed bovine papilloma virus genomes by tumour promotors. Nature 296:675.
15. Southern PJ, Berg P (1982). Transformation of mammalian cells to antibiotic resistance with a bacterial gene under control of the SV40 early region promotor. J Mol & Appl Genetics 1:327.
16. Rogers S, Rous P (1951). Joint action of chemical carcinogen and a neoplastic virus to induce cancer in rabbits. J Exp Med 93:459.

**Papillomaviruses: Molecular and Clinical Aspects, pages 501–511**


# LOCALIZATION OF HPV-5 TRANSFORMING FUNCTIONS[1]

Susan L. Watts*[2], Louise T. Chow*[3], Ronald S. Ostrow#, Anthony J. Faras#, and Thomas R. Broker*[3]

*Cold Spring Harbor Laboratory, Cold Spring Harbor, NY 11724
#Dept. of Microbiology, University of Minnesota, Minneapolis, MN 55455

ABSTRACT Based on electron microscopic heteroduplex analysis indicating regions of homology between HPV-5 and HPV-1 DNAs, we estimated the approximate locations of the putative open translation frames of the HPV-5 genome. Mutant HPV-5 subgenomic species represent deletions within the proposed late region of the virus genome, yet retain the abilities to transform C127 cells and to replicate as persistent episomes within the transformed cells. Subgenomic fragments corresponding to portions of the proposed early genomic region also transform cultured cells but integrate into the host cell chromosome.

## INTRODUCTION

Several distinct types of human papillomaviruses (HPV) have been found in the multiple persistent flat warts of patients with the familial disease syndrome epidermodysplasia verruciformis (EV) (1,2,3,4). HPV-5 in particular has been associated with the progression of sun-exposed lesions to primary and metastatic squamous cell carcinomas, multiple episomal copies of HPV-5 DNA being found in both benign and

[1]This work was supported by grants R23-CA39775 and P01-CA13106 from the National Cancer Institute.
[2]Current address: Dept. of Surgery, University of North Carolina, Chapel Hill, NC 27514
[3]Current address: Dept. of Biochemistry, University of Rochester, Rochester, NY 14642

malignant lesions. Furthermore, subgenomic species of HPV-5 DNA have been identified in carcinomas of EV patients (5). We have demonstrated previously that molecularly-cloned HPV-5 DNA is able to induce morphological transformation of cultured mouse C127 cells and to persist as an episome in these transformed cells (6). Accordingly, we chose to investigate the functional organization of the HPV-5 genome by determining whether naturally-occurring deletion mutants and fragments of molecularly-cloned HPV-5 DNA were able to transform cells in culture and to replicate episomally.

## METHODS

### Recombinant Vectors.

HPV-5 and HPV-1a viral DNAs were cloned at the Bam HI site of pBR322 and HPV-5 was also cloned into the Bam HI site of a poison-minus pBR322 derivative (pML) (7). The Bam HI (03) - Hind III (71) fragment of HPV-5 DNA was ligated to Bam HI - Hind III cut "pML" and the Bgl II (03) - Bgl II (62) fragment of HPV-5 DNA was ligated into the Bam HI site of pML.

Subgenomic species of HPV-5 from EV patients were cloned by cleaving total cellular DNA extracted from the tumors with Sac I or Bam HI and ligating into the respective cloning site of bacteriophage λCharon 16A or λCharon 27. Following packaging and screening of recombinant clones, three separate subgenomic species as well as wild-type HPV-5 DNA were identified: λCh16A clones of 5.0 Md, 4.0 Md, 3.7 Md, 3.5 Md species of HPV-5 DNA and λCh27 clones of 5.0 Md and 3.5 Md species. Restriction endonuclease analyses of the cloned species corresponded with the viral subgenomes detected by Southern blot analysis of carcinoma DNAs.

Plasmids and phage were amplified in *E. coli* HB101 or LE392, respectively, by standard procedures.

### Electron Microscopic Analysis of DNA Heteroduplexes.

Cloned DNAs of HPV-5 and HPV-1 were allowed to anneal under less stringent hybridization conditions of 30% (v/v) formamide, 0.1 M Tris-HCl, pH 7.2, 0.01 M EDTA, 0.07 M Na for 30 min at 22 $^0$C. Hybrids were examined by electron microscopy after spreading in cytochrome c monolayers using a hyperphase containing 30% formamide and a hypophase containing 5% formamide.

Hybrids of wild-type and subgenomic HPV-5 cloned DNAs were formed under stringent hybridization conditions of 50% formamide for 30 min at 22$^0$C. Samples were spread for electron microscopy with a hyperphase of 40% formamide and a hypophase of 10% formamide (8).

Transfection of C127 Cells and Isolation and Analysis of Cellular DNAs from Transformed Foci.

Mouse C127 cells were maintained and transfected with cloned DNAs as described previously (9) using intact plasmid-HPV DNA, λ phage-HPV DNA cleaved with the insertion site enzyme, or purified fragments of HPV-5 DNA isolated by elution from agarose gels. Transformed foci were picked using cloning cylinders, propagated, and analyzed for virus-specific DNA by Southern blot hybridization of total cellular DNA (6,9).

## RESULTS

Electron Microscopic Heteroduplex Analyses.

Genomic arrangement of HPV-5 DNA. The complete nucleic acid sequence of HPV-5 DNA has not yet been determined. Therefore, to infer the approximate locations of the functional regions of the HPV-5 genome, we annealed HPV-5 DNA to DNA of HPV-1a, for which the complete DNA sequence and the organization of open translation frames is known (10), and examined the heteroduplexes by electron microscopy. Under low stringency hybridization conditions, partial hybrids were formed between HPV-5 and HPV-1 DNAs in two regions, the major one representing portions of the E1-E2 open reading frames and another, less homologous region, representing a portion of the L2 open reading frame of the HPV-1 genome (Fig. 1A). Partial homologies of these particular regions have been seen consistently between many pairs of papillomavirus genomes annealed under conditions of reduced stringency. By measurement of the partially hybrid molecules, we determined that the Sac I site of HPV-5 was 5% permuted with respect to the Hpa I site of HPV-1 DNA, relative to the total DNA length of 7800 base pairs for both DNAs. This allowed us to estimate the approximate positions of the early and late open reading frames within HPV-5 DNA relative to its alignment to HPV-1 DNA (Fig. 2A,C).

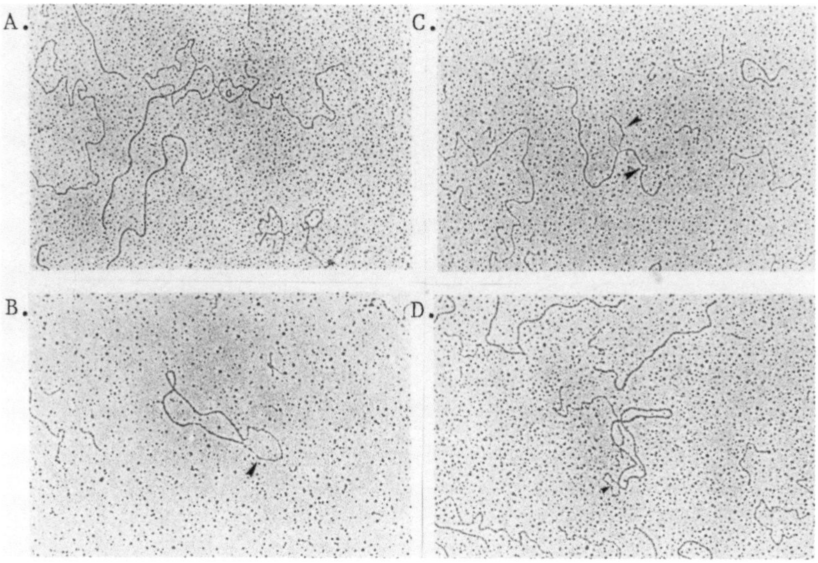


FIGURE 1. Electron microscopic analyses of DNA-DNA heteroduplexes. (A) Partial hybrid of pBR322-HPV-1 (Bam HI) and pBR322-HPV-5 (Bam HI) DNAs linearized by partial Bam HI digestion and annealed under less stringent hybridization conditions. (B) Hybrid of Sac I-excised 3.5 Md subgenomic HPV-5 DNA cloned in λCh16A and wild-type HPV-5 DNA excised with Bam HI from pBR322-HPV-5. An arrowhead marks the deleted sequences not present in the subgenomic species. (C) Hybrid of 3.7 Md subgenomic HPV-5 and wild-type HPV-5 DNAs both cloned in λCh16A and excised with Sac I. (D) Hybrid of 4.0 Md subgenomic HPV-5 DNA excised with Sac I from the cloning site in λCh16A and pBR322-HPV-5 DNA linearized by cleavage at the Cla I site in pBR322.

Mapping of HPV-5 subgenomic species. Restriction endonuclease mapping of the subgenomic species of HPV-5 DNA from EV carcinomas indicated that some restriction sites of wild-type HPV-5 were missing. Thus, from the size of these subgenomic species, we expected that they represented deletion mutants of wild-type HPV-5. In order to precisely map

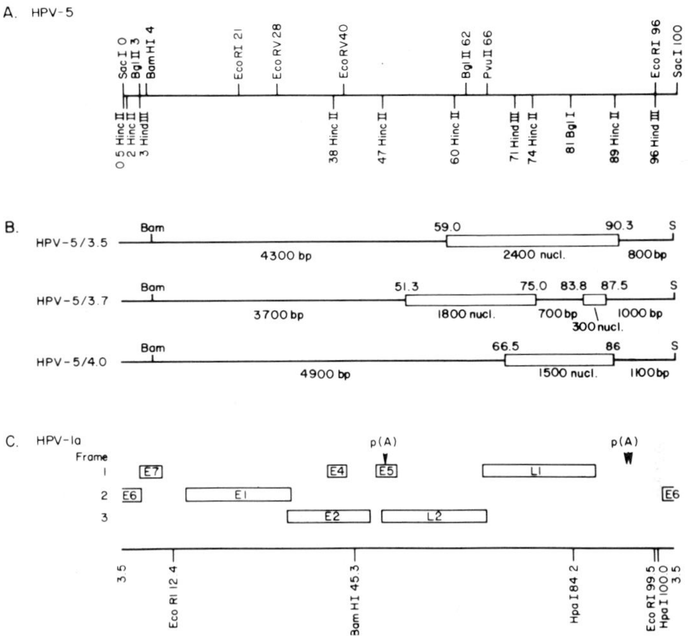


FIGURE 2. Physical mapping of the DNAs of HPV-5 wild-type and subgenomic species relative to the DNA of HPV-1. (A) Restriction endonuclease map of HPV-5 DNA. (B) Maps of the 3.5 Md, 3.7 Md, and 4.0 Md subgenomic species relative to wild-type HPV-5 DNA. The open boxes represent deleted segments not present in the subgenomic species. (C) Alignment of HPV-1 DNA and its open translation frames relative to HPV-5 DNA.

the deletions, we annealed each subgenomic cloned DNA with cloned wild-type HPV-5 DNA and examined the heteroduplexes by electron microscopy (Fig. 1B,C,D). Single deletion loops were seen with the 3.5 Md and 4.0 Md subgenomic species, while the 3.7 Md species lacked two segments of DNA present in wild-type HPV-5. The 3.5 Md, 3.7 Md, and 4.0 Md species lacked segments of 2400, 1800 plus 300, and 1500 nucleotides, respectively, which were present in 5.0 Md HPV-5 DNA. With respect to the genomic alignment of HPV-5 and HPV-1, the deleted segments mapped in the proposed late region of the HPV-5 genome, spanning in sum most of the L2 and L1 open reading frame regions (Fig. 2).

Cellular Transformation by Subgenomic Species and by Fragments of HPV-5 DNA.

C127 cells were transfected with 2 μg of recombinant DNA consisting of λ-HPV-5 wild-type or subgenomic species cleaved with the cloning site enzyme. Transformed foci appeared on monolayers transfected with each subgenomic species of HPV-5 with transformation efficiencies somewhat less than that of wild-type HPV-5 DNA.

Fragments of HPV-5 DNA were obtained by cleavage of pBR322 or λ recombinant DNAs with the restriction endonucleases whose sites are mapped in Fig. 2A, alone or in combination. Fragments larger than 1 Md in size were purified by elution from agarose gels and used for transfection. Two fragments exhibited transforming activity: 3.3 Md Bam HI (04)-Hind III (71) and 2.9 Md Bgl II (03)-Bgl II (62). No fragments assayed spanned the Sac I or Bam HI cloning sites, therefore none covered the entire early genomic region.

Analyses of Cellular DNAs from Transformed Foci.

Cellular DNAs from propagated foci induced by transfection with molecularly-cloned DNA of wild-type and subgenomic species as well as with fragments of HPV-5 DNA were analyzed by Southern blot hybridization to determine the state of virus-specific sequences. In the transformants from each of the HPV-5 subgenomic species, the viral DNA persisted in a small number of episomal copies per cell, which could be identified by restriction endonuclease mapping (Fig. 3).

Cellular DNAs from foci induced by transfection with the purified fragments Bam HI-Hind III and Bgl II-Bgl II contained virus-specific DNA species comigrating with chromosomal DNA upon electrophoresis (Fig. 4, channels c,k,n,o). Restriction endonuclease digestion of these cellular DNAs indicated a limited number of integrated copies of these viral sequences per cell (Fig. 4, channels d,e,f,g,h,l,m,p). In addition, these two HPV-5 fragments were each cloned into a pML-2-derivative plasmid. Transformed foci induced by each of these plasmid recombinants also contained integrated virus-specific DNA (Fig. 5).

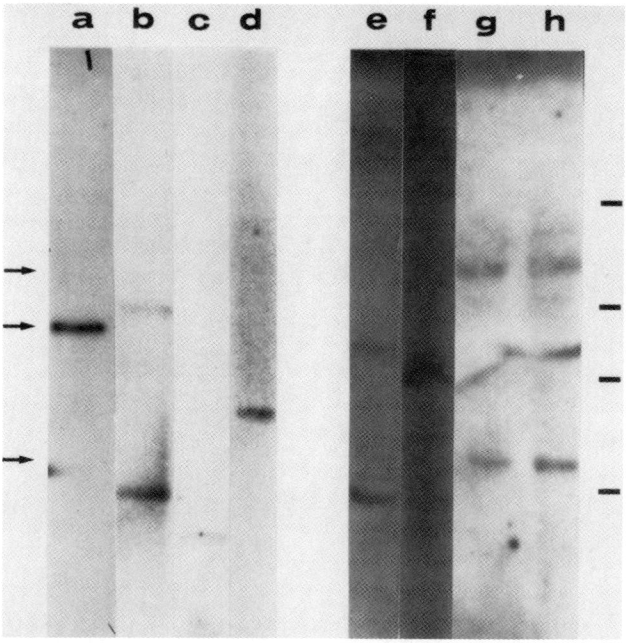


FIGURE 3. Southern blots of cellular DNAs from foci induced by transfection with wild-type and subgenomic species of HPV-5 DNA hybridized to $^{32}$P-HPV-5 DNA. (a) pBR322-HPV-5 plasmid DNA; (b) focus C417-8-2 from transfection with Sac I-cleaved λCh16A-4.0 Md HPV-5; (c) focus C526-9-2 from Sac I-cleaved λCh16A-3.5 Md HPV-5; (d,e) focus C526-10-1 from Bam HI-cleaved λCh27-3.5 Md HPV-5; (f) focus C526-7-2 from Sac I-cleaved λCh16A-3.7 Md HPV-5; (g) focus C21-4-3 from Sac I-cleaved λCh16A-5.0 Md HPV-5; (h) focus C21-4-2 from Sac I-cleaved λCh16A-5.0 Md HPV-5. DNAs in channels (a), (d), and (f) were digested with Bam HI. Arrowheads denote the migration positions of forms I, II, and III wild-type viral HPV-5 DNA. Dashes mark the migration positions of Hind III-cleaved phage λ DNA fragments, 14.7 Md, 5.85 Md, 4.09 Md, and 2.63 Md.

## DISCUSSION

Studies with HPV-5 subgenomic species and genomic fragments have delineated the genomic regions sufficient or necessary for in vitro transformation and episomal replication and are consistent with the organization of the genome which we propose as a result of heteroduplex mapping relative

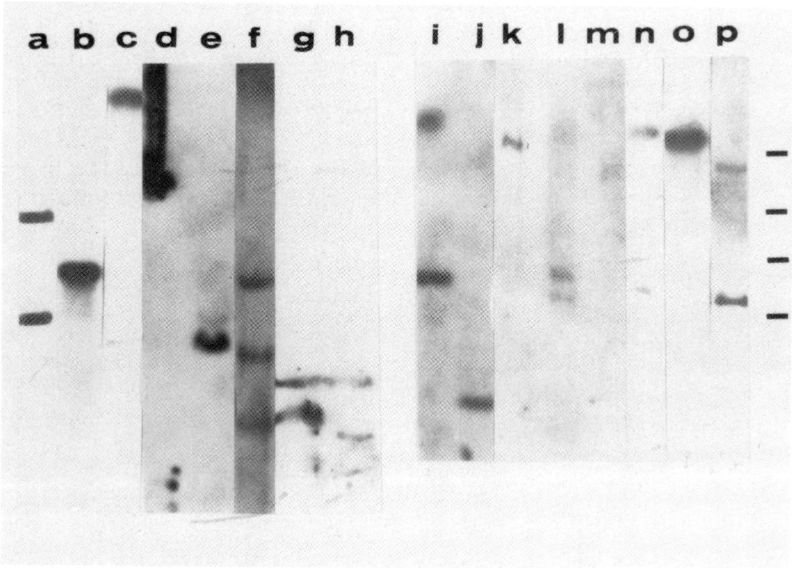


FIGURE 4. Southern blots of cellular DNAs from foci induced by fragments of HPV-5 DNA hybridized to $^{32}$P-pBR322-HPV-5 DNA. (a) pBR322-HPV-5 plasmid DNA, Bam HI cut; (b) purified Bam HI-Hind III fragment of HPV-5 DNA; channels (c-h) from foci induced by transfection with Bam HI-Hind III fragment: (c) focus C21-3-2, (d) focus C216-7-8, Eco RI cut, (e) focus C216-7-8, Hinc II cut, (f) focus C216-7-7, Eco RI cut, (g) focus C216-7-2, Eco RI cut, (h) focus C216-7-1, Eco RI cut; (i) purified Bgl II-Bgl II fragment of HPV-5 DNA; (j) same fragment, Eco RI cut; channels (k-p) from foci induced by transfection with Bgl II-Bgl II fragment: (k,l,m) focus C216-8-5, (k) Sal I cut, (l) Eco RI cut, (m) Hinc II cut, (n) focus C216-8-4, (o-p) focus C21-2-1, (p) Eco RI cut.

to HPV-1 DNA. That the HPV-5 DNA sequences deleted in the subgenomic species from EV carcinomas span the late region open reading frames L2 and L1 is consistent with the ability of the species to express the early functions of in vitro transformation and episomal replication, since they retain the complete early region intact. The Bam HI-Hind III and Bgl II-Bgl II transforming fragments lack part of the early region (the noncoding region and parts of the E6 and/or E7 open reading frames). Since these fragments integrate into

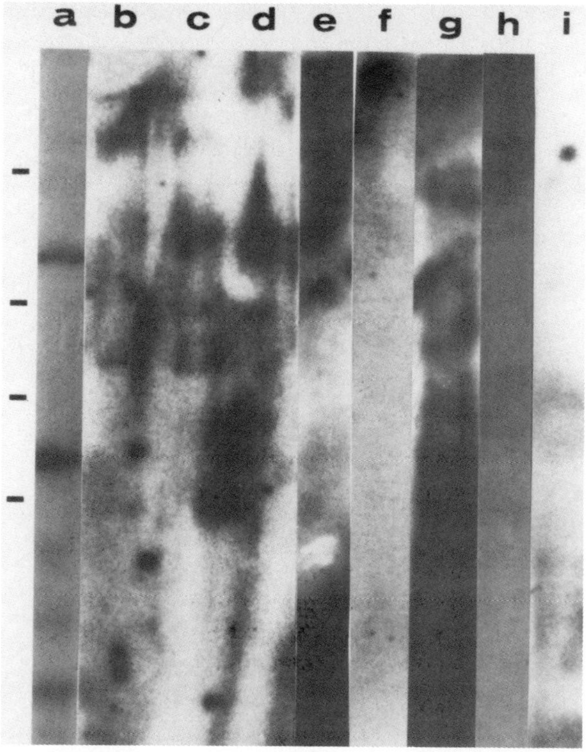


FIGURE 5. Southern blots of cellular DNAs from foci induced by recombinant plasmid-HPV-5 DNAs hybridized to $^{32}$P-pBR322-HPV-5 DNA. (a) pML-Bgl II-Bgl II HPV-5 plasmid DNA; (b) and (c) foci C124-3-1 and C124-3-2, respectively, from pML-HPV-5; (d) focus C124-6-1 from pML-Bgl II-Bgl II HPV-5; (e) and (g) focus C124-6-3 from pML-Bgl II-Bgl II HPV-5; (f), (h), and (i) focus C312-13-1 from pML-Bam HI-Hind III HPV-5; channel (g) was cleaved with Eco RI, (h) with Sal I, and (i) with Hinc II.

the transformed cell chromosome, these additional early sequences must be necessary for episomal replication (11). However, these fragments do express the transforming function likely encoded by open reading frames E2/E4/E5 considering results with BPV-1 DNA (12, 13). That they lack the major early promoter upstream of the E6 open reading frame may indicate that a downstream sequence is promoting expression of the transformation function, a promoter not identified in BPV-1 transcripts previously (14,15). The generation and analysis of further defined mutants will be necessary to clarify the functions of the HPV-5 genome.

## REFERENCES

1. Orth G, Jablonska S, Favre M, Croissant O, Jarzabek Chorzelska M, Rzesa G (1978). Characterization of two types of papillomaviruses in lesions of epidermodysplasia verruciformis. Proc Nat Acad Sci, USA 75:1537.
2. Kremsdorf D, Jablonska S, Favre M, Orth G (1983). Human papillomaviruses associated with epidermodysplasia verruciformis. II. Molecular cloning and biochemical characterization of human papillomavirus 3a, 8, 10, and 12 genomes. J Virol 48:340.
3. Pfister H, Gassenmaier A, Nurnberger F, Stuttgen G (1983). Human papillomavirus 5-DNA in a carcinoma of an epidermodysplasia verruciformis patient infected with various human papillomavirus types. Cancer Res 43:1436.
4. Tsumori T, Yutsudo M, Nakano Y, Tanigaki T, Kitamura H, Hakura A (1983). Molecular cloning of a new human papillomavirus isolated from epidermodysplasia verruciformis lesions. J Gen Virol 64:967.
5. Ostrow RS, Bender M, Niimura M, Seki T, Kawashima M, Pass F, Faras AJ (1982). Human papillomavirus DNA in cutaneous primary and metastasized squamous cell carcinomas from patients with epidermodysplasia verruciformis. Proc Nat Acad Sci, USA 79:1634.
6. Watts SL, Phelps WC, Ostrow RS, Zachow KR, Faras AJ (1984). Cellular transformation by human papillomavirus DNA in vitro. Science 225:634.
7. Mellon P, Parker V, Gluzman Y, Maniatis T (1981). Identification of DNA sequences required for transcription of the human α1-globin gene in a new SV40 host-vector system. Cell 27:279.
8. Davis RW, Simon M, Davidson N (1971). Electron microscope heteroduplex methods for mapping regions of base sequence homology in nucleic acids. In Grossman L, Moldave K (eds): "Methods in Enzymology," vol 21, Pt D, p 413.
9. Watts SL, Ostrow RS, Phelps WC, Prince JT, Faras AJ (1983). Free cottontail rabbit papillomavirus DNA persists in warts and carcinomas of infected rabbits and in cells in culture transformed with virus or viral DNA. Virology 125:127.

10. Danos O, Katinka M, Yaniv M (1982). Human papillomavirus 1a complete DNA sequence: a novel type of genome organization among Papovaviridae. EMBO J 1:231.
11. Lusky M, Botchan M (1984). Characterization of the bovine papillomavirus plasmid maintenance sequences. Cell 36: 391.
12. Nakabayashi Y, Chattopadhyay SK, Lowy DR (1983). The transforming function of bovine papillomavirus DNA. Proc Nat Acad Sci, USA 80:5832.
13. Sarver N, Rabson MS, Yang Y-C, Byrne JC, Howley PM (1984). Localization and analysis of bovine papillomavirus type 1 transforming functions. J Virol 52:377.
14. Engel LW, Heilman CA, Howley PM (1983). Transcriptional organization of bovine papillomavirus type 1. J Virol 47:516.
15. Heilman CA, Engel L, Lowy DR, Howley PM (1982). Virus-specific transcription in bovine papillomavirus-transformed mouse cells. Virology 119:22.

# IX. VIRAL VECTORS

**Papillomaviruses: Molecular and Clinical Aspects, pages 515–527**


# SUSTAINED HIGH-LEVEL EXPRESSION OF RECOMBINANT HUMAN GAMMA INTERFERON USING A BOVINE PAPILLOMAVIRUS VECTOR

Nava Sarver, George A. Ricca, Margaret Hood, John Link
G. Criss Tarr, and William N. Drohan

Department of Molecular Biology,
Revlon Health Care Research & Development
Springfield, Virginia 22151

**ABSTRACT:** We have obtained a sustained high-level expression of recombinant human gamma interferon ($\gamma$-IFN) by employing a cDNA cloned into a bovine papillomavirus (BPV) shuttle vector. Analysis of gene expression in several foci of C127 mouse cells transformed with the recombinant molecule indicated considerable heterogeneity in the levels of $\gamma$-IFN secreted into the medium. In contrast, single-cell clones derived from a single $\gamma$-IFN producing focus exhibited a more uniform level of expression closely reflecting that of the original parental line.

Immunoprecipitation of extracellular protein with a $\gamma$-IFN antiserum demonstrated the presence of a homogeneous peptide comigrating in SDS-polyacrylamide gels with natural $\gamma$-IFN marker. Crude preparations of the recombinant-derived protein (a) conferred protection against EMC infection of WISH cells, (b) was neutralized by monoclonal antibodies against $\gamma$-IFN, (c) competed with natural $\gamma$-IFN in an immunoprecipitation reaction, and (d) induced expression of the class II major histocompatibility complex antigens in fibroblasts and in endothelial cells. Greater than $10^5$ U/ml of $\gamma$-IFN was secreted from $10^6$ cells in 24 hours. This rate has been sustained by a single culture for at least 85 days. Moreover, recombinant $\gamma$-IFN is stable in the medium for up to five days. Large-scale purification of the recombinant protein from extracellular medium resulted in 77% recovery of highly purified human $\gamma$-IFN (>$10^8$ U/mg).

## INTRODUCTION

The use of bovine papillomavirus (BPV) DNA as a viral vector is well documented (3, 6, 17, 19, 24) and was originally based on the observation that the viral genome persists as an extrachromosomal plasmid in transformed cells (10). Exogenous DNA, cloned in a BPV vector, is maintained in the uniform sequence environment of the BPV minichromosome. This eliminates potential problems associated with the integration of the exogenous DNA into inactive regions of host chromosomes and with insertion mediated inactivation of functions required for cellular viability. This property was fully exploited in the establishment of BPV shuttle vectors capable of replicating in both prokaryotic and eukaryotic cells (4, 7, 18). Such vectors are efficient in directing regulated expression from inducible promoters (6, 14, 16, 24) and in expressing foreign gene products destined for either an intracellular or an extracellular location (3, 9, 19).

γ-IFN is a glycoprotein whose synthesis in cells is primarily induced by viruses or mitogens. It possesses potent antiviral, anticellular, antitumor, and immunoregulatory activities (22 and references cited therein). Interferon treatment of cancer and viral infections in animals has met with some success. Consequently, γ-IFN is of potential clinical and pharmacological application.

Using γ-IFN as a test gene, we explored whether the ability of BPV DNA to immortalize cells and to exist as a multicopy plasmid in transduced cells can be adapted for prolonged expression of a foreign protein.

## MATERIALS AND METHODS

### Cells and DNA Transfections:

DNA transfections were performed using the calcium phosphate co-precipitation method (5) followed by enhancement with 25% dimethylsulfoxide (23) as described previously (19). Phenotypically transformed foci were isolated and established as cell lines. Single cell cloning was achieved by plating at limited dilution into 96 well plates (Co-star), visual identification of wells containing a single cell and propagation of these cells into established lines.

Cells were maintained in either complete medium (Dulbecco modified Eagle medium supplemented with 100 U/ml penicillin, 100 μg/ml streptomycin, and 10% heat inactivated fetal calf serum) or in defined medium lacking fetal calf serum (medium 199 containing 10 μg/ml insulin, 10 μg/ml transferrin, 10 ng/ml epidermal growth factor, 2 ng/ml bovine serum albumin, 150 μg/ml bovine brain extract, 1.4 μM hydrocortisone and 1 nM 3,3',5-triiodo-D-thyronine) (12).

### γ-IFN Bioassay

γ-IFN activity was measured by a cytopathic effect inhibition assay using 3-fold serial dilutions of the sample on human WISH cells which were then challanged with encephalomyocarditis virus (EMC) (1).

## RESULTS

The γ-IFN cDNA clone employed in this study is described in detail elsewhere (Lee, et al., submitted). Briefly, polyA selected RNA was isolated from A23187 and mezzarine induced human peripheral blood lymphocytes (1). The RNA was converted into double-stranded cDNA and cloned into the PstI site of pBR322 by G-C tailing using standard procedures (13). A γ-IFN cDNA clone was identified by hybridization with a synthetic oligonucleotide, and an 843 base pair Sau 3A fragment containing the coding region for γ-IFN signal peptide, the mature protein, and the translation termination codon, was cloned into a BPV shuttle vector to be described elsewhere (Sarver, et al., in preparation). The resulting construct, p8-4, is shown in Figure 1. Following transformation of mouse C127 cells with the p8-4 DNA, the cells were incubated at 37°C and observed for the formation of foci. Foci (designated NS8-4-A to NS8-4-P) were isolated and established as cell lines.

Southern DNA analysis (21) of transformants expressing high levels of γ-IFN (>$10^5$ U/ml/$10^6$ cells/24 hours) revealed that the transferred DNA is maintained as an episome and for the most part is unrearranged. (Data not shown.)

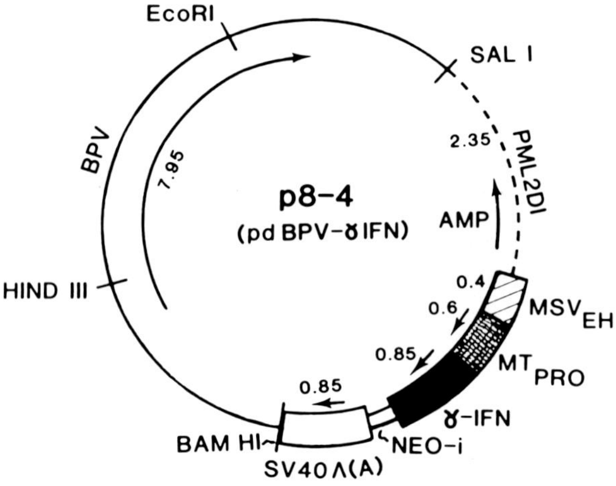


**Figure 1:** Physical map of pdBPV-human γ-IFN (p8-4) DNA. The plasmid consists of the following structural elements, described in a clockwise direction. The complete BPV genome (solid line) is joined to the pML2dl (dashed line) sequence which contains the pBR322 origin of replication and a functional ß-lactamase gene (11). The moloney murine sarcoma virus enhancer (MSV) (striped box) was originally obtained from the proviral LTR (2) as a HinfI/XbaI fragment (141-525, respectively). Both termini had previously been converted to BamH1 sites with synthetic linkers (provided to us by L. Laimins). The mouse metallothionein I promoter (gray box) is the KpnI to BglII fragment (approximately 600 base pairs) of the promoter described by Pavlakis and Hamer (17). The KpnI site was previously modified to a BglII site to facilitate cloning. Downstream from the promoter is the human gamma interferon cDNA (black box) obtained as a Sau3A fragment. The fragment designated as neo-i (thin box) is a remnant of the 3' region of the Tn5 gene and does not confer resistance to G418. The 3' processing signals are contained within an 850 base pair fragment derived from SV40 DNA (open box) (15).

## γ-IFN Expression in Isolated Foci and in Single Cell Clones

As an initial characterization of the transformed cells, tissue culture media, derived from 16 individual foci (NS8-4-A to NS8-4-P), was collected and assayed for the presence of biologically active γ-IFN. The biological assay measures a reduction in the cytopathic effect of encephalomyocarditis virus on WISH cells (1). The results in Figure 2A demonstrate a considerable heterogeneity in the amount of biologically active γ-IFN recovered from different foci (<42 U/ml to >$10^4$ U/ml). However, when the analysis was performed on 24 single-cell clones derived from a single high-level expressor (NS8-4-G), the amounts of biologically active γ -IFN produced varied over a much smaller range and were similar to levels obtained from the original parental line (Figure 2B).

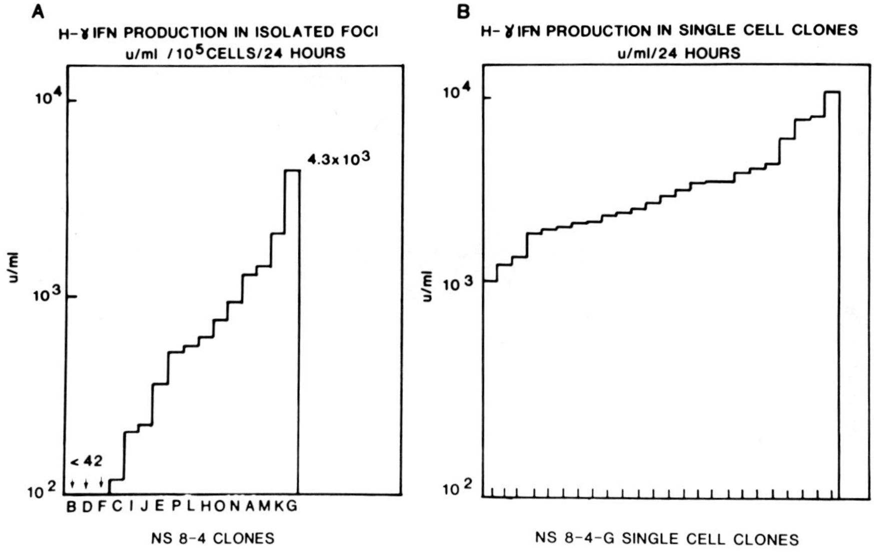


**Figure 2A & 2B:** Expression levels of human γ-IFN in transformed C127 cells. γ-IFN activity was measured as described in Materials and Methods.

A. Expression levels in 16 isolated foci (NS8-4-A to NS8-4-P) derived from p8-4 transformed C127 cells.

B. Expression levels in 24 single cell clones derived from parental line NS8-4-G.

## Requirement for Fetal Calf Serum in Long-Term Expression of Recombinant γ-IFN

Expression of γ-IFN was then examined as a function of the serum concentration in the medium. Duplicate cultures of NS8-4-G-4 transformants were grown in the presence or absence of FCS, the media harvested daily, and assayed for the presence of biologically active γ-IFN. The data in Figure 3 demonstrate that approximately 10-fold more γ-IFN is produced in cells maintained in the presence of 2.5% FCS when compared with cells maintained in defined medium lacking FCS. Moreover, in the experimewnt presented in Figure 3, a constant expression level of γ-IFN was maintained for 38 days. Additional experiments have extended this period to 85 days (data not shown).

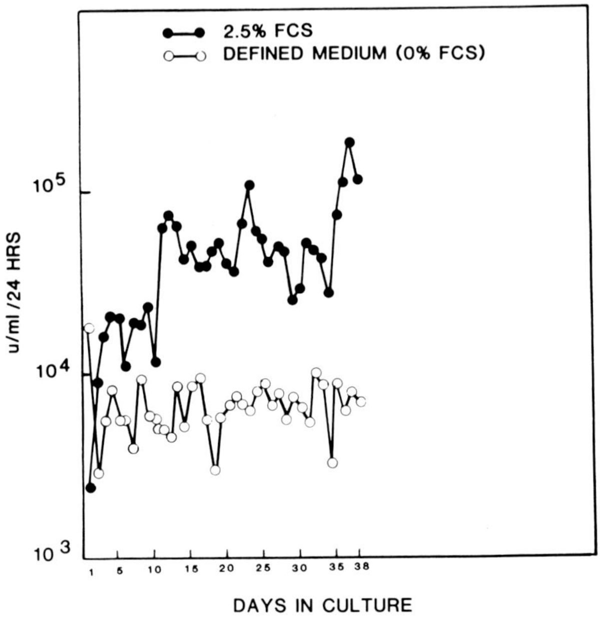


**Figure 3:** Long-term expression of human γ-IFN in NS8-4-G-4 transformants. C127 transformed cells (NS8-4-G-4) were seeded in 850 $cm^2$ roller bottles containing 40 ml of either complete medium containing 10% FCS or in defined medium lacking fetal calf serum as described in Materials and Methods. The medium was changed every 24 hours and assayed for γ-IFN activity.

## Protein Analysis

Having identified γ-IFN biological activity in tissue culture media from BPV transformed cells, the nature of the polypeptide product was further characterized. Cells were labeled with $^{35}S$-methionine, and extracellular media was harvested and immunoprecipitated with a goat anti-γ-IFN serum. The immunoprecipitated proteins were then analyzed on SDS polyacrylamide gels as described (19). Analysis of the extracellular media from BPV transformed cells demonstrated the presence of a prominent band identical in electrophoretic mobility to native γ-IFN (Figure 4). This band was absent from immunoprecipitated media obtained from non-producing cells transformed by a recombinant molecule in which the γ-IFN cDNA is placed in a transcriptional direction opposite that of the metallothionein promoter. In a competitive binding study, samples were incubated with antiserum previously neutralized with 2 µg of γ-IFN. Under these conditions, there was a considerable reduction in the amount of γ-IFN that was immunoprecipitated.

## Purification of Recombinant Human γ-IFN

In order to obtain sufficient material for biochemical characterization, approximately 50 liters of crude tissue culture medium was collected and used for large-scale protein purification. The purification procedure used was as described previously (1) for the purification of natural γ-IFN. The protocol consists of essentially 5 steps that are summarized in Table 1.

Material obtained from the entire 50 liters of media was processed through Sephadex G-100 chromatography. This resulted in an 85% recovery of the γ-IFN activity present in the starting material. Approximately one-third of the Sephadex G-100 fractions were further processed on a CM-Biogel column. Peak fractions of the CM-Biogel column had a specific activity of $1.2 \times 10^8$ IU per mg. The specific activity of the recombinant γ-IFN is similar to that reported for the natural protein (1). Thus, the purified recombinant material is indistinguishable from native γ-IFN in terms of size and specific activity.

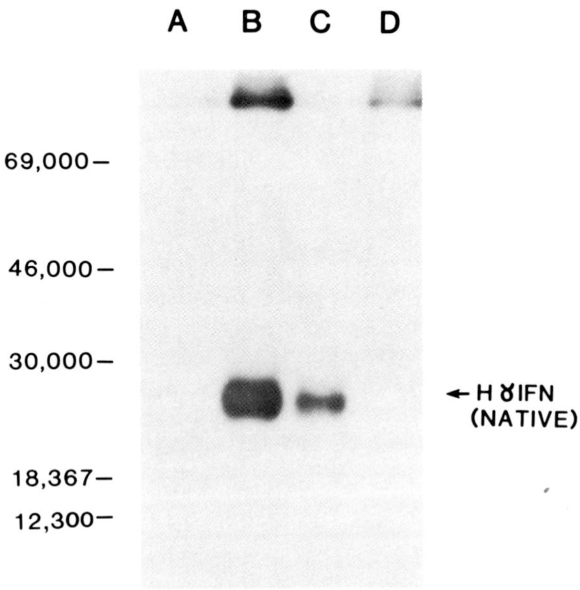


**Figure 4**: Immunoprecipitation of extracellular γ-IFN secreted from NS8-4-G-4 transformants. Cells in 100 mm plates were washed with methionine-free medium (GIBCO) containing 2% dialyzed fetal calf serum (FCS) and labeled in 3 ml of the same medium with 400 μCi/ml of L-$^{35}$-S-methionine (1063.6 Ci/mmol; New England Nuclear) for 4 hours at 37°C. Proteins in the extracellular medium were immunoprecipitated with anti-human gamma interferon serum as described previously (19). For competition studies, the antiserum was first preincubated with 2 μg of human γ-IFN after which the complex was added to the samples. Analysis of the immunoprecipitated proteins was performed on a 10% SDS-polyacrylamide gel after which the gels were treated with En$^3$Hance (New England Nuclear) and fluorographed as described (8, 20).

Lane A: Normal goat serum
Lane B: Goat anti-γ-IFN serum
Lane C: Goat anti-γ-IFN serum neutralized with 2 μg of γ-IFN prior to immunoprecipitation.
Lane D: Extracellular medium is from transformants harboring a recombinant DNA in which the γ-IFN cDNA is in a transcriptional direction opposite that of the metallathionein promoter. The sample was treated with goat anti-γ-IFN serum.

Table 1

## PURIFICATION OF RECOMBINANT HUMAN GAMMA INTERFERON BY SEQUENTIAL CHROMATOGRAPHY

| Step† | Volume (ml) | IFN (IU) X $10^{-8}$ | Protein (mg) | Specific Activity (IU/mg) | Total Fold Purification | Total % Recovery |
|---|---|---|---|---|---|---|
| **CPG** | | | | | | |
| Input | 50,000 | 7.85 | 81,500 | 9.63 X $10^3$ | -- | --- |
| Output | 2,300 | 7.85 | 3,772 | 2.08 X $10^5$ | 22 | 100 |
| **ConA/S** | | | | | | |
| Output | 1,370 | 7.85 | 356 | 2.20 X $10^6$ | 228 | 100 |
| **H/S** | | | | | | |
| Output | 65 | 6.64 | 115 | 5.77 X $10^6$ | 599 | 85 |
| **Sephadex G-100** | | | | | | |
| Output | 92 | 6.64 | 48 | 1.38 X $10^7$ | 1.433 | 85 |
| **CM-BGA** | | | | | | |
| Input* | 36* | 3.22* | 11* | 2.93 X $10^7$* | -- | --- |
| Output | 60 | 2.43 | 4 | 6.08 X $10^7$ | 6,314 | 77+ |

† The abbreviations used are CPG, Controlled Pore Glass; ConA/S, concanavalin A-Sepharose; H/S, heparin Sepharose; CM-BGA, carboxymethyl-Bio-Gel-agarose.

* Selected fractions from the Sephadex G-100 output were processed on CM-BGA.

\+ Recovery assuming all the Sephadex G-100 was processed.

## DISCUSSION

The ability of BPV DNA to immortalize cells and to persist as a multicopy plasmid in transformed cells makes it a particularly attractive system for continuous, amplified expression of exogenous genes. In this study, we demonstrate the utility of a BPV vector for the continuous expression of human γ-IFN. Human γ-IFN engineered C127 cells secrete greater than $10^5$ IU/ml in 24 hours from $10^6$ cells, a rate that is sustained by a single culture for at least 85 days. The recombinant protein is also very stable as evidenced by the fact that during 5 days of continuous incubation, no detectable loss in biological activity was observed (data not shown).

Interestingly, isolated foci harboring the recombinant DNA manifest considerable heterogenity in the level of γ-IFN expression. This contrasts sharply with the more homogenous levels of expression observed with single-cell clones derived from the same parental line. Since neither the DNA copy number nor the extent of molecular rearrangements appear to be a contributing factor, the observed heterogenity may depend on a yet unidentified variation in the individual host cells.

The recombinant protein is biologically indistinguishable from natural γ-IFN in that it confers antiviral protection on appropriate host cells, induces the expression of class II major histocompatibility (MHC) antigens in HeLa and endothelial cells (F. Sekaly, personal communication), and is neutralized by anti-human γ-IFN serum. Its identity with authentic human γ-IFN is further illustrated by the fact that a monoclonal antibody (provided by Rebesh Rubin, New York Blood Center) which recognizes natural γ-IFN isolated from induced peripheral blood leukocytes, but not bacterially produced recombinant human γ-IFN, completely neutralizes the γ-IFN obtained from the engineered C127 cells (data not shown).

Greater than 80% of the recombinant protein is found extracellularly (data not shown), indicating efficient transport across the cell membrane. The reported amino acid sequence of γ-IFN accounts for a peptide of 17,000 daltons. The apparent size of 22,000-25,000 daltons of crude (Figure 4) and purified γ-IFN (data not shown), coupled with the observation that it binds to the ConA sepharose column, strongly suggests that it contains carbohydrate moieties. Thus, post-translational modifications of the γ-IFN protein, including removal of the signal peptide and glycosylation of the protein (22), appear to be faithfully carried out in transformed C127 cells.

We have thus demonstrated the applicability of the BPV vector system to achieve a sustained amplified expression of a foreign protein of potential pharmacological use.

## ACKNOWLEDGEMENTS

We are grateful to Dr. William Terry for his continued support and to Drs. Ing-Ming Chiu, Francine Eden-McCutchan and Michael Jaye for critical reviewing of the manuscript. Our sincere thanks to Ms. Nancy Mode for excellent editorial preparation of the manuscript.

## REFERENCES

1. Braude, I.A., Purification of Human γ-Interferon to Essential Homogeneity and Its Biochemical Characterization. Biochemistry, 23:5603-5609, 1984.
2. Dhar, R., W.L. McClements, L.W. Enquist, and G.F. Vande Woude, Nucleotide sequences of integrated Maloney sarcoma provirus long terminal repeats and their host and viral junctions. Proc. Natl. Acad. Sci USA, 77:3937-3941, 1980.
3. DiMaio, D., V. Corbin, E. Subley, and T. Maniatis, High level expression of a cloned HLA heavy chain gene introduced into mouse cells on a bovine papillomavirus vector. Mol. Cell. Biol., 4:340-350, 1984.
4. DiMaio, D., R. Treisman, and T. Maniatis, A bovine papilloma-virus vector which propagates as an episome in both mouse and bacterial cells. Proc. Natl. Acad. Sci. USA, 79:4030-4034, 1982.
5. Graham, F.L., and A.J. van der Eb, A new technique for the assay of infectivity of human adenovirus 5 DNA. Virology, 52:456-461, 1973.
6. Karin, M., G. Cathala, M.C. Nguyen-Huu, Expression and regulation of a human metallothionein gene carried on an autonomously replicating shuttle vector. Proc. Natl. Acad. Sci. USA, 80:4040-4044, 1983.
7. Kushner, P.J., B.B. Levinson, H.M. Goodman, A plasmid that replicates in both mouse and E. coli cells. J. Mol. Appl. Genet., 1:527-538, 1982.

8. Laemmli, U.K., Cleavage of structural proteins during the assembly of the head of bacteriophage $T_4$. Nature, 227:680-685, 1970.
9. Law, M.-F., B. Howard, N. Sarver, and P.M. Howley, Expression of selective traits in mouse cells transformed with a BPV DNA derived hybrid molecule containing E. coli gpt. Viral Vectors, Cold Spring Harbor Laboratories, Cold Spring Harbor, New York, 1982.
10. Law, M.-F., D.R. Lowy, I. Dvoretzky, and P.M. Howley, Mouse cells transformed by bovine papillomavirus contain only extachromosomal viral DNA sequences. Proc. Natl. Acad. Sci. USA, 78:2727-2731, 1981.
11. Lusky, M., and M. Botchan, Inhibitory effect of specific pBR322 DNA sequences upon SV40 replication in simian cells. Nature, 293:79-81, 1981.
12. Maciag, T., R.E. Nemore, R. Weinstein, and B.A. Gilchrest, An endocrine approach to the control of epidermal growth: Serum free cultivation of human keratinocytes. Science, 211:1451-1454, 1981.
13. Maniatis, T., E.F. Fritsch, and J. Sambrook, In T. Maniatis and E.F. Fritsch (ed.), Molecular cloning: a laboratory manual. Cold Spring Harbor Laboratory, Cold Spring Harbor, New York, 1982.
14. Mitrani-Rosenbaum, S., L. Maroteaux, Y. Mory, M. Revel, P.M. Howley, Inducible expression of the human interferon beta 1 gene linked to a bovine papillomavirus DNA vector and maintained extrachromosomally in mouse cells. Mol. Cell Biol., 3:233-240, 1983.
15. Mulligan, R.C., and P. Berg, Expression of a bacterial gene in mammalian cells. Science, 209:1423-1427, 1980.
16. Ostrowski, M.C., H. Richard-Foy, R.G. Wolford, D.S. Berard, G.L. Hagar, Glucocorticoid regulation of transcription at an amplified, episomal promoter. Mol. Cell Biol., 3:2045-2057, 1983.
17. Pavlakis, G.N., D.H. Hamer, Regulation of a metallothionein-growth hormone hybrid gene in bovine papilloma virus. Proc. Natl. Acad. Sci. USA, 80:397-401, 1983.
18. Sarver, N., J.C. Byrne, and P.M. Howley, Transformation and replication in mouse cells of a bovine papillomavirus--pML2 plasmid vector that can be rescued in bacteria. Proc. Natl. Acad. Sci. USA, 79:714771-51, 1982.

19. Sarver, N., P. Gruss, M.-F. Law, G. Khoury, and P.M. Howley, Bovine papilloma virus deoxyribonucleic acid: a novel eucaryotic cloning vector. Mol. Cell. Biol., 1:486-496, 1981.
20. Sarver, N., M.S. Rabson, Y.C. Yang, J.C. Byrne, and P.M. Howley, Localization and analysis of bovine papillomavirus type 1 transforming functions. J. Virol., 52:377-388, 1984.
21. Southern, E.M., Detection of specific sequences among DNA fragments separated by gel electrophoresis. J. Mol. Biol., 98:503-517, 1975.
22. Stewart, W.E., II, The interferon system. (Springer, Berlin) 1979.
23. Stowe, N.D., and N.M. Wilkie, An improved technique for obtaining enhanced infectivity with Herpes simplex type 1 DNA. J. Gen. Virol., 33:447-458.
24. Zinn, K., P. Mellon, M. Ptastne, T. Maniatis, Regulated expression of an extrachromosomal human beta-interferon gene in mouse cells. Proc. Natl. Acad. Sci. USA, 79:4897-4901, 1979.

Papillomaviruses: Molecular and Clinical Aspects, pages 529–544


# USE OF BOVINE PAPILLOMA VIRUS VECTORS TO STUDY METALLOTHIONEIN GENE EXPRESSION

Michael Karin, Heidi Holtgreve, Simon Ford,
Adriana Heguy and Alois Haslinger

Department of Microbiology
University of Southern California School of Medicine
2011 Zonal Avenue, Los Angeles, CA. 90033

ABSTRACT Plasmid vectors derived from Bovine papilloma virus (BPV) are useful tools to study the regulation of gene expression in mammalian cells. Such vectors are capable of autonomous replication as low copy number episomes in rodent fibroblasts. We have used this system to investigate the function and expression of the human metallothionein (MT) gene family. This multigene family codes for a group of low molecular weight, heavy metal binding proteins, implicated in the control of trace metal metabolism and protection against free hydroxyl radicals. Expression of the hMT-$I_A$ and hMT-$II_A$ genes carried on BPV derived vectors is regulated by cadmium ions. The induction of the hMT-$II_A$ gene is mediated by metal dependent enhancer elements found in its 5' flanking region. We present evidence to suggest that these elements also lead to metal dependent increase in BPV early gene expression and consequently allow the vector to replicate even in the presence of "poison sequences" contributed by pBR322. The inhibitory effect of such "poison sequences" is probably due to a transcriptional block caused by increasing the distance between BPV enhancer and promoter elements.

## INTRODUCTION

Metallothioneins (MT's) are ubiquitous low molecular weight proteins with an unusually high cystein content (30%) and a selective capacity to bind heavy metal ions such as zinc (Zn), cadmium (Cd) and copper (Cu). In mammals MT's are encoded by a multigene family whose products can be separated according to their electrophoretic and chromatographic properties. On that basis, the proteins are classified into two groups referred to as MT-I and MT-II (1). While MT-II, the major form of the protein, is a unique molecular species encoded by a single functional gene (2), the MT-I group contains several different isoforms encoded by many functional genes, referred to as MT-$I_A$, MT-$I_B$, etc. (3).

The MT genes make up an interesting model system for studying the control of transcription in animal cells. Their transcription is directly induced by heavy metal ions (4,5), glucocorticoid hormones (4,6), interferon (7) and phorbol esters (P. Angel and P. Herrlich, personal communication). As a first step toward complete understanding of the mechanisms which control MT gene expression, we have determined that the 5' flanking regions of these genes contain promoter and regulatory elements which govern their response to various inducers (3,8). Next we have mapped the exact location of these elements within the 5' flanking region of the hMT-$II_A$ gene. Three regulatory elements were identified: The first one, lying between nucleotide positions -270 to -240, is responsible for induction by glucocorticoid hormones and therefore is named GRE for glucocorticoid responsive element. The next element, responsible for metal induction and referred to as MRE for metal responsive element, exists in three copies present at positions -154 to -140, -78 to -65 and -50 to -37. The third element is responsible for the basal level of expression referred to as BLE for basal level element, is present between -100 to -80 (9,10).

Footprinting experiments have shown that the GRE is coincident with the DNA binding site for the glucocorticoid hormone receptor (9) and by analogy we assume that the MRE's and the BLE, which show a high degree of evolutionary conservation (9,10), also serve as binding sites for DNA binding proteins. However, further understanding of the mechanisms which are responsible for induction of MT gene transcription will require the identification of these regulatory factors and determining how their interaction with specific DNA sequences is translated into a signal leading to increased transcription by RNA polymerase II. One possible mechanism is that the binding of regulatory proteins to DNA induces a change in the chromatin structure of the regulatory/promoter region which either increases its accessibility to RNA polymerase or increases the binding of that enzyme to the protein DNA complex. One approach which we hope would allow the elucidation of these steps as they occur *in vivo* is the construction of minichromosomes containing MT genes in a state which allows regulation of their transcription by exogenous agents. Such minichromosomes can be easily constructed utilizing the unique properties of Bovine papilloma virus (BPV). BPV derived vectors replicate autonomously as low copy number episomes in rodent fibroblasts (10), without leading to cell lysis like other viruses. Therefore, studying the expression of genes carried on BPV vectors alleviates many of the complications inherent to studying the expression of genes stably integrated into the genome after transfection and whose expression is effected by the sites of integration (8). The low copy number of BPV compared to SV40 and polyoma is another advantage as it is likely not to exhaust the available supply of regulatory factors.

Properties of hMT-II-BPV Vectors.

A HindIII restriction fragment carrying the $hMT\text{-}II_A$ gene was inserted into the HindIII site of $pBPV_{69T}$ (11) to generate two plasmids: pMT-II-BPV+ and pMT-II-BPV-, which differ in the orientation of the MT-II gene relative to the BPV subgenomic fragment (Figure 1). Rodent fibroblasts transformed with this vector become resistant to the cytotoxic effects of Cd, due to the high level of expression of the human MT-II gene. The expression of this gene, now carried on an episome, is still subject to regulation by heavy metal ions. Increasing the Cd concentration from 10 to 100 $\mu$M leads to 5 fold induction of hMT-II mRNA, which is initiated from the normal start sites of the $hMT\text{-}II_A$ gene (12).

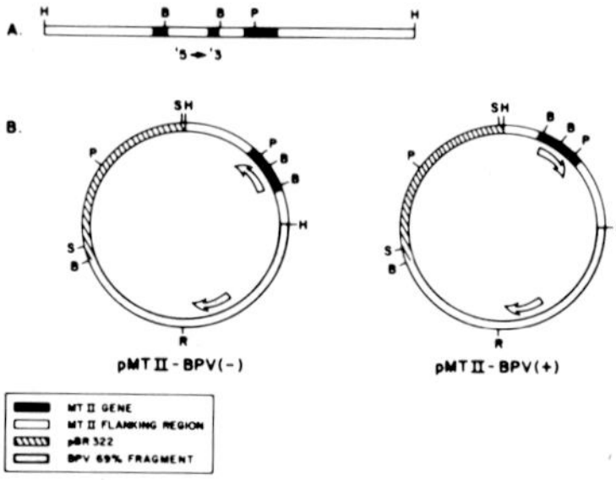


FIGURE 1: Structure of MTII-BPV vectors.

A. Structure of the hMT-$II_A$ gene. Black boxes denote exons.

B. Structure of pMTII-BPV vectors. The arrows indicate the direction of transcription of the hMT-$II_A$ gene and the BPV subgenomic fragment. Restriction sites are indicated as follows: B, BamHI; H, HindIII; P, PvuII; S, SalI, R, EcoRI.

Interestingly, the presence of the hMT-$II_A$ gene allows the MT-II-BPV vectors to be maintained as episomes even though they contain an intact pBR322 sequence. Normally the physical linkage of bacterial plasmid sequences to the $BPV_{69T}$ fragment leads to a significant reduction (2-3 orders of magnitude) in its transformation frequency (11). However, this reduction can be overcome by the insertion of additional sequences into the vector. In addition to the hMT-$II_A$ gene such sequences are present on the human $\alpha$ globin gene (13), the rat growth hormone gene (14) and the late region of BPV (15). The copy number of the hMT-II-BPV episomes is low (10-20 copies/cell) and does not seem to be affected by the presence or absence of plasmid sequences.

We have attempted to further characterize and identify the specific sequences, present within the hMT-$II_A$ gene responsible for the ability of MTII-BPV vectors to replicate in presence of plasmid sequences. We first compared the ability of pMT-II-BPV- to form cadmium resistant ($Cd^r$) colonies to its ability to induce the formation of transformed foci in C127 cells. As shown in Table 1, in the absence of plasmid sequences pMT-II-BPV has almost equal specific activity for either focus formation or the induction of $Cd^r$ colonies, however in the presence of plasmid sequences this vector does not give rise to transformed foci. Therefore the ability of the MT-II gene to counteract the inhibition exerted by plasmid DNA on BPV replication probably requires the induction of MT gene transcription by Cd ions present in the selective medium.

TABLE 1
EFFECT OF BACTERIAL PLASMID SEQUENCES ON TRANSFORMATION FREQUENCIES OF MTII-BPV-

| | pMTII-BPV +SalI | pMII-PBV- -SalI | Carrier DNA |
|---|---|---|---|
| Foci per plate | 110 | 2 | 1 |
| $Cd^r$ colonies per plate, 30 μMCd | 182 | 125 | 1 |
| $Cd^r$ colonies per plate, 50 μMCd | 110 | 70 | 1 |

3T3 cells were seeded at an approximate density of $5x10^5$ cells/100mm plate and 24 hours later were transfected with a calcium phosphate coprecipitate containing 1 μg of pMTII-BPV- either digested or not digested with SalI (to remove plasmid sequences) and 10 μg of carrier DNA alone. The precipitate was left on the cells for 18 hours, at which time the medium was changed. Twenty four hours later the cells were placed in selective medium containing 50 μM of $Zn^{++}$ and either 30 or 50 μM of $Cd^{++}$, or were split at 1:3 ration and were left on normal growth medium. Two weeks later the number of transformed foci or $Cd^r$ colonies per plate was determined. Shown are averages for three different plates.

To further narrow down the DNA sequences capable of "neutralizing" the inhibitory effect of plasmid sequences we have constructed a series of nested 5' deletion mutants of the hMT-II$_A$ gene using Bal31 and inserted them into the HindIII site of pBPV$_{69T}$ to generate the following vectors: pBPV-MT-II $\Delta$-268, pBPV-MT-II $\Delta$-242, pBPV-MT-II $\Delta$-92 and pBPV-MT-II $\Delta$-80. To our disappointment, all of them were able to form Cd$^r$ colonies in the presence of plasmid sequences. Since the transcriptional activity of all the mutants is Cd inducible (9) we were not able to dissociate between the heavy metal responsive elements (MRE's) of the hMT-II$_A$ gene and the sequences required for counteracting the inhibitory effect of plasmid sequences. In other experiments to be published elsewhere (Haslinger, et al., in preparation), we found that the regulatory region of the hMT-II$_A$ gene contains at least two metal responsive enhancer elements. These elements can lead to metal activated transcription from heterologous promoters regardless of their position and orientation. The activity of these elements is not limited to a single adjacent promoter and they can lead to the activation of two promoters placed in tandem (8). Based on these observations we would like to propose the following model to explain the inhibition of BPV replication by plasmid sequences and its relief by hMT-II$_A$ gene. As shown by Lusky et al. (16) BPV replication and maintenance require the expression of several viral encoded early gene products. Therefore, these functions are dependent on transcription. Expression of the BPV early promoter is controlled by an enhancer element located at the 3' end of the early transcription unit (17). It is likely that when plasmid sequences are separating it from the early promoter, the activity (of the enhancer) is inhibited, leading to diminished expression of the early genes and consequently to inhibition of replication. On the other hand, if another transcriptional enhancer element is placed upstream to the early promoter, the activity of the latter is restored even though plasmid sequences are present on the same molecule. Since the enhancer elements associated with the hMT-II$_A$ gene are metal dependent, then replication of pMT-II-BPV vectors carrying pBR322 sequences is metal dependent as well.

The level of hMT-$II_A$ transcriptional activity drops several fold when promoter sequences present upstream to position -80 are deleted (9). However, the levels of hMT mRNA expressed in cells carrying the various pPBV-MT-II deletion mutants do not seem to vary considerably (Figure 2A). This is probably due to the fact that all of these cell lines were selected to be resistant to the same level of Cd (30 μM). On the other hand, the copy number of the different mutant vectors does vary (Figure 2B). As shown in Table 2, the copy number of pBPV-MT-II-80 is 2-3 times higher than that of pPBV-MT-II-242. Thus, the vector's copy number seems to adjust in order to compensate for its reduced transcriptional activity and maintain the required level of the gene product being selected for, i.e. MT.

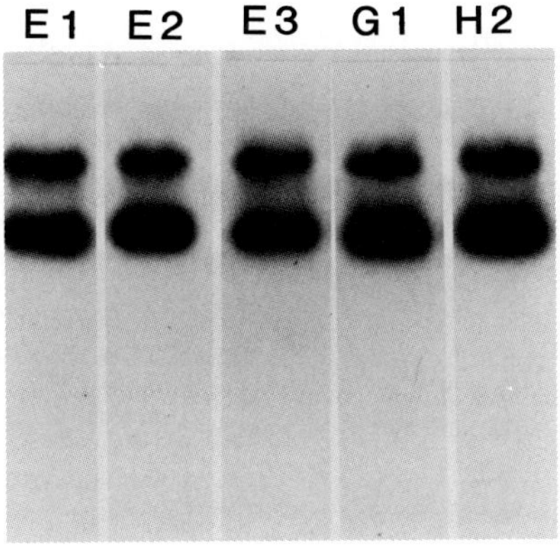


FIGURE 2A: Expression and copy number of pBPV-MTII 5' deletion mutants.

Expression of MTIImRNA in cell lines transformed with pBPV-MTII-80 (E1, E2 and E3), pBPV-MTII-242 (G1) and pBPV-MTII-268 (H2). 20 μg of total RNA were separated on 1.5% agarose gel, transferred to nitrocellulose and hybridized to a human MTII specific probe and to an actin probe (for normalization). The upper band is actin mRNA and the lower band is hMTII-mRNA.

FIGURE 2B: Expression and copy number of pBPV-MTII 5' deletion mutants.

Copy number of pBPV-MII 5' deletion mutants. 10 μg of total genomic DNA prepared from cells harboring pBPV-MTII-80 (E1, E2 and E2), pBPV-MTII-242 (G1) or pBPV-MTII-268 (H2) and digested with EcoRI was separated on 1% agarose gel, transferred to nitrocellulose and hybridized to an hMT-$II_A$ specific probe. The first three lanes on the left are copy number standards of pBPV-MTII-268 digested with EcoRI.

TABLE 2
CORRELATION BETWEEN COPY NUMBER AND mRNA EXPRESSION FOR BPV-MTII 5' DELETION MUTANTS

| Mutant | Line | MTmRNA/actin mRNA | Copy number |
|---|---|---|---|
| pBPV-MTII-80 | E1 | 1.7 | 27 |
| | E2 | 1.4 | 26 |
| | E3 | 1.5 | 22 |
| pBPV-MTII-242 | G1 | 1.4 | 11 |
| pBPV-MTII-268 | H2 | 1.5 | 11 |

The relative amount of MTmRNA expressed in the various cell lines was determined by densitometry of the autoradiogram shown in figure 2A and was normalized to the amount of actin mRNA. The copy number was determined by densitometry of the autoradiogram shown in figure 2B and comparison to the copy number standards.

Transformation of 293 Cells to a Cadmium Resistant Phenotype.

In the past we attempted to transform various cell lines to cadmium resistance using the pMT-II-BPV(-) vector. Only mouse and rat fibroblast lines such as C127, NIH3T3, Rat 1 and Rat 2 were found to be efficiently transformed to a $Cd^r$ phenotype and harbour the vector as a free replicating episome. A possible cause for the inability to transform many other cell lines including human fibroblast and HeLa cell lines (M.K., unpublished observations), is the limited host range of the BPV transcriptional apparatus. A possible way to circumvent this limitation is to construct a vector capable of expressing a transacting transcriptional factor which could lead to its increased expression in every cell type. Such factors can be supplied by the EIA gene of adenovirus which codes for two transacting transcriptional activators known as the 12S and the 13S gene products (18). These factors are expressed in the human cell line 293 which is stably transformed by a fragment of the adenovirus 5 genome. To test whether the EIA gene products can activate BPV expression and allow it to replicate in this human cell, pMT-II-BPV(-) DNA was introduced into 293 cells by a calcium-phosphate mediated transfection and cells were selected for resistance to 15 $\mu$M of Cd. After two weeks 15 colonies of $Cd^r$ cells appeared on each plate transfected with 1 $\mu$g of pMT-II-BPV(-) DNA, while transfection with $pBPV_{69T}$ did not give rise to colonies. Eight of the colonies were expanded to mass cultures and were analyzed for the presence of unintegrated vector DNA by the Hirt extraction procedure (20). Most of the clones analyzed exhibited a low copy number (2-8 copies/cell) of unintegrated vector DNA (data not shown). Since the 293 line is the only human cell line capable of supporting BPV replication thus far, we believe that this capacity is due to the expression of the EIA proteins. To carry these studies a step further we have constructed a BPV-EIA chimeric plasmid. However, all of our attempts to transform mouse fibroblasts with this vector have failed, probably due to the cytotoxicity of the overexpressed proteins. This assumption is supported by the fact that, early (3-5 days) after transfection, small foci appear in the culture, but after a few more days they disappear.

Expression of human MT Genes using BPV vectors.

The human MT gene family is quite complex, consisting of 12-15 different genes including several pseudogenes. There are no easily recognized biochemical functions associated with these genes except heavy metal binding. We have used this property to characterize the genes and define whether they are active or not. Our assay consists of inserting a cloned MT gene into a BPV vector and transfection into NIH3T3 cells. The cells are placed in Cd containing medium and the frequency of $Cd^r$ colonies is determined two weeks later. A functional MT gene is judged by its ability to give rise to $Cd^r$ colonies. Recently we have determined the nucleotide sequence of two "MT-I like" genes, $MT\text{-}I_A$ and $MT\text{-}I_B$ (ref. 3 and our unpublished results). The amino-acid sequences predicted for these putative proteins are different from the amino-acid sequence determined by direct sequencing of a mixture of several human MT-I subtypes. Because of this disagreement we were concerned about the functionality of these genes; and therefore we introduced them into BPV vectors. Transfection of 3T3 cells with either MT-$I_A$-BPV or MT-$I_B$ -BPV gives rise to $Cd^r$ colonies, indicating that the genes are expressed and code for a functional protein. On the other hand MT-$II_B$-BPV, a vector which contains the hMT-$II_B$ processed pseudogene (2) does not give rise to $Cd^r$ colonies, even though this gene has the potential to code for a normal MT-II protein.

We have compared MT-II-BPV(-) and pMT-$I_A$-BPV (figure 3) in their ability to protect cells against Cd toxicity. As shown in figure 4, the vector which contains the MT-$II_A$ genes is 2-3 times more efficient in protecting cells against Cd than the vector containing the MT-$I_A$ gene. These differences are due to the different levels of MTmRNA expressed by the two vectors. The MT-$II_A$ gene which has a more efficient promoter element than the MT-$I_A$ gene (A.H. and M.K., unpublished results) and gives rise to 2-3 fold higher levels of MTmRNA (figure 5) and protein (figure 6). These results indicate that the proteins encoded by the two different genes have a similar Cd binding activity.

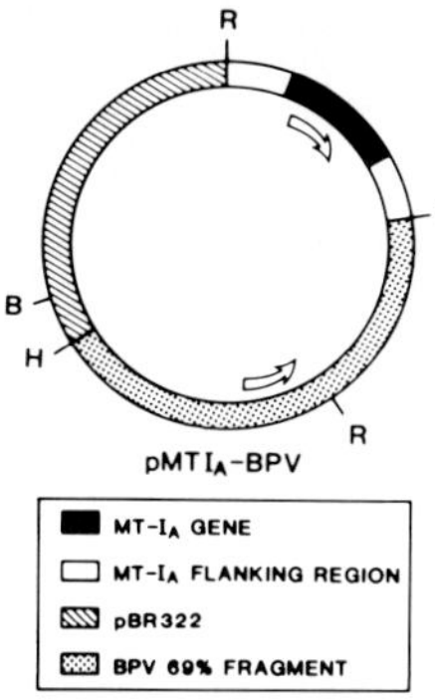


FIGURE 3: Structure of pMT$I_A$-BPV.

Restriction sites are indicated as in the legend to figure 1.

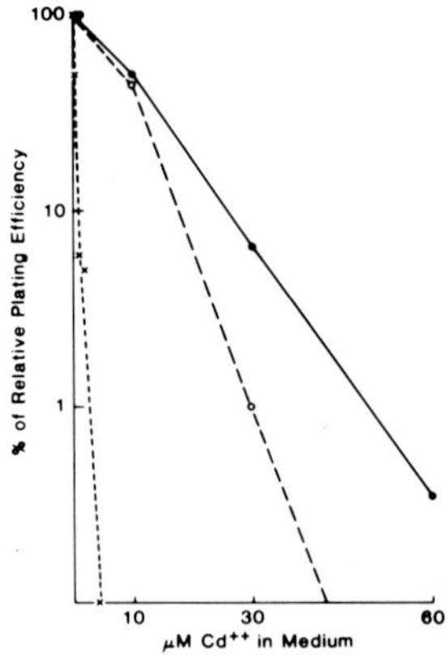


FIGURE 4: Protection of NIH3T3 cells against $Cd^{++}$ toxicity by $pMTI_A$-BPV and pMTII-BPV.

Mixed populations of NIH3T3 cells containing $pMTI_A$-BPV (0) or $pMTII_A$-BPV (0) were originally selected for survival in 10 μM $Cd^{++}$. These cells and the parental NIH3T3 (x) cells were plated in various dilutions and grown for 2 weeks in increasing $Cd^{++}$ concentrations. The number of surviving colonies was determined and converted to percentage of the plating efficiency in the absence of $Cd^{++}$.

FIGURE 5: Expression of MTmRNA by $pMTI_A$-BPV and pMTII-BPV transformed cells.

Twenty μg of RNA extracted from cells transformed with either $pMTI_A$-BPV or $pMTII_A$-BPV and grown in the presence of the indicated concentrations of $Cd^{++}$ were analyzed by blot hybridization as described in legend to figure 2A.

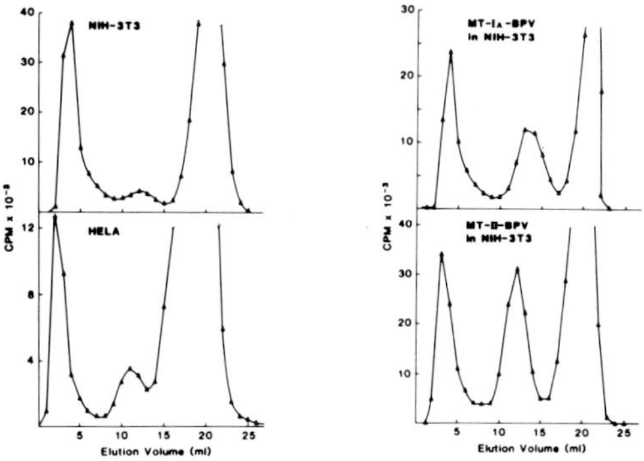


FIGURE 6: Expression of MT protein.

Confluent cultures of HeLa, NIH3T3 and two transformed NIH3T3 lines carrying either pMTI$_A$-BPV or pMTII-BPV were grown in the presence of 5 μM Cd (HeLa and NIH3T3 cells; optimal inducing concentration for these cell lines) or 50 μM Cd (pMT-I$_A$-BPV and pMTII-BPV transformed cells; optimal inducing concentration) and labelled for four hours with 10 μCi of $^{35}$S-cystein. Cytoplasmic extracts were prepared and analyzed by chromatography on Sephadex G-75 columns.

## SUMMARY

The introduction of cloned transcriptionally regulated genes into BPV derived vectors offers a unique opportunity to study the molecular events involved in the control of gene expression. The studies described in this manuscript on the regulation of human MT genes carried on BPV vectors by heavy metal ions are only the first steps we are taking toward elucidation of the molecular mechanisms controlling the expression of this unique gene family.

Having established an experimental system in which the expression of the hMT-II$_A$ gene carried on an autonomously replicating episome, can be easily manipulated by external stimuli, we next plan to examine the effects of the inducer on the structure of the episome. Increased transcriptional activity is likely to be accompanied by changes in the conformation of the DNA template making it more accessible to RNA polymerase. Examining the structure of the MT-BPV minichromosomes before and after induction should give us some clues about these events. We are currently developing techniques which will allow us to determine the effect of inducers on the topology of the minichromosome. In addition to being useful for studying the transcriptional control of MT genes, the BPV system is also very useful in obtaining large amounts of the different MT gene products, studying their protective properties in vivo, and characterizing their chemical properties in vitro.

## ACKNOWLEDGMENTS

The work described was supported by grants from The National Institutes of Health (ES03222), the Environmental Protection agency (R811284) and the Department of Energy (DE-F603-84ER60271). M. Karin is also supported by the Searle Scholar program and A. Haslinger by an EMBO longterm fellowship.

## REFERENCES

1. Karin M (1985). Metallothioneins, proteins in search of function. Cell, in press.
2. Karin M, Richards RI (1982). Human metallothionein genes - primary structure of the metallothionein-II gene and a related processed gene. Nature 299:797-802.
3. Richards RI, Heguy A, Karin M (1984). Structural and functional analysis of the human metallothionein-$I_A$ gene: differential induction by metal ions and glucocorticoids. Cell 37:263-272.
4. Karin M, Andersen RD, Slater E, Smith K, Herschman HR (1980). Metallothionein mRNA induction in HeLa cells in response to zinc or dexamethasone is a primary induction response. Nature 286:295-297.
5. Durnam DM, Palmiter RD (1981). Transcriptional regulation of the mouse metallothionein-I gene by heavy metals. J Biol Chem 256:2268-2272.
6. Hager LJ, Palmiter RD (1981). Transcriptional regulation of mouse liver metallothionein I gene by glucocorticoids. Nature 291:340-342.

7. Friedman RL, Manly SP, McMahon M, Kerr IM, Stark, GR (1984). Transcriptional and posttranscriptional regulation of interferon induced gene expression in human cells. Cell 38:745-755.
8. Karin M, Haslinger A, Holtgreve H, Cathala G, Slater E, Baxter JD (1984). Activation of a heterologous promoter in response to dexamethasone and cadmium by metallothionein gene 5' flanking DNA. Cell 36:371-379.
9. Karin M, Haslinger A, Holtgreve H, Richards RI, Krauter P, Westphal HM, Beato M (1984). Characterization of DNA sequences through which cadmium and glucocorticoid hormones induce human metallothionein $II_A$ gene. Nature 308:513-519.
10. Law MF, Lowry DR, Dvoretzky J, Howley PM (1981). Mouse cells transformed by bovine papilloma virus contain only extra chromosomal viral DNA sequences. Proc Natl Acad Sci USA 79:6453-6456.
11. Lowry DR, Dvoretzky J, Shaber R, Law MF, Engel L, Howley PM (1980). In vitro tumorigenic transformation by a defined subgenomic fragment of bovine papilloma virus DNA. Nature 287:72-74.
12. Karin M, Cathala G, Nguyen-Huu MC (1983). Expression and regulation of a human metallothionein gene carried on an autonomously replicating shuttle vector. Proc Natl Acad Sci USA 80:4040-4044.
13. DiMaio D, Treisman R, Maniatis T (1982). Bovine papilloma virus vector that propogates as a plasmid in both mouse and bacterial cells. Proc Natl Acad Sci USA 79:4030-4034.
14. Kushner PJ, Levenson BB, Goodman HM (1982). A plasmid that replicates in both mouse and E. coli cells. J Mol Appl Genet 1:527-539.
15. Sarver N, Byrne JC, Howley P (1982). Transformation and replication in mouse cells of a bovine papilloma virus/pML2 plasmid vector that can be rescued in bacteria. Proc Natl Acad Sci USA 79:7147-7151.
16. Lusky M, Botchan MR (1984). Characterization of the bovine papilloma virus plasmid maintenance sequences. Cell 36:391-401.
17. Lusky M, Berg L, Weiher H, Botchan M (1983). Bovine papilloma virus contains an activator of gene expression at the distal end of the early transcription unit. Mol Cell Biol 3:1108-1122.

18. Imperiale MJ, Feldman LT, Nevins JR (1983). Activation of gene expression by adenovirus and herpesvirus regulatory genes acting in trans and by a cis-acting adenovirus enhancer element. Cell 35:127-136.
19. Hirt B (1967). Selective extraction of polyioma DNA from infected mouse cell cultures. J Mol Biol 26:365-369.

**Papillomaviruses: Molecular and Clinical Aspects, pages 545–555**


# RETROVIRAL VECTORS FOR GENE TRANSFER[1]

M. Jacqueline Johnson, A. Dusty Miller[2], Ming Fan Law[3], Ronald M. Evans and Inder M. Verma

Molecular Biology and Virology Laboratory, The Salk Institute
San Diego, California 92138

ABSTRACT We describe the advantages of using retroviral vectors for gene transfer and as a possible means of introducing genes into bone marrow cells for somatic gene therapy treatments. Several types of vector constructs are described--those containing only selectable genes and those containing a selectable and a non-selectable gene. In vitro experiments in which these constructs were used to transfect or infect cells are described.

## INTRODUCTION

Knowledge of the mechanisms of eukaryotic gene regulation and expression has been greatly increased with the ability to introduce these genes into mammalian cells. Commonly used methods of introduction include: i) $CaPO_4$ precipitation of foreign DNA which is inefficient and limited to tissue culture cells (1,2,3); ii) microinjection, which is laborious and requires sophisticated instrumentation (4); or iii) the use of viral vectors, some of which can be used to introduce DNA via infective routes. In this latter category, the papovaviruses such as SV40 are commonly used viral vectors. However, they are limited in the length of foreign DNA which can be inserted, as well as in their host range (5,6)

[1]This work was supported by NCI and ACS

[2]Present address: Fred Hutchinson Cancer Center, Seattle, Washington 98104

[3]Present address: Sibia, La Jolla, California 92037

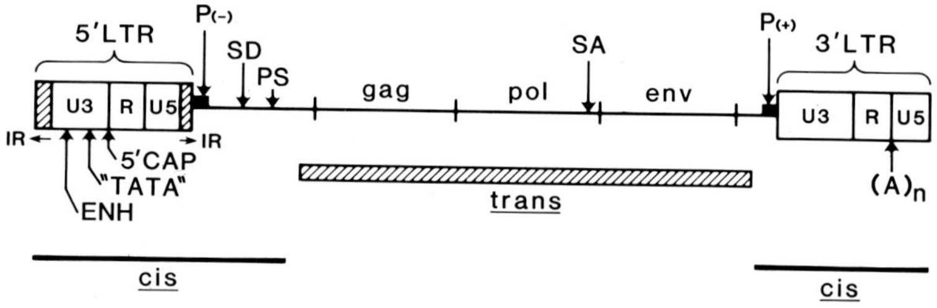


FIGURE 1. Diagram of typical murine proviral DNA. The provirus consists of LTR (long terminal repeat), <u>gag</u> (group specific antigen), <u>pol</u> (reverse transcriptase), <u>env</u> (envelope proteins), U3 (unique 3' sequences), R (genomic terminal redundancy), U5 (unique 5' sequences), IR (inverted repeat), ENH (transcriptional enhancer element), "TATA" (promoter), 5' CAP (first nucleotide of the genomic RNA), P(-) (tRNA primer for initiation of -ve strand viral DNA), SD (splice donor), PS (packaging signal sequences), SA (splice acceptor sequence), P(+) (primer for +ve strand synthesis), $(A)_n$ (presumed polyA addition signal). <u>CIS</u> refers to regulatory sequences which must be supplied in CIS for viral replication, while <u>TRANS</u> indicates those functions which can be supplied by another virus present in the same cell.

It is the emerging consensus that retrovirus based vectors may serve as excellent vehicles for gene transfer. The structure and important features of these viruses are shown in Figure 1. There are numerous advantages to using retroviral vectors including i) their ability to infect a wide variety of species; ii) their integration into the host chromosome in an efficient, defined manner; iii) their regulatory sequences are contained within the viral long terminal repeats (LTRs) which provide efficient signals for transcript initiation and termination; iv) their lack of strict size requirements for packaging allows DNA segments of 1-7 Kb to be inserted; v) their ability to grow in a wide variety of cell types; and vi) their ability to infect both embryos and stem cells.

Our interest in retroviral vectors is two-fold. They may be used for efficient transfer of genes into a wide variety of recipient cells to study expression, and to introduce genes into human somatic cells as a means of gene therapy treatment. Below we describe some of the retrovirus based vectors generated in this and other laboratories.

## RESULTS AND DISCUSSION

### Selectable Genes.

Several research groups have developed vectors containing selectable genes. Cell lines have been established which produce high titers of retrovirus containing the human hypoxanthine phosphoribosyltransferase (HPRT) gene (7), the bacterial neomycin resistant gene (8), the E. coli guanine phosphoribosyltransferase gene (gpt)(9,10), the Herpes thymidine kinase gene (11,12,13) and the mouse dihydrofolate reductase (DHFR) gene (14). As a model system, much of the initial work in our laboratory was done with the retroviral vector containing the HPRT cDNA sequence ( 7,15). This gene was chosen for two reasons: its function in purine biosynthesis is well understood and the genetic disease, Lesch Nyhan's is the result of a defect in this gene (16).

Two retroviral constructs made with HPRT cDNA are shown in Figure 2. One, (pLPAL) contains the poly A signal of the HPRT gene while in the second construct (pLPL) this sequence was removed. Results of a Northern blot illustrate that with pLPAL two transcripts are seen representing the entire retrovirus transcript as well as an HPRT specific transcript. In the pLPL construct, only the full length retroviral length transcript is seen, presumably because there is no premature termination following the HPRT gene. A Southern blot analysis shows that each cell contains only a single fragment, corresponding to the 3.9 Kb full length retrovirus. Enzymatic assays were done to illustrate that the protein is made in the Lesch-Nyhan cells which were infected with either construct.

### Non-selectable Genes.

A second type of viral construct in which the vector contains both a selectable and non-selectable gene has also been developed. An example of such a vector is shown in Figure 3 where the rat growth hormone gene was inserted in either orientation in a retrovirus containing the HPRT gene (17). Table 1 summarizes transfection experiments with these two vectors. The growth hormone gene retained its inducibility regardless of the orientation, suggesting that sequences in the growth hormone promoter remain responsive

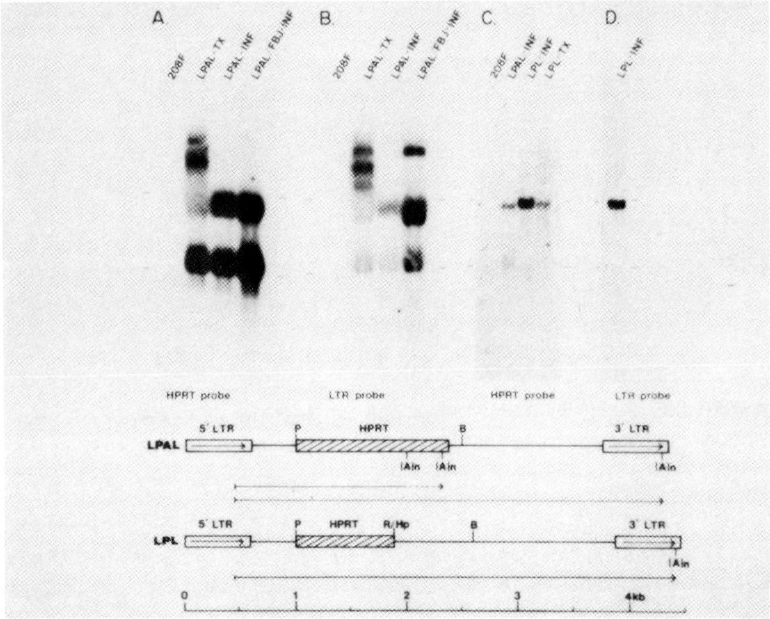


FIGURE 2. RNA blot analysis of rat 208F cells transfected (TX) or infected (INF) with either of the HPRT constructs shown. The probes used are indicated below the autoradiograms. Dashes indicate position of 28S and 18S RNA (4.5 and 1.8 Kb, respectively).

to induction despite the presence of the viral LTRs. These experiments also prove the feasibility of expressing non-selectable genes in retroviral vectors. Again, results from a Northern blot show that two growth hormone transcripts are made - one corresponding to the full length retrovirus and a second corresponding to the 1.1 Kb growth hormone transcript (Figure 4). S1 mapping studies following induction with dexamethasone show that the growth hormone gene transcript is initiated correctly. Such experiments also emphasize another advantage of retroviral vectors as only a single linear genome is integrated in the recipient cell - studies of transcript initiation are possible.

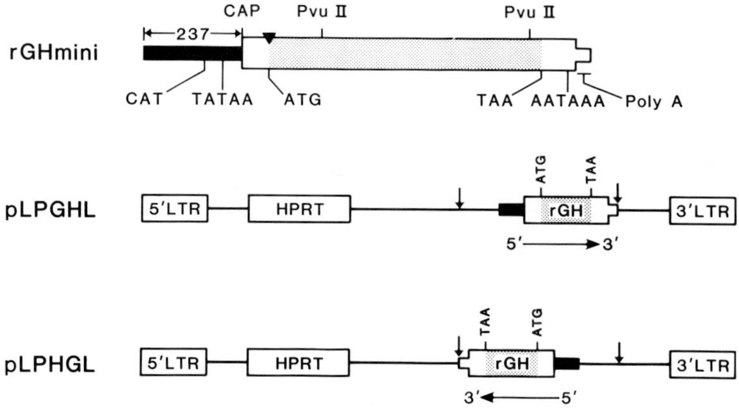


FIGURE 3. Retroviral constructs which contain both the selectable HPRT gene and the rat growth hormone gene. The uppermost construct shown is the rat growth hormone "minigene" which contains its own promoter and poly A site.

As previously mentioned, one of the advantages of retroviral vectors is their efficient infection of a wide variety of cell types. This may be the only plausible method of infecting rare cells such as pluripotent stem cells which constitute less than .1% of the bone marrow. The HPRT-GH construct was used to infect bone marrow, then given to a recipient animal and eventually spleen and bone marrow were assayed for the presence of the HPRT. Recombinant HPRT virus were also rescued from the bone marrow and spleen cells.

To fully exploit the potential of this system for somatic gene therapy vectors containing the mutant DHFR gene were constructed. This gene, isolated by Simonsen and Levinson (18), confers resistance to methotrexate as it has 1/270th the affinity for this folate analogue as compared to the wild type gene. Therefore, this construct can be used in any cell type as it contains a dominantly selectable marker, obviating the need for biochemically deficient cell lines. Additionally, the presence of the DHFR gene allows for amplification in response to increased methotrexate concentrations.

A problem to be addressed for future application in gene therapy treatment was the use of helper virus to package the recombinants. This was solved by making cell lines containing integrated copies of a packaging deficient

TABLE 1
INDUCTION OF GROWTH HORMONE IN RETROVIRAL CONSTRUCTS[a]

| Transfected DNA | Growth hormone production (ng/ml) | | | Induction | Virus recovery | |
|---|---|---|---|---|---|---|
| | Control | Dex | Dex + $T_3$ | | HPRT$^+$ ($10^2 \times$ cfu/ml) | MoMLV ($10^4 \times$ pfu/ml) |
| pLPGHL | | | | | | |
| Experiment 1 | 11 | 23 | 24 | 2.2 | 6.5 | 8 |
| Experiment 2 | 22 | 102 | 99 | 4.5 | 3.2 | 8 |
| pLPHGL | | | | | | |
| Experiment 1 | 29 | 83 | 101 | 3.5 | 2.4 | 7 |
| Experiment 2 | 35 | 70 | 75 | 2.1 | 2.3 | 8 |
| No DNA | <2 | <2 | <2 | | | |

[a]Results of induction experiments using the HPRT-rat growth hormone retroviral constructs. Growth hormone production was measured after induction with dexamethasone and $T_3$, and compared to growth hormone levels of uninduced cells. Recombinant virus was recovered and assayed for its ability to confer HAT resistance to 208F HPRT cells and by PFU.

retrovirus. Mann et al. (9) made an ecotrophic packaging cell line while Miller et al. (14) developed an amphotropic packaging cell line which has a broad host range enabling the infection of human cells. The scheme of this latter construct is shown in Figure 5. Such cell lines will theoretically only package the recombinant virus and not an active retrovirus due to the lack of a packaging signal in the replication competent retrovirus. In experiments where mouse cells were infected with the DHFR virus, Miller et al. (14) show that titers of recombinant virus are quite high, with no production of helper virus (Table 2).

Numerous vector constructs are now in use for both in vitro and in vivo experiments in this and other laboratories. Examples of these (shown in Fig. 6) are HPRT and DHFR retroviral constructs containing the adenosine deaminase gene (19,20), the nucleoside phosphorylase gene (21), as well as the factor IX gene (22). It is hoped that in the future these will prove to be useful in correcting single gene defects which now have such devastating effects as well as to further studies of gene expression.

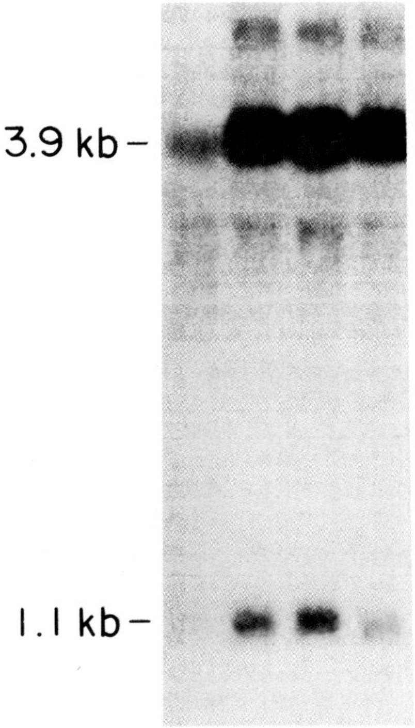


FIGURE 4. A Northern blot analysis of RNA from cells infected with the HPRT-growth hormone retrovirus constructs. When a growth hormone sequence was used as a probe, two transcripts were seen: a 3.9 Kb band corresponding to a full length retrovirus transcript and a 1.1 Kb band corresponding to the rat growth hormone transcript.

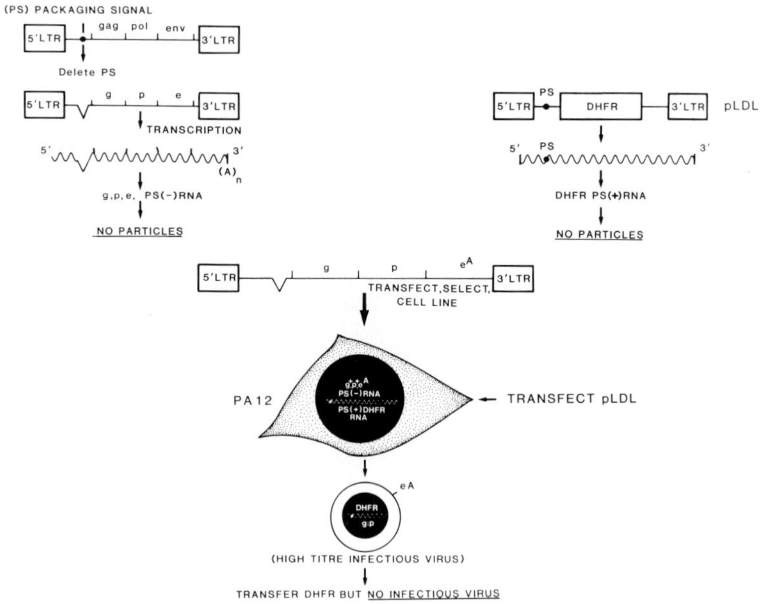


FIGURE 5. Diagram of the scheme used to construct a helper-virus free amphotropic packaging cell line.

TABLE 2
ASSAY OF HELPER-FREE DHFR TRANSDUCING VIRUS[a]

| Clone number | $Mtx^r$ colonies/ml medium | helper virus/ml medium |
|---|---|---|
| PA-LDL1 c6 | $1.6 \times 10^6$ | <2 |
| PA-LDL1 c7 | $3.5 \times 10^6$ | <2 |
| PA-LDL1 c9 | $4.2 \times 10^6$ | <2 |

[a]Assay of recombinant retrovirus containing the mutant DHFR gene. In three different clonal cell lines, methotrexate resistant colonies were found, indicating high virus titers with no helper virus present.

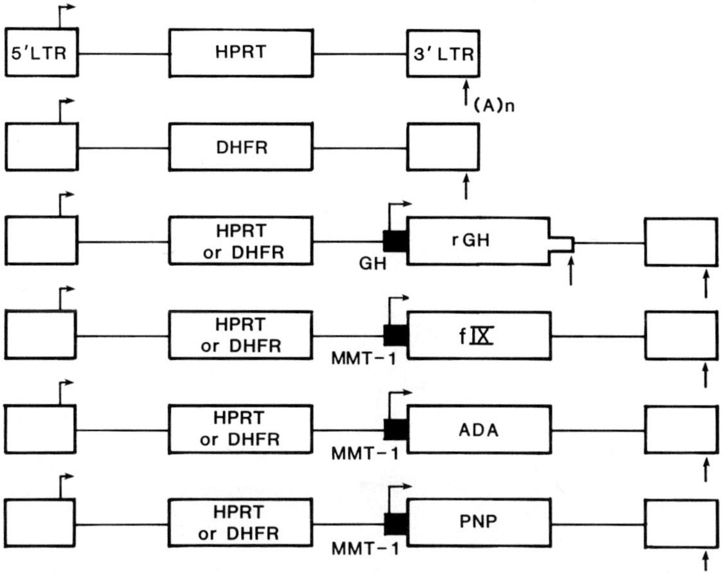


FIGURE 6. Diagram of several retroviral constructs presently being used for in vitro and in vivo experiments. All constructs contain either HPRT or DHFR as the selectable gene, followed by a second gene which may be useful for somatic gene therapy treatments.

## REFERENCES


1. Cursaro CM, Pearson ML (1981). Enhancing the efficiency of DNA-mediated gene transfer in mammalian cells. Somat Cell Genet 7:603.
2. Graham FL, van der Eb AJ (1973). A new technique for the assay of infectivity of human adenovirus 5 DNA. Virology 52:456.
3. Wigler, M, Sweet R, Sim GK, Wold B, Pellicer A, Lacy E, Maniatis T, Silverstein S, Axel R (1979). Transformation of mammalian cells with genes from procaryotes and eucaryotes. Cell 16:777.
4. Capecchi MR (1980). High efficiency transformation by direct microinjection of DNA into cultured mammalian cells. Cell 22:479.
5. Gluzman Y (1982)."Eukaryotic viral vectors". Cold Spring Harbor Laboratory, Cold Spring Harbor New York, p 1.

6. Mulligan RC, Howard BH, Berg P (1979). Synthesis of rabbit β-globulin in cultured monkey kidney cells following infection with a SV40-β-globin recombinant genome. Nature 277:108.
7. Miller AD, Jolly DJ, Friedmann T, Verma I (1983). A transmissible retrovirus expressing human hypoxanthine phosphoribosyltransferase (HPRT): Gene transfer into cells obtained from humans deficient in HPRT. PNAS 80: 4709.
8. Cepko CL, Roberts BE, Mulligan RC (1984). Construction and applications of a highly transmissible retrovirus shuttle vector. Cell 37: 1053.
9. Mann R, Mulligan RC, Baltimore D(1983). Construction of a retrovirus packaging mutant and its use to produce helper-free defective retrovirus. Cell 33:153.
10. Stuhlmann H, Cone R, Mulligan RC, Jaenisch R (1984). Introduction of a selectable gene into different animal tissue by a retrovirus recombinant vector. PNAS 81: 7151.
11. Shimotohno K,Temin HM (1981). Formation of infectious progeny virus after insertion of herpes simplex thymidine kinase gene into DNA of an avian retrovirus. Cell 26: 67.
12. Wei CM, Gibson M, Spear PG, Scolnick EM (1981). Construction and isolation of a transmissible retrovirus containing the src gene of Harvey murine sarcoma virus and the thymidine kinase gene of herpes simples virus type 1. J. Viorl. 39: 935.
13. Tabin CJ, Hoffmann JW, Goff SP, Weinberg RI (1982). Adaptation of a retrovirus as a eucaryotic vector transmitting the herpes simplex virus thymidine kinase gene Mol.Cell.Biol. 2:426.
14. Miller AD, Law MF, Verma IM (1985). Generation of helper-free amphotropic retroviruses that transduce a dominant acting, methotrexate-resistant dihydrofolate reductase gene Mol.Cell.Bio. 5: 431.
15. Jolly DJ, Okayama H, Berg P, Esty AC, Filpula D, Bohlen P, Johnson GG, Shively JE, Hunkapillar T, Friedmann (1983). Isolation and characterization of a full-length expressible cDNA for human hypoxanthine phosphoribosyltransferase PNAS 80: 477.
16. Miller AD, Ong ES, Rosenfeld MG, Verma IM, Evans RM (1984). Infectious and selectable retrovirus containing an inducible rat growth hormone minigene. Science 225: 993.
17. Simonsen CC and Levinson AD (1983). Isolation and expression of an altered mouse dihydrofolate reductase cDNA. PNAS 80: 2495.

18. Valerio D, Duyvesteyn MGC, Khan PM, Kessel AGvan, de Waard A, van der Eb AJ (1983). Isolation of cDNA clones for human adenosine deaminase. Gene 871.
19. Valerio, D, McIvor RS, Williams SR, Duyvesteyn MGC, Ormondt H, van der eb AJ, Martin DW (1984). Cloning of human adenosine deaminase cDNA and expression in mouse cells. Gene 31: 147.
20. McIvor RS, Goddard JM, Simonsen CC, Martin DW (1985). Expression of a cDNA sequence encoding human purine nucleosede phosphorylase in rodent and human cells. Mol.Cell.Bio. 3.
21. Anson DS, Choo KH, Rees DJG, Giannelli F, Gould K, Huddleston JA, Brownlee GG (1984). The gene structure of human anti-haemophilic factor IX. EMBO 3: 1053.

# Index